Entrepreneurship in Livestock and Agriculture

Entrepreneurship in Livestock and Agriculture

Editors

MC SHARMA
MVSc, PhD (Vet. Med.)
Director, Central Institute for Research on Goats
Makhdoom, Farah, Mathura 281 122 (UP)

RUPASI TIWARI
MSc, PhD (Exten Educ.)
Senior Scientist and Incharge, ATIC
Joint Directorate of Extension Education
Indian Veterinary Research Institute
Izatnagar 243 122 (UP)

JP SHARMA
MSc (Ag. Exten and Commun), PhD (Ag. Exten)
Principal Scientist and Incharge, ATIC
Indian Agriculture Research Institute
Pusa, New Delhi 110 012

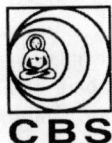

CBS

CBS Publishers & Distributors Pvt. Ltd

New Delhi • Bengaluru • Chennai • Kochi • Kolkata • Mumbai
Hyderabad • Uttarakhand • Nagpur • Patna • Pune • Jharkhand

Entrepreneurship in Livestock and Agriculture

ISBN: 978-81-239-1774-0

First Edition: 2010
Reprint: 2012, 2014, 2019

Published by **Satish Kumar Jain** and produced by **Varun Jain** for
CBS Publishers & Distributors Pvt. Ltd.,
4819/XI Prahlad Street, 24 Ansari Road, Daryaganj, New Delhi - 110002
delhi@cbspd.com, cbspubs@airtelmail.in • www.cbspd.com
Ph.: 23289259, 23266861, 23266867 • Fax: 011-23243014

Corporate Office: 204 FIE, Industrial Area, Patparganj, Delhi - 110 092
Ph: 49344934 • Fax: 011-49344935
E-mail: publishing@cbspd.com • publicity@cbspd.com

Branches:
- **Bengaluru:** 2975, 17th Cross, K.R. Road, Bansankari 2nd Stage, Bengaluru - 70 • Ph: +91-80-26771678/79 • Fax: +91-80-26771680
  E-mail: cbsbng@gmail.com, bangalore@cbspd.com
- **Chennai:** No. 7, Subbaraya Street, Shenoy Nagar, Chennai - 600030
  Ph: +91-44-26681266, 26680620 • Fax: +91-44-42032115
  E-mail: chennai@cbspd.com
- **Kochi:** Ashana House, 39/1904, A.M. Thomas Road, Valanjambalam, Ernakulum, Kochi • Ph: +91-484-4059061-65
  Fax: +91-484-4059065 • E-mail: cochin@cbspd.com
- **Kolkata:** 6-B, Ground Floor, Rameshwar Shaw Road, Kolkata - 700014
  Ph: +91-33-22891126/7/8 • E-mail: kolkata@cbspd.com
- **Mumbai:** 83-C, Dr. E. Moses Road, Worli, Mumbai - 400018
  Ph: +91-9833017933, 022-24902340/41 • E-mail: mumbai@cbspd.com

Representatives:

- Hyderabad: 0-9885175004
- Pune: 0-9623451994
- Nagpur: 0-9021734563
- Jharkhand: 0-9811541605
- Patna: 0-9334159340
- Uttarakhand: 0-9716462459

Printed at: Neekunj Print Process, Delhi (India)

Foreword

E MPLOYMENT and INCOME GENERATION are the buzzwords in all the developmental sectors. With the increasing population, there seems to be an extreme scarcity of employment in the government sectors, and further the government is also burdened thus trying to cutoff the already existing posts in various departments to meet the financial burden. In such a scenario, the youth employment has become the major cause of concern. The scenario is similar worldwide and the unemployment rates have been growing annually at more than 15% all over the world. According to a United Nations 2000 report on youth unemployment, the problem is worse in Asia. This region accounts for 54 percent of world's unemployed youth population and major portion of this population is in India. In next coming years it is estimated that only 25–30 percent could be absorbed in the labour force. Simultaneously, there has been a marked decrease in the number of jobs on offer from the organized sector (less than 10 percent). As a result, the emphasis on job creation has shifted to the informal sector. In the present era of shrinking landholdings and increasing unemployment of youth in rural areas, agribusiness and micro-enterprise promotion has evolved as an answer to the employment crisis facing the world.

Animal husbandry is one of the most important components of agriculture system and plays a pivotal role in the overall growth of agrarian economy of India. In India, livestock sector remains one of the mainstays of agriculture which is a source of livelihood for over 68 percent of the population. If Indian economy has to grow at a sustainable growth of 8 percent, agriculture needs to grow at a rate of 4 percent wherein livestock sector will contribute considerably.

Our country is now the topmost producer of milk and the third largest producer of eggs in the world. We have also made very significant advances in poultry production and the other animal products. It is due to animal products that India has been on the world map of animal husbandry since a long time. These improvements have been possible with the use of scientific methods, the need for which will continue to grow in the years to come. For this, it is essential that the various opportunities in the agriculture and livestock sector and the underlying concepts behind enterprise setting be communicated to the researchers, educationists, planners and developmental workers so as to facilitate entrepreneurship generation in this sector. More specifically, the information regarding the various types of diverse micro-enterprises, including dissemination of loans, insurance, value-added products, WTO concerns, GMP, etc. need to be provided to the students seeking education in the agricultural universities so as to make them job providers from the job seekers. There is a need to discuss and deliberate in detail the issues listed above by the policy planners and experts entrusted to develop government programmes. In this prevailing scenario this book "Entrepreneurship in Livestock and Agriculture" provides a very good exposure to the students and educationists in the field of agricultural sciences and will motivate them to set up their own enterprises, thus helping themselves as well as reducing the burden on the government also.

The present compilation of 38 chapters in the form of a book written by scientists, educationists, bankers and developmental workers from various fields of agricultural sciences is indeed a timely effort in this direction. The book would be highly relevant for policy planners, executors at field level, researchers, academicians, students and entrepreneurs.

CD Mayee
Chairman, ASRB
KAB-I, PUSA, New Delhi

Preface

Unemployment and underemployment are becoming a global concern and the situation is getting more serious with the continuous rise in the population. More than half of the world's unemployed youth are present in the region and majority of Asia's unemployed youth are Indians. Only a limited number of unemployed youth in India could be engaged in the coming time. The number of jobs in organized sector is decreasing every year due to which the gravity of unemployment among the youth is increasing. At this juncture it is the duty of all the responsible organizations of the country to explore newer avenues to provide the employment to a larger number of eligible youth for fruitful utilization of their potential. Development of rural areas can bring about holistic national development, which is sustainable. Poverty alleviation can be addressed by generating employment opportunities and creating an entrepreneurial environment. Micro-enterprise development in rural areas is envisaged as the first step towards employment generation. Work force in our country is mostly (92 percent) engaged in the nonformal sector while only about 8 percent is in the organized sector. Recent initiatives related to employment generation made it clear that the nonformal sector has enormous potential and must be targeted. Rural areas are indeed looking for a comprehensive initiative for self-promoted employment through micro-enterprise development. Increasing population, urbanization and income in a developing country are catalyzing a massive global increase in demand for food of animal origin. The present scenario indicates the animal protein requirement would rise faster than the cereals in the consumption pattern of Indian people mainly due to increase in income and demand for quality food. Such a demand-driven growth, taking place mostly in developing countries, will call for greater emphasis on harvesting, storing and processing facilities. Government and the industry must prepare themselves for long-term policies and investment that will satisfy consumer demand for food of animal origin, improve nutrition, income and employment opportunities. Generation and dissemination of appropriate technologies to enhance production and productivity should be given greater attention.

We should take the advantage of the emerging trade opportunities in various livestock, poultry and agriculture-based commodities, services and animal products. India has the advantage of having diverse agroclimatic conditions, rich biodiversity, competent professional's work force and cheap labour apart from huge number of livestock population. Emphasis should be laid down on those commodities in which particular country has the cost advantage and also on the export of value-added products rather than on the primary products for increasing share in the world livestock-based exports. Many initiatives and efforts have been directed towards this aspect in the recent years and the present book is documentation of research experiences and strategies for entrepreneurship promotion in livestock and agriculture sector. In this book, an attempt has been made to explain the basics of entrepreneurship, the underlying concepts, communication acumen, interpersonal communication strategies, agribusiness ventures, WTO and IPR issues, banking and insurance facilities, and various other aspects related to the promotion of livestock and agriculture enterprises, especially in the rural areas.

We sincerely thank Dr NN Pathak, Dr Chinmay Joshi, Dr AK Goel, Dr Puneet Kumar, Dr Ashok Kumar, Dr PK Rout and Dr Gunjan Das for their endeavour in bringing out this publication. We express our thanks to all the contributing authors, without their support, it would have not been possible to bring this book in the present shape. The secretarial assistance provided by Mr JP Singh, Deepak Sheel and Gaurav Singh is deeply acknowledged.

MC Sharma
Rupasi Tiwari
JP Sharma

Contributors

Rashmi Singh
Senior Scientist
Division of Agricultural Extension
IARI, New Delhi

JP Sharma
Principal Scientist and Incharge
ATIC, IARI, New Delhi

NN Pathak
Former Director
CIRB, Hisar
Haryana

Amresh Kumar
Director General
KCM.T, Bareilly (UP)

MC Sharma
Director, Central Institute for
   Research on Goats,
Makhdoom, Farah
Mathura (UP)

Rupasi Tiwari
Senior Scientist and Incharge ATIC
Joint Directorate of Extension
   Education
Indian Veterinary Research
   Institute
Izatnagar, Bareilly (UP)

Debashish Sengupta
Professor
Alliance Business Academy
Bangalore

Simmi Tomar
Senior Scientist
Central Agricultural Research
   Institute
Port Blair

K Dhama
Senior Scientist
Division of Avian Diseases
Indian Veterinary Research
   Institute
Izatnagar, Bareilly (UP)

Mahesh Mahendran
Research Scholar
Division of Avian Diseases
Indian Veterinary Research
   Institute
Izatnagar, Bareilly (UP)

JM Kataria
Director
Animal Health Institute
Bagpat, Meerut (UP)

R Prasad
Zonal Coordination Unit (ICAR)
Rawatpur, Kanpur (UP)

C Singh
Training Organiser
KVK
Chitrakoot (UP)

RA Rawat
Training Associate (LPM) KVK
Gonda (UP)

Shahaji Phand
Assistant Professor
Jabalpur Veterinary College
Jabalpur (MP)

Sapna Gautam
Research Scholar
Department of Clothing and
   Textile
College of Home Science
GBPUAT, Pantnagar
Uttarakhand

Alka Goel
National Fellow
Department of Clothing and
   Textile
College of Home Science
GBPUAT, Pantnagar
Uttarakhand

KL Jeengar
Assistant Professor (Entomology)
KVK, Bhilwara
MPUAT, Udaipur
Rajasthan

Prakash Panwar
Assistant Professor (Home Science)
KVK, Bhilwara, MPUAT, Udaipur
Rajasthan

PM Khan
Chief Scientist-cum-Head
KVK, Bhilwara
MPUAT, Udaipur
Rajasthan

AK Thakur
Associate Professor and Head
Department of Dairy Extension
SG Institute of Dairy Technology
Patna

Prakash Singh
Department of Extension
   Education
ND University of Agriculture and
Technology, Kumarganj
Faizabad (UP)

Anupam
Department of Extension
   Education
ND University of Agriculture and
Technology, Kumarganj
Faizabad (UP)

B Mishra
Head
Department of Extension
   Education
ND University of Agriculture and
   Technology, Kumarganj
Faizabad (UP)

Nirmal Kaur
PhD Scholar
Department of Family Resource
Management
College of Home Science
GB Pant University of Agriculture
   and Technology
Pantnagar (US Nagar)
Uttaranchal

Deepa Vinay
Professor
Department of Family Resource
   Management
College of Home Science
GB Pant University of Agriculture
   and Technology
Pantnagar (US Nagar)
Uttaranchal

Shalini Agarwal
PhD Scholar
Department of Family Resource
   Management,
College of Home Science
GB Pant University of Agriculture
   and Technology
Pantnagar (US Nagar), Uttaranchal

Sanjeev Kumar Singh
Assistant Professor
Veterinary and Animal Husbandry
  Extension
College of Veterinary Sciences
Pt DDU University of Veterinary and
  Animal Sciences
Mathura (UP)

Pankaj Kumar
Scientist, Division of Medicine
Indian Veterinary Research
  Institute
Izatnagar, Bareilly (UP)

Umesh Dimri
Senior Scientist
Division of Medicine
Indian Veterinary Research
  Institute
Izatnagar, Bareilly (UP)

D Swarup
Principal Scientist and Head
Division of Medicine
Indian Veterinary Research
  Institute
Izatnagar, Bareilly (UP)

HP Dwivedi
Research Scholar
Department of Epidemiology and
  Preventive Medicine
GB Pant University of Agriculture
  and Technology
Pantnagar

Mahesh Kumar
Professor and Head
Department of Epidemiology and
  Preventive Medicine
GB Pant University of Agriculture
  and Technology
Pantnagar

Lal Ji Singh
Chief Manager
Agriculture, State Bank of India
Regional Head Quarter
Bareilly (UP)

VK Bhasin
Admn. Officer
Department of Marketing
Oriental Insurance Co Ltd
Rampur Garden, Bareilly (UP)

Shubha Johri
Assistant Professor
Lal Bahadur Shastri Institute of
  Management and Technology
Bareilly (UP)

Richa Bahadur
Lecturer
Lal Bahadur Shastri Institute of
  Management and Technology
Bareilly (UP)

Rajendra P. Bharti
Director
Lal Bahadur Shastri Institute of
  Management and Technology
Bareilly (UP)

Chinmay Joshi
Lecturer in Zoology
Govt PG College
Dwarahat (Almora)
Uttaranchal

Manish Sharma
University of Aberdeen
Scottland (UK)

Shalini Agarwal
PhD Scholar
Department of Family Resource
  Management
College of Home Science
GB Pant University of Agriculture
  and Technology
Pantnagar (US Nagar)
Uttaranchal

SK Mendiratta
Senior Scientist
Division of Livestock Products
  Technology
Indian Veterinary Research
  Institute
Izatnagar, Bareilly (UP)

N Kondaiah
Head and Principal Scientist
Division of Livestock Products
  Technology
Indian Veterinary Research
  Institute
Izatnagar, Bareilly (UP)

Gunjan Das
Assistant Professor
Clinical Veterinary Medicine
CVSc and AH, CAU
Selesih, Aizawl
Mizoram

Kundan Singh
In-Charge, Communication
  Centre
Indian Veterinary Research
  Institute
Izatnagar, Bareilly (UP)

PN Kaul
Ex. Principal Scientist
Indian Veterinary Research
  Institute
Izatnagar, Bareilly (UP)

GS Bisht
Principal Scientist and In-Charge
  ARIS-Cell
Indian Veterinary Research
  Institute
Izatnagar, Bareilly (UP)

YP Singh
Scientist (Sr. Scale)
ARIS-Cell
Indian Veterinary Research
  Institute
Izatnagar, Bareilly (UP)

Sanjay Kumar
Senior Scientist
ARIS-Cell
Indian Veterinary Research
  Institute
Izatnagar, Bareilly (UP)

Shahnawazul Islam
Scientist, Division of Computer
Applications, IASRI
New Delhi

Hari Om Agarwal
Scientist SG, Division of Computer
  Applications
IASRI, New Delhi

Mohd. Samir Farooqui
Scientist, Division of Computer
Applications, IASRI
New Delhi

Hemant Yadav
Asstt. Director (CS & IT), KCMT
Bareilly (UP)

BP Singh
Senior Scientist, Joint Directorate
  of Extension Education
Indian Veterinary Research
  Institute
Izatnagar, Bareilly (UP)

Contents

1

Entrepreneurial Need and Inculcation

Rashmi Singh, JP Sharma

Entrepreneurship is usually described as the whole process of finding opportunities, mobilising and acquiring resources, managing the production process and marketing the products. Entrepreneurs are architects of every conceivable material project and are motivated force behind development of any nation. Entrepreneurial spirit and defining characteristics of entrepreneurs have generated a lot of interest among researchers and academicians since long.

Many research studies have contributed to the literature on the characteristics of entrepreneurs. From an economist's point of view, an entrepreneur is one who brings resources, labour, materials and other assets into combinations that make their value greater than before. The one who brings about changes, innovations and a new order, from psychologists' viewpoint, an entrepreneur is a person typically driven by certain wishes and forces within self to achieve certain goals to make experiments or to gain independence. A sociologist views entrepreneurship as a combination of strong achievement motivation in an individual along with certain conditions of social structure and culture strongly favouring the individual to pursue economic pursuits.

Despite these differing emphases of different disciplines, an entrepreneur has been described as an especially talented person, as he/she possesses certain qualities and characteristics which make entrepreneurial behaviour possible. Some of them are listed below.

Need for Achievement

Most people dream of success and achievement, but do not take any action towards achieving these dreams. People with entrepreneurial qualities, on the other hand, have a strong desire to achieve a higher goal and make their dreams come true. For them winning is achievement.

Capacity to Assume Risk

A successful entrepreneur prefers a situation where there is moderate challenge, which can be overcome by his/her efforts. All the pros and cons for a decision are taken into account but neither a very high-risk endeavor nor something which is not having any challenge at all is preferred. This is one of the most important characteristics since success or failure of business depends on how decisions are made.

Taking Initiative

The entrepreneurs are independent and highly self-reliant. Studies have also shown that effective entrepreneurs actively seek and take initiatives. When they undertake a task, they make sure to complete it. They prefer situations where the result depends on their ability or efforts rather than a chance or other factors beyond their control.

Seek Feedback of Own Efforts

Entrepreneurs are very concerned about their performance. They prefer to gauge their achievement objectively and take corrective action immediately. Constant feedback is stimulating and satisfying to them and they use it to modify and improve their efforts at appropriate levels.

Long-term Involvement and Possess Drive

These characteristics differentiate between an entrepreneur and a promoter. They make commitment for a long-term project and to working towards goal that may be quite distant in the future. Successful entrepreneurs also know building of a business, a total treatment to attain a distant goal. They possess drive to excel and attain their goal with enthusiasm and passion.

Self-confidence

Studies have also shown that successful entrepreneurs have high level of self-confidence. They have confidence in their own capabilities to achieve the goal set by them. They also believe that events in their lives are mainly self-determined, and they have major influence on their own destinies and have little faith in fate.

Money as Measure of Performance

Money is the tool to judge the performance. Profits, gains, net worth are seen as measures of how well an entrepreneur is doing. The entrepreneur is always involved in process of making money, going out and investing it in another venture and then starting all over again.

Orientation towards Future Goals

Entrepreneurs are goal and action oriented. They have an ability to set goals and commitment to work towards them. They have high need for achievement. They set clear, measurable goals and accordingly they set priorities, measures and guide their time allocations.

Persistent Problem Solving

Successful entrepreneurs are not afraid by difficult situations. They possess intense level of determination and desire to overcome blocks. Researches have also shown that while entrepreneurs are extremely persistent, they are also realistic in recognizing their own abilities, and from where they can get help to solve difficult but necessary tasks. They believe in solving problems, navigating through other routes if faced with hurdles and are not problem avoiders.

Resource Utilization

Successful entrepreneurs are always aware about the resources, outside as well as inside, and understand when and how to utilize them efficiently. They seek expertise and assistance in achieving their goals. They are not so ego invalid in purely individual achievement of goals and independent accomplishment that they will not seek aid from others or refuse others offer of help.

Set High Standard for Themselves

High performing entrepreneurs also possess internalized competitive spirit in which they continuously engage in competition with themselves to best performance. They are always bettering themselves.

Tolerance to Ambiguity

Successful entrepreneurs are better able to tolerate ambiguity and uncertainty. They do not require complete structuring of a situation in order to function and in making of decisions. Job security and permanency are less preferred by entrepreneurs than other managerial counterparts.

Creative and Innovators

Entrepreneurs always try different alternatives to achieve their goals at their disposal. They tend to be creative and innovators for methods of choice, which will work best. They are ingenious at adopting and modifying whatever is at hand to solve the problems or to achieve objective.

Some Prevalent Myths about Entrepreneurs

Despite the fact that the entrepreneur has been defined and redefined by historians, economists, sociologists, psychologists and behavioural scientists, we find some misconceptions prevalent with respect to entrepreneurs in the developmental process. Examining the misconception/myths is one way of clarifying our concept in this regard.

Entrepreneur's Primary Motivation is a Desire for Wealth

The most misunderstood aspect of the entrepreneur is his/her relationship to money. Popular opinion generally holds that entrepreneurs are driven by greed, which is fundamental to their character. They work just for money that drives them to do things which ordinary people would not do. But, the fact is that money is very rarely the primary driving force for successful entrepreneur (Gifford Pinchot, 1985). Their attitude towards money is complex and intimate. They do care about it and work for it but it is not the chief goal in their life. As Hallmark card's founder J.C. Hall (1965) stated "he (the entrepreneur) does not seem to be galvanized into activity by the prospect of profit, it is people with low achievement need who require money incentives to make them work harder. The person with high need for achievement work hard anyway, provided there is an opportunity for achieving something. He is interested in money rewards or profits primarily because of the feedback they give him as to how well he is doing. Money is not the incentive to efforts but rather a measure of the success for the real entrepreneur."

Entrepreneurs are High Risk-takers

Popular belief holds the entrepreneur as a daring, devil-may-care risk-taker. The common saying—no risk no gain—is often viewed as implying that a very high order of risks required establishing an enterprise where fortune and chance play a vital role. The term 'risk' commonly refers to as outcome, which leads to losses or deviations of realization from expectation. This simple meaning of risk, however, does not seem to be applicable in context of entrepreneurial behaviour. Risk taking willingness in case of an entrepreneur indicates a challenge in his activity where there reasonable chance of success. Success depends not on chance but on one's own efforts. McClelland (1985) argued "one of the striking characteristics of an entrepreneur is their willingness to take calculated risk to innovate in ways that have reasonable change of success." Studies show that successful entrepreneurs avoid high-risk situations; rather they seek and enjoy calculated moderate risk. They choose challenging goals, but they also do everything they can, to reduce the risk. Part of the entrepreneur's strategy for reducing risk is anticipating barriers and remaining open to feedback, both positive and negative. One who cannot see problems or imagine how anything might go wrong may be more aptly called a 'promoter' not a real entrepreneur.

Entrepreneurs are Amoral

Perhaps the most striking similarity of all venture capitalist' description of the entrepreneur is their insistence that honesty and integrity are characteristics of the successful entrepreneur. Some may find this surprising because in the popular mind entrepreneurs are often seen as willing to sacrifice morals for profit. But it is less surprising when one considers that entrepreneurs are generally deeply committed to what they consider to be worthwhile purpose. Their need to achieve produces flexibility with the rules, not a loss of integrity.

One venture capitalist described his idea of successful entrepreneurs like this "they are darned honest with themselves. If there is a problem, they tend to get it out in the open fast and then stick with it until it is solved." Another said of entrepreneurs "all are extremely honest with themselves and will not tolerate untruthfulness or dishonesty".

Since entrepreneur often has to handle dozens of functions that they know little about, this ability to steer through truthfully is essential.

Entrepreneurs are Power Hungry Empire Builders

Watching entrepreneurs build large organizations with themselves at the helm. It is easy to imagine that they are driven by the need to tell others what to do. But it turns out that the need for power is not an important part of the entrepreneurial motivation. Power driven people are satisfied to achieve things by getting others to do them. However, we may find it quite reserve in case of entrepreneurs.

Lying behind motivation, McClelland felt, are the fantasies every person has of what he or she wants to be or do. Based on his extensive studies of entrepreneurs he concludes that entrepreneurs are not driven by need for power, instead, their motivation stems from a very high need of achievement. Entrepreneurs, he found, are not so concerned with the corner offices, large number of people to tell what to do and imposing possessions. They are not satisfied with rising in the hierarchy and having the esteem of their peers. Instead, entrepreneurs are driven by the need to achieve behind their mark by accomplishing things that have never been done before. Therefore the myth of the power-motivated than executive and the facts that they are achievement oriented instead explains both their strength as business starters and their potential weakness as executives.

Entrepreneurs are Inventors

It is commonly believed that an entrepreneur is basically an intelligent person and has a definite ability to create something new to prove his worthiness. On the basis of the existing profile of a successful entrepreneur, it has been found clearly that entrepreneurs are innovators, not inventors. Invention and innovation are two entirely different aspects. Invention provides the initial insight or discovery that as scientific or technological problem can be solved, whereas 'innovation' is the socio-managerial process by which new products and techniques are introduced into a socio-economic system. It has been established that not all inventors are good innovators. Henry Ford is a good example. He did not invent a thing. He drew upon the ideas of others and put them together on the assembly line of his automobile industry. There was nothing new in these techniques. But Ford was an innovator and entrepreneur. On the other hand, Thomas Edison was an inventor. He went bankrupt once, and though he survived the disaster, he could not make money in his lifetime. He was not an innovator and entrepreneur. To give yet another example, Chester Carlson, the physicist, invented a document-copying device in 1930, based on his knowledge of photoconductivity, carrying out his experiment in his own kitchen. But it was only in 1960 that a creative group under Joseph C. Wilson of the Haloid Corporation exploited the invention fully to bring about a major revolution in the field of giving us Xerox copying. Thus enterprises require not only brilliant ideas but also creative ideas harnessed to a productive drive in order to workout the invention into a product.

Entrepreneurs are Born

A common belief that the entrepreneurs are born has been another block in understanding fully the key element in developing entrepreneurship. Emergence of entrepreneurs in a few restricted castes and regions of people more often than others perhaps made the belief stronger even among those promoting entrepreneurship. People belonging to some of the castes like Marwari, Sindhi, Punjabi, etc. are generally believed to have inborn entrepreneurship qualities viewed objectively, it is not difficult to accept that those who take birth in these castes are definitely in advantageous position as they get an opportunity to be aware about business environment more than those from other castes. However, it has been clearly established that emergence of entrepreneurs is independent of caste/region. Any one with certain entrepreneurial characteristics at least to a minimum level qualifies to be an entrepreneur.

Some of the important characteristics of an entrepreneur are psychological in nature. These characteristics can be influenced through training. The kind of influencing that is attempted in training, perhaps, also takes place as the process of socialization of the 'child and the youth' in the family and the community for the traditional entrepreneurial caste groups. In other words, the characteristics in an individual are heightened to a required level which finally gives rise to a unique kind of manifestation that may be termed as entrepreneurial behaviour. Some people have gone far in oversimplifying by saying that "entrepreneurs can be manufactured" which no doubt does equal disservice to the cause of entrepreneurship development.

The misconception stated earlier seems to have implications in promoting entrepreneurship in any society. Since the entrepreneurs are the key factors in developing entrepreneurship, any misunderstanding about this key element may create a basic problem of integrating other aspect like support facilities with them. Even worse, problem may arise in terms of treating the entrepreneurs in the right spirit. It is established fact that the entrepreneur does seek positive recognition in the society and therefore, would not like to be treated like any venture capitalists or businessmen. To preserve the dignity and prestige it appears to be important that all those engaged in promoting entrepreneurship understand the entrepreneurs as what they are rather than what they are not.

Intrapreneur

Another term often we come across is intrapreneur. An intrapreneur is a person who wants and accesses to corporate resources. Goal oriented and self-motivated, but also respond to corporate rewards and reorganization. He is very much like the entrepreneur but situation demands greater ability to prosper within the organization. He dislikes the shortcomings of the system but learns to manage it for reaching excellence and works out problem within the system.

Entrepreneurship

Entrepreneurship is a function of at least four sets of factors, which mainly influenced it, could be identified. In the first place, entrepreneurship is generated in a society by individuals who for some reasons, initiate, establish, maintain and expand new enterprises. It is observed that entrepreneurs grow in the traditions of their families and the society, and internalized certain values and norms from these sources. The second factor thus constitutes the socio-cultural traditions emanating from these sources. The contribution from this socio-cultural factor in the process of transmission, however, gets filtered through the individuals get more influenced than others. The influence of these factors, on entrepreneurship is, thus, only indirect.

In addition to these two indirectly influencing factors, two other aspects directly influence entrepreneurship. The socio-political and economic policies of the government and other financial institution; and the opportunities available in a society as a result of such policies; may be considered to play a crucial role in exerting direct influence on entrepreneurship.

This factor, in practice, operates as one of the major given constraints for the effective functioning of the support system, which work for the development of the entrepreneurs. The support system would include consultancy services as well as large industrial units interested in developing ancillary industries.

Figure 1.1 shows that these factors interacting and influencing entrepreneurship. While the individual, the environment, and the support systems directly influenced entrepreneurship, socio-cultural milieu contributes through the individual. In this sense, the individual directly contributes to entrepreneurship. Socio-cultural factors, in addition to influencing the individual, exert influence on the support systems as well. The support systems, by and large, reflect the values of the socio-cultural traditions, and take shape accordingly.

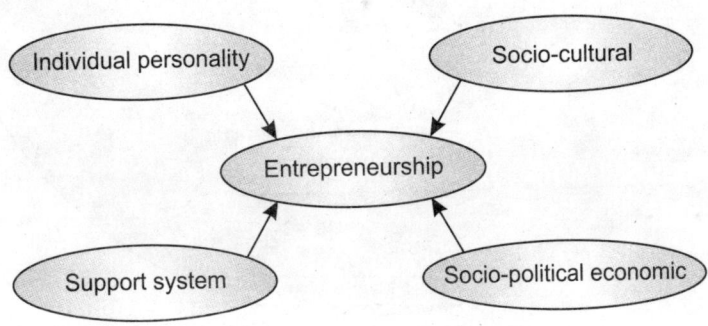

Fig. 1.1: Dynamics of entrepreneurship

Even though entrepreneurship is viewed here as a dependent variable, with all the four sets of factors influencing and contributing to it, it also functions as an independent variable because of the influence of the individual entrepreneur is likely to exert on the socio-cultural factors like norms, values, and behaviour, the entrepreneurs tend to behave differently on several dimensions, and they help in creating new norms and values in their own families, and eventually in the society.

In the context of employment generation, the three terms, i.e. entrepreneurship, self-employment and income generation are often used interchangeably (Fig. 1.2). Although there are a lot of commonalties among these concepts, yet the three terms are not the same. Self-employment refers to full time involvement in one's occupation or pursuits in which one may or may not have to take any risk to mobilize inputs and other resources to organize total production and services or to market the product and services. Income generating activities on the other hand are often part time and casual and practised for the purpose of

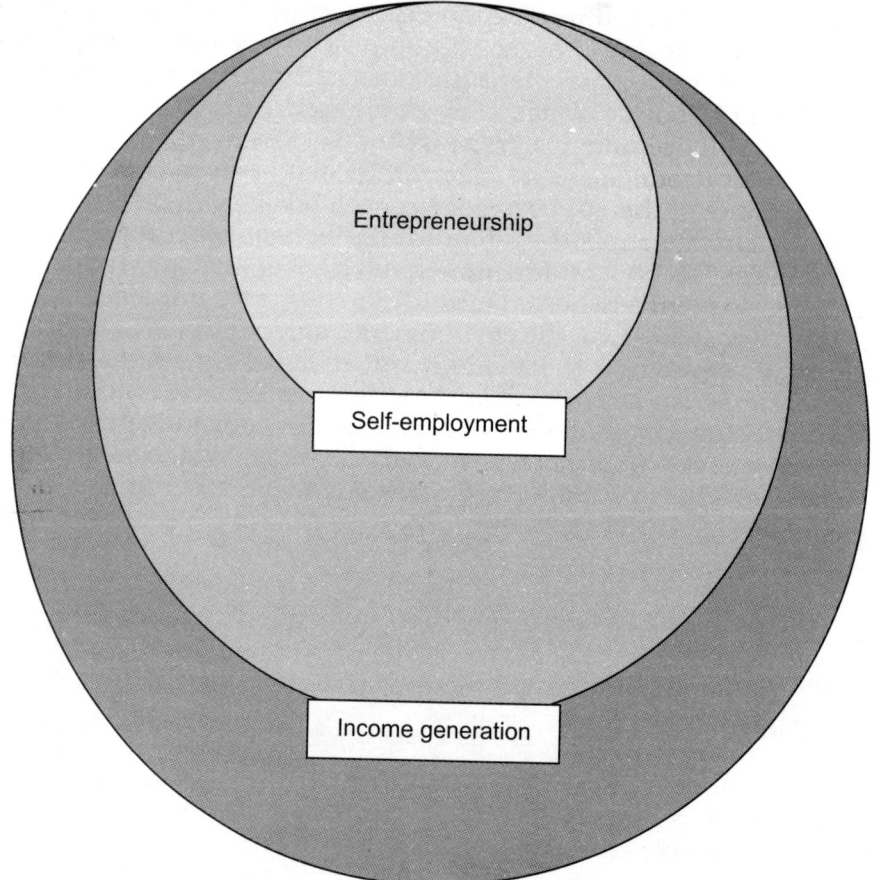

Fig. 1.2: Entrepreneurial growth process

raising additional income. The functions of entrepreneurs, as explained earlier, suggest that all entrepreneurs are self-employed and income generating persons. But all self-employed and income generating persons may not necessarily be entrepreneurs.

Accordingly, all the three may be useful means for employment generation in terms of their scope and impact with others.

The three, however, can be viewed as initial, middle and terminal stages in entrepreneurship growth process. With the conception, the plan of entrepreneurial development in late 1960's, the initiation of the self-employment programme by the Government of India, mooted along with the concept of entrepreneurship training. Until 1972-73, self-employment programme was equated with the implementation of the entrepreneurial development (ED) programme in most of the states. Ironically, many of the industrial change agents still consider entrepreneurship as a substitute for self-employment. In consequence, the aforesaid two terms have been used interchangeably during the implementation of the several ED programmes. A farmer, barber, or blacksmith may not be called as an entrepreneur, though he is self-employed. Entrepreneurship generates self-employment and additional employment but all those self-employed cannot be entrepreneurs.

An entrepreneurial spirit implies a commitment to certain ends, adherence to self-fulfillment and vision towards progress and means of realizing certain ends. The Schumpeterian model suggests that notwithstanding the infrastructural or community conditions, the entrepreneur dares to take risk to realize these goals and individual's emergence as entrepreneur in any set up is a complex process. Though the process is a blend of environmental variants and their socio-personal matrices, the person 'entrepreneur' becomes the product of overall management of the entrepreneurial development programme (EDP), mentioned or geared by the various local institutions in the state.

The various concepts and theories propounded by the past researchers seem to indicate that the emergence of entrepreneurs in a society depends upon closely interlinked economic, social, religious, cultural and psychological variables. Studies in India and abroad have strongly supported that achievement motivation has been a strong manifestation in one form or the other to the entrepreneurial pursuits. Some sociologists have found that the niter-group relationship cluster of ethical communities, occupational groups for the economic activities get charged through entrepreneurs alone. Economists have been suggesting incentives for entrepreneurial development such as appropriate monetary systems, balance of payment policy, removal of market uncertainty, stimulation of demand, local import tariffs or government subsidies programme, etc. A question arises, therefore, can we integrate the approach while envisaging the EDP for a particular client system? How, the best management development strategy can be employed during implementation of the above programmes to enable the local institutions, generate, mobilize and sustain the human resources.

Development process: Experiences have shown that two major factors have played significant role in developing entrepreneurship. One of them is the development of human factor—the entrepreneurship himself, another major factor is the development of environment where entrepreneurial activities can flourish and grow.

The human factors refer to the attitude, desire and motivation of an individual, his capability to perceive the environment changes and opportunities as well as his ability to solve the problems which he is likely to face. The training is effective in developing all these aspects of human factor provided it is planned well with balanced emphasis on all the aspects. Training has played crucial role for all such strategies in initiating and accelerating the process of entrepreneurship development. The training targets, however, have been both entrepreneurs and promoters of self-employment/entrepreneurship.

An analysis of the entrepreneurship development process (that helps in the emergence of people opting for entrepreneurial career) reveals that it follows a sequence of development of individual personality, capabilities and abilities.

The first generation of entrepreneurs requires developing:

a. Entrepreneurial quality/motivation;
b. Capability for enterprise launching/resourcing;

c. Ability for enterprise management; and

d. Sense of responsibility to the society that promotes/supports them.

a. Entrepreneurial quality/motivation: Generally, we find people opt for wage-earning career, society, by and large, spreads and popularizes such orientation. Social institutions such as the family as well as school, more or less support and development of qualities like conformity and compliance which are not conducive to the growth of entrepreneurial values. As a result of this, creativity, risk taking, perseverance, innovativeness and problem-solving orientation which are some of the accepted entrepreneurial qualities, are not encouraged. Whenever efforts are made to induct people to entrepreneurial career, such entrepreneurial qualities are generally found lacking or dormant. These are required to be aroused to an extent that people may start opting for entrepreneurial career. This is a basic requirement and much needed force, which drives people to their new ventures. Left to them, such qualities and motivation will be developed in only very few. Accordingly, as part of the planned programme of entrepreneurship development, the inputs have to be thought out and administered effectively to ensure development of the minimum entrepreneurial qualities/motivation adequate enough to drive them to entrepreneurial pursuits.

b. Capability for enterprise launching/resourcing: This opportunity exists in the society but not all of us are sensitive to it. Most of us in the society can perceive only the apparent and traditional openings for earnings. Similarly, resources are also available but very few make the efforts to make use of these. Together with economic insight for sensing opportunities in the area, prospective entrepreneurs may have to develop capability for selecting suitable project, formulating project report, arranging plant machinery, etc. and availing facilities and resources relevant to the launching of their enterprises. These are to be developed through training interventions.

c. Ability for enterprise management: The enterprise may be small or big, but it demands good management abilities in its owner/manager. Various factors of management such as production, marketing, financial management, etc. are crucial for enterprises. These have direct influence on the results and, are therefore, necessary determinants for sustenance of an enterprise. The management inputs to the potential entrepreneurs also raise their expectancy for success. However, the intensity of these inputs may vary depending upon the size of enterprise that is selected by an entrepreneur/self-employed person.

d. Social responsibility and entrepreneurial discipline: The entrepreneurs who are developed and promoted at the social cost have certain responsibility to the society that promotes, and supports them. The Government and other public institutions that invest on them also expect something in return. In order to sustain the efforts of developing entrepreneurship, it is necessary that a sense of responsibility towards the society in general and towards the entrepreneurial movement in particular needs to be developed among the potential entrepreneurs, especially those belonging to the younger generation. These entrepreneurs need to follow certain discipline, which is useful for entrepreneurial career. Such discipline may cover subjects like repayment behaviour, response to tax and statutory requirements, progressive outlook towards labour and above all care for ecology and environment.

These aspects related to individual behaviour, abilities and capabilities follow a logical sequence of development, which ultimately drives prospective youth to actual self-employment/entrepreneurial career.

Entrepreneurial Awareness in a Society can be Created/Generated

A society or community can be said to possess entrepreneurial awareness when most of its members are conscious of the importance that the entrepreneurs play in accelerating the growth of the economy and in enriching the quality of life in the society. When it is generally realized that man is not necessarily the creature of his environment, he is potentially to be the creator; that change not by what people desire but by what they endeavour to do and are concerned with. The entrepreneurial awareness of the community must lead to detect and appreciate the personality characteristic of entrepreneurs it must help by action the rise of entrepreneurial sprit and in leaders and community institutions to participate in the process of prolific emergence and healthy growth of genuine entrepreneurs.

Integrated Strategy

Entrepreneurship development strategy follows a cycle consisting of stimulatory, support and sustaining activities. The stimulatory activities ensure the supply of entrepreneurs ready to take initiative and organize their enterprises even if it involves risking their career. The support activities provide infrastructure facilities, resources, ability and skill to entrepreneurs for enterprise launching and management. Sustaining activities refer to all such efforts that facilitate growth and continuity through expansion, modernization, diversification and technology up-gradation of on-going healthy enterprises and opportunity for rehabilitation of sick units. Each group of activities is highly interacting, supplementary and crucial to each other. The absence/negligence/overemphasis of anyone may render the whole effort infructuous.

The entrepreneurship growth process can be further accelerated. The experimentations have amply demonstrated that entrepreneurship can be developed through planned efforts. Such planned efforts may require integration of stimulatory, supportive and sustaining activities. Training has been accepted and found very effective intervention in motivating and developing entrepreneurial qualities; capabilities and abilities for enterprise launching and management.

Entrepreneurship development is a process comprising essentially three phases, stimulatory, support and sustenance.

Stimulatory

Entrepreneurship refers to enterprising or achieving attitude. The question arises how this is enterprising or "need for achievement" attitude to be developed and fostered. Motivation through stimulation and training psychologically prepares an individual to take the entrepreneurship. The stimulatory phases require a well-designed training programme based on experiential learning. On the part of trainer also it is very important that he/she should have deep knowledge about psychology and interested genuinely in the people.

Entrepreneurship development centres have sprung all over country in recent years since initial effort during 1971. Universities have also started introducing entrepreneurship development as a subject in their syllabi at the graduate and postgraduate level assuming that it is possible to stimulate the entrepreneurial attitude and competencies in the persons who have potential through specific training and teaching programmes.

Support

An entrepreneur does need, no doubt a sport of enterprise in him to be handled but to actually start an industry, he equally needs the timely help from various corners and concerns such as skill training, financial assistance, technical know-how and locating institutions to get training and facilities which involve huge costs, such as physical infrastructure, (power transport, communication at a cheaper rate).

Sustenance

Small is beautiful but sensitive also, small business is such a sensitive thing. In India and many developing countries, development agencies pay too much attention to the "start up phase" but too little to the operational stage of an industry during the course of its operation, it is essential to follow-up and to, help sustain their on endeavour. Examples of sustaining activities undertaken by the promotional agencies may include:

Promotion	Diversification
Expansion	Competition
Modernization	Consultancy
Marketing	Policy measures
Reservation of items, etc.	

2

Basics of Entrepreneurship for Livestock-based Enterprises

NN Pathak

Udiyoginah Singh Mupait Lakshi Takee Cheri means wealth is the maid of entrepreneur. This has been emphasized in ancient literature of India thousands of years ago. Similar expression has been put forward in a Latin phrase *Audaces fortuna Juvat* means fortune favours entrepreneur. Entrepreneur is a French word means to undertake but in today's context of entrepreneur this meaning does not provide complete information about the main characteristics of an entrepreneur. The meaning of an entrepreneur given in the new Encyclopedia Britannica defines entrepreneur as a person capable of bearing the risk of undertaking a business without taking the note of performance and future condition.

CHARACTERISTICS OF AN ENTREPRENEUR

1. A person with confidence.
2. Capable to take initiative without hesitation.
3. Possesses skill of managing available resources in hand and also capable of mobilizing resources from potential sources.
4. Have courage to take risk in utilizing the invention or newer technologies for commercial exploitation.

Characteristics of an Entrepreneur in Livestock Business

Most of the graduates even with rural background are not exposed to the risk involved in livestock enterprises. Despite high level of scientific advancement it is very difficult to forecast the performance of a particular animal because production performance of livestock is influenced by several socio-environmental factors. Therefore, it is important to acquire adequate knowledge about the production and marketing which are highly variable due to high variation in the types of products, their self-life, class of consumers and economic status. Under such situation, an entrepreneur venturing for livestock enterprise should have the following characteristics:

1. Should have well-defined objective for the production (qualitative and quantitative) of livestock and livestock products.

2. Determination of dimension of production units. This will depend on the objective, i.e. (i) small scale for supplementing family income, (ii) a larger unoit for earning livelihood and (iii) commercial enterprise of various sizes.
3. Management of resources for development of infrastructure, purchase of livestock, feeds, utensils and appliances, processing of products and marketing of products.
4. Should be prepared to take risk because most of the livestock products are highly perishable items.
5. Should develop skill for the alternate method of disposal viz. excess or surplus milk left unsold should be utilized for the production of khoa, paneer, etc.

Prerequisites for Livestock Farming Enterprise

Before proceeding for the establishment of any enterprise of livestock production, it will be very useful to acquire the followings:

1. The entrepreneur should have basic knowledge of selected animal husbandry.
2. Availability of market within the approachable limits.
3. Seasonal fluctuations for the demand of products.
4. Scope of sale of value added products.
5. Availability of unskilled and skilled manpower.
6. Availability of land and natural water sources.
7. Scope of seasonal purchase and storage of feedstuffs.
8. Cycle of occurrence of natural calamities, if any.
9. Insurance facility for farm commodities and livestock will provide protection against unforeseen mishaps.

Selection of Livestock for Farming

In Indian society, there are inherited limitations for the selection of animal species for rearing. This is significantly influenced by religion, region, economic status, educational background and availability of markets.

Effect of Religion

Rearing of certain specific species of farm animal is strictly prohibited in some of the religions like even sight of pigs is prohibited in the followers of Islam, cattle for beef in Hindu and protection of all kind of living mammals, birds, other animals and even some species of vegetation is strictly observed by Bishnoi community of Hindu. Therefore, this aspect be kept in mind for the selection of livestock species and products.

Effect of Region

Some of the Indian societies are still highly arthodox and do not accept families opting for non-acceptable animal husbandry like swine farming by Brahmins, Agravanshi and Jain, etc. These groups also do not associate themselves with any kind of animal rearing for slaughter in most part of the country. Consumption of meat and meat products is negligible in these communities. Therefore, animal husbandry practice for meat production should be avoided in areas populated by these families.

Economic Status of the Population

Although families of highly diversified economic groups live in almost all parts of the country but in certain large areas in some of the states of India, proportion of economically weaker class is quite high. In such areas, demand of food of animal origin like milk, meat and their processed products is very low and establishment of a small scale livestock production for local population may not be even sustainable. However, livestock production for marketing in areas of demand and export may be taken up in such areas, if resources like land, feeds and fodders are available at reasonable rates, because man power will be easily available on the payment of low wages. Establishment of large scale livestock production projects in such area may be in the interest of both the entrepreneur and the local economically weaker class of people. The cost of production of former will be less and later will get remunerative employment needed for their livelihood.

Educational Background

Proliferation of higher and technical education particularly the education of veterinary sciences and agriculture during the past over half century has brought significant changes in the outlook of even many orthodox classes of Hindu community in India. These changes are now reflected in the acceptance of restricted animal husbandry enterprises of older years. Educated unemployed youth of many upper strata of society is now adopting swine rearing, rabbit farming, poultry farming, goat farming and fisheries in addition to diary farming. In some areas, fattening of male buffalo calves for meat production has been accepted by the livestock owners irrespective of social inhibitions.

Availability of Markets

Dimension of exploration of marketing of livestock and livestock products has shown a rising trend. This is mostly the effect of increased communication facilities. Now pigs fattened in Uttar Pradesh are marketed in the remunerative markets of north-eastern states, and male buffaloes fattened in some parts of northern states are marketed in Mumbai.

Similarly, producers of milk products like khoa and paneer have extended marketing covering up to 200–300 km in many parts of the country. For example, khoa produced in Ghazipur district is marketed mostly in Varanasi and Allahabad, whereas ghee produced in Chandausi, Aligarh, Hathras, Bulandshahar and Meerut is famous in north India.

Development of information systems, availability of fast transport facilities and availability of cold tankers have enlarged the marketing facilities.

Seasonal Fluctuations in the Demand of Livestock Products

Although some milk, meat and egg products are being marketed round the year, indeed there is distinct seasonal influence on the demand of certain products. Consumption of milk and milk products like khoa, chhenna, paneer and curd is increased many fold during the marriage season. This increase is quite high in the northern states. On the other side, such increase is more in the demand of meat, fish and poultry in the eastern and north-eastern regions.

Similarly demand of milk products, poultry products and fish increases in hotels and restaurants of all ranges during the tourism season and festivals in all parts of country. Therefore, it would be beneficial for the entrepreneurs to develop facilities for the safe conservation of perishable products, maintaining their quality, for marketing during the remunerative period of higher demand.

Need of Information Supply in Remote Areas for the Availability of Markets

Despite great increase in information systems, entrepreneurs engaged in production and sale of milk products are not aware of the great difference in the cost of products even within the radius of less than 50 km. For example, some sweets of chhenna marketed at the rate of Rs 40 to 50 per kg in Mahaban town of Mathura district are sold at Rs 80 to 150 per kg at Mathura, Agra, Vrindavan and Bhartpur towns. Although, consumers sometimes mention difference in the quality of products, but main effect appears to be that of brand name, decorated shop and good packaging in attractive containeRs The economic status of such entrepreneurs can be improved significantly by providing them short duration training on manufacture of products of desired quality and their good packaging along with increased hygienic conditions.

Nomenclature of Value-added Products

In modern society, a craze has been developed for show off and presenting oneself elevated in the society. Persons of these newer class of society prefer things different from commonly available in the market. In this direction, the good examples are the sweets of khoa and chhenna. All types of sweets available in the market are prepared from the use of khoa and sugar or chhenna and sugar, but the altering ratio of the khoa or chhenna and sugar, form and saturation of syrup, altering the shape and size of the products, use of some dry fruits in different forms, use of edible colours in different concentrations and decoration with silver leaves, etc. have increased the apparent number of several products. Similar technologies are being applied for the value addition of other products.

There is also a trend of naming these products with link of ancient and medieval royals. These approaches are successfully used for attracting the consumers and increasing the margin of profit. Some examples are Shahi paneer, Nawabi makhan, Lal dahi or Misti dahi, Gulab jamun and Kalajam, etc.

Revival and Introduction of Old and Forgotten Recipe

With the emergence of newer economically sound families, a large number of young persons are developing fancy for show and craze for presenting themselves more elite in their circle. The possession of costly watches, latest model of motor vehicles and regular visit to hotels, restaurants, café and even modern dhabas on high ways. A good number of such persons feel elevated by discovering newer food items of past. A good restaurant manager now use prefixes like Shahi, Muglai, Continental, Chinese and so on. On similar line there is great scope of reviving pauranik and ancient names of milk products like Jayur, haviya, payasm, sajaw dahi, sweet dahi bada and many others. While bringing such products in the market it is important to standardize the recipe for quality control, prepare a nutritional chart depicting content of important nutrients per unit of product, a good advertisement pamphlet and attractive shape and packing, etc.

Development of Demand in Consumers

Once a revived product of olden days has become popular among the consumers there will be need of modification in marketing strategies. This can be achieved by several ways but more effective will be creation of artificial shortage of product at a time when there is great demand for that product at a particular time. This approach may not be considered ethical, but such practice for a short time after intervals may be helpful in increasing the craze for the products in consumers. Such artificial shortage in market often indicates the higher liking and consumption of the product. In this regard, an example of sale of dahi bada at Gautam Budh Marg opposite the dairy about half century ago shown the effective impact of limited supply. Panditji used to prepare only 100 pieces of dahi bada with high quality dough, good curd, sonth (sweet chatani of tamarind pulp) and greens chatani of coriander, etc. He was a good sales maneger as he was able to maintain the quality of his single product and desire of eating in consumer by limiting the supply of his product for a short duration of 2–3 hours in evening.

Present Status of Supply of Foods of Animal Origin and Future Scope

The average availability of milk and milk products in India is only 214 g against the minimum daily requirement of about 250 g. Similarly availability of meat and meat products, eggs, chicken and fishes is much less than the requirement. Number of newer products as well as consumers are increasing, and for many products demand is much more than the production, therefore, there is tremendous scope of opting livestock enterprises. Selection aspect of production of a raw material and value-added product will depend on the skill and interest of an entrepreneur.

3

Career Opportunities for Veterinary Graduates

Amresh Kumar

Veterinary education in India has registered an incredible and tremendous growth. Veterinary profession has also undergone metamorphic changes in accordance with society's requirements during recent years.

VETERINARY PROFESSION

It is one of the old professions. It has reference in Atharveda (1500-500 BC) on horse management and treatment, elephant management and health care, etc. Emperor Ashoka, the great son of Chandra Gupta Maurya provided a new turn to veterinary science in India. It is described that world's first veterinary hospital on record existed in Ashoka's regime. During his period human and animal hospitals existed side by side. Medicines and herbs were regularly supplied to both human and animal hospitals, when needed. Hospitals had well-defined wards, where patients were treated indoors. The period of renaissance saw a decline of veterinary science. Around 1791-99 due to long scale epidemics and economic losses the interest in veterinary science aroused. The first training school came into existence in 1862 in Pune. In 1882, the first veterinary college was established at Lahore. This was followed by establishment of other colleges, viz. Bombay in 1884, Bengal in 1893, Madras in 1902-03 and Bihar in 1930. At the time of independence, there were nine veterinary colleges in India.

Importance of Veterinary Profession

The old objectives of veterinary education for producing graduates to undertake practice of veterinary medicine is no longer relevant in the present context. The contribution of livestock sector towards national gross domestic product has shown an increasing trend during the last two decades whereas the agriculture sector is facing a decline in GDP. Livestock not only caters to the food production but also contributes for draught power and organic manure. Thus, livestock has emerged as an important source for both income and employment generation of millions of people. The 90% of our livestock is being held by landless, small and marginal farmers which have made better distribution of livestock wealth compared to agricultural land.

Apart from the well recognized role in the prevention, diagnosis and treatment of diseases in animals, a veterinarian plays a critical role in number of areas including human health, research and development. Veterinarians also play important role in drug development and pharmaceutical industry, food industry, government and regulatory affairs, teaching and research; civil services, etc.

VETERINARY EDUCATION IN INDIA

Veterinary education in India today forms an integral component of Land Grant System of education. There are 41 veterinary colleges which offer recognized graduate veterinary qualifications. They are affiliated to either state agricultural universities or veterinary universities. At present, there are 7 veterinary universities and 37 state agricultural universities and 2 deemed universities (IVRI and NDRI) dealing with postgraduate qualifications in veterinary and animal sciences. The veterinary colleges produce more than 2500 veterinary graduates per annum. All veterinary colleges have implemented minimum standard of veterinary education regulation 1993 of Veterinary Council Act, 1984. Considering the increase in importance of veterinary profession in the country, Veterinary Council Act, 1984 was enacted by Parliament. The registration at the Veterinary Council became a legal mandate for a veterinary graduate to practice veterinary medicine. For registration with the Council, a person should possess a recognized veterinary qualification.

As per minimum standard of veterinary education, there are 17 teaching departments in addition to a teaching veterinary hospital complex in every veterinary college. The minimum admission in-take capacity as prescribed by Veterinary Council of India in a veterinary college is 60 per annum. The students admitted to BVSc and AH. Degree programmes have to undergo nine semesters of course work followed by 6 months compulsory internship programme. Besides prescribing minimum standard of education in veterinary colleges, Veterinary Council of India, a statutory body of Govt. of India, i.e. India Veterinary Council Act, 1984 (52 of 1984) regulates veterinary practice. Veterinary student receives a well rounded basic education. Veterinarians acquire a broad understanding of how a living organism works and impart their skills in many areas.

CAREER OPPORTUNITIES FOR VETERINARY GRADUATES

There are many avenues open to a graduate veterinarian and some of the important organizations/establishments/agencies engaging veterinary graduates are given below.

Animal Husbandry Departments of State Governments

Various state governments recruit the veterinary graduates to the post of veterinary officers/veterinary surgeons. These recruitments are made through the respective State Public Service Commissions and the basic qualification required for the posts is graduate degree in veterinary sciences. The veterinarians in the state departments may have to look after animal health cover, animal reproduction, veterinary and animal husbandry extension, meat inspection and cattle, buffalo, sheep, goat, pig and poultry production, breeding farms, etc.

Some of the veterinary graduates are engaged in the disease diagnostic laboratories of the state Government, while a few are recruited in the biological production units. The various developmental programmes of government agencies are also taken care of by these veterinary officers.

Pradeshik Co-operative Dairy Federation (PCDF)

PCDFs work through co-operative societies and are involved in production/ procurement of milk and milk products and the upliftment of dairy animals. It provides animal's health care, veterinary extension and animal reproduction facilities to the livestock farmers. It employs a large number of veterinary graduates. The job is quite challenging and entails hard work.

Entrepreneurship

The establishment of one's own veterinary clinic is the best bet for an aspiring, forward looking, competent, confident and hard working young veterinarian. He is his own master in this venture. The private clinics have been established in large numbers in metropolitan cities and towns. In cities, veterinarians are confined to small animal practice but in towns, they are engaged in mixed practice. The canine breeding is also practised by some of these practitioners, which is quite rewarding since there is great demand of pedigreed pups in the society.

Pharmaceutical Companies

A large number of Indian and multinational pharmaceutical companies have entered into the production of veterinary drugs and pharmaceuticals. They employ veterinary graduates for production, quality control and marketing of drugs and vaccine. The job is quite challenging, demanding and involves professionalism.

Remount Veterinary Corps (RVC)

RVC of the Indian Army offers a very rewarding career to an aspiring and dedicated veterinary graduate who is interested in a disciplined and active life. Veterinary graduates are selected in short service commissions or for permanent commission and recruitment is done through Services Selection Board. The job requires breeding, feeding, management, disease control and treatment of animals maintained by army, managing breeding centres, remount depots, slaughter houses and military dairy farms, etc.

Paramilitary Forces

A limited number of veterinary graduates are recruited by the Indo-Tibetan Border Police (ITBP), Boarder Security Force (BSF) and other paramilitary forces to manage dog and equine breeding centres and provide animal health cover and surveillance.

Bank and Insurance Companies

Most of the nationalized banks and insurance companies also recruit limited number of veterinary graduates to supervise and monitor sanctioning/awarding of funds for the purchase of milch animals under various loan schemes, preparation and screening of various project proposals, etc. The veterinarians engaged in these organizations do not get opportunity of rendering professional services in the area of treatment and control of diseases in animals.

Private Poultry Production and Dairy Farms

Many prestigious private poultry and dairy farms and private hatcheries also offer lucrative jobs to veterinary graduates having adequate experience in that area. The job requires a high degree of professional efficiency and devotion to duty.

Stud Farms/Race Course

The stud farms also recruit veterinarians to look after the breeding, feeding and management of equines. The job is quite challenging so are the emoluments. The veterinarians having interest and aptitude for equines are engaged by different race courses in metropolitan cities as consultant and for treatment of animals.

Diagnostic Laboratories

Some of the reputed organizations particularly the hatcheries and poultry farm owners have established the disease investigation facilities with an aim to provide the quick diagnostic facilities. Such laboratories also recruit veterinarians to undertake disease diagnostic work.

Zoo and National Parks

Though the zoo and national parks get veterinary assistance through respective animal husbandry departments, but some of them recruit their own veterinary officers to provide health cover to their animals. The job is quite challenging and rewarding.

Slaughter Houses

Some slaughter houses particularly those located in big cities and managed by municipal corporations as well as large slaughter houses in private sector also recruit veterinary graduates to look after the slaughtering, their management and for meat inspection work. They also help in preparation/utilization of slaughter house byproducts.

Teaching and Research Organizations

The veterinary graduates who have acquired higher qualifications, viz. MVSc, PhD, etc. are engaged by various academic and research institutes of different state universities/colleges, UPSC, ICAR, etc. They undertake teaching, research and extension work.

Research and Development Wings

Most of the pharmaceutical and other organizations have research and development wings for carrying out trials or developing protocols for clinical trials. They also recruit few veterinary graduates. However, they prefer the Masters/PhD degree holders in their respective specialization to undertake challenging task.

Thus broadly career opportunities for veterinarians can be grouped as per employment agencies, viz. state govt. centralized sectors, local bodies/municipalities/panchayats, private sector and in self-employment in private practice.

State Government

- Veterinary hospitals/primary veterinary centres.
- Organized state farms for managing livestock forms.
- Semen banks/sperm stations, where proven bulls are kept.
- Poultry farms for managing egg farms, hatcheries, chick rearing units.
- Meat/milk processing plants for supervising of hygienic production of meat, collection and distribution of milk.
- Polyclinics-where specialized service like surgery, special diagnostics and treatment, etc. are given.
- Disease investigation centres—survey disease profile and investigation work.
- Biological products or vaccine institutions prepare quality control and distribute vaccines, biologicals.
- Disease eradication schemes/check posts/vaccination camps.
- Public health labs—investigation of disease transmissible from animals to man and *vice versa*.

Centralized Sectors

- Army (Remount veterinary corps)—to train and look after horses, dogs, camel, etc. in the forces.
- BSF/police—to look after horses, dogs, camels, etc. in the forces.
- ICAR—co-ordination and funding of animal based research programmes.
- Department of Animal Husbandry and Dairying, Ministry of Agriculture—for administrative management and co-ordination of veterinary service.
- Quarantine units—these are international check posts preventing entry of exotic diseases like mad cow disease or fowl influenza, etc.
- Central farms—same as state farms and sperm stations.
- Academic/research/extension wing of veterinary colleges in state agricultural universities, state veterinary universities, or universities having veterinary faculty.
- Para-veterinary staff training schools.
- Experimental and germ-free animal facilities attached to veterinary and medical institutions, drug research institutions.
- Experimental animal unit, (animal model preparation for experimentation, etc.)
- Clinical, diagnostic and investigation centres attached to veterinary colleges and research institutes.

Local Bodies/Municipalities/Panchayats

- Slaughter houses/cattle farms/public health laboratories.
- Zoo and wildlife centres.
- Animal resource development under Panchayati Raj.

Private Sector

- Pharmaceuticals.
- Commercial dairy and poultry farms; breeding farms, hatchery, etc.
- Race club, stud farms.
- Veterinary instruments/equipment industry.
- Biological products and vaccine product plants.
- Insurance companies, banks, corporate bodies, e.g. National Dairy Development Board, Milk Board, Milk Unions, etc.
- Feed processing industry.
- Self-employment.

Private Practice

- Consultancy.
- Practising veterinarian for small and large animal; zoo animals.
- Entrepreneur in livestock farms, poultry farms, etc.
- Diagnostic laboratories (pathology, biochemistry, microbiology).
- X-rays, ultrasound facility.

Thus, the graduate veterinarians have a bright future. They have multiple job opportunities. They should not look only for the government job as there is vast scope and ample opportunities in other organizations too. The veterinary curriculum in veterinary institutions has been so structured that can shoulder the responsibility with great competence and ability.

4

Avenues of Entrepreneurship in Public and Private Sector

MC Sharma, Debashish Sengupta, Rupasi Tiwari, Manish Sharma

Planning in India focused at realizing a high rate of growth of output in the long term. A basic assumption was that shortage of capital goods in relation to employable persons constituted a fundamental constraint on growth in the economy. Therefore, the planning process made no attempt to define an independent employment strategy; the focus on economic growth was viewed as essential for improving the employment situation. Initially, labour force expansion was not seen as a problem to be contented with. Thus, in the Five Year Plans, the generation of employment was viewed as part of the process of development and not as a goal in conflict with, or to be pursued independently of economic development.

GLOBAL EMPLOYMENT AND UNEMPLOYMENT SITUATION

The global employment and unemployment situation according to the World Employment Report 1998-99, was as follows:

- Out of an estimated 6 billion population in the year 1997 around 3 billion was in the labour force.
- 160 million persons have been estimated to be fully unemployed.
- 25 to 30% of the employed labour force is under employed.
- A large number of young people in the age group of 15 and 24 (around 60 million in 1997) are continuously in search of work, i.e. unemployed.

A few important conclusions which emerge from the above report are:

- Limited demand for unskilled and less skilled labour.
- Increase in demand for skilled labour on account of technological development and upgradation and changes in the organization of work.
- Problems in maintaining the continued employability of labour force.
- Demand for multi-skilling.

Some of the important strategies recommended in the World Employment Report are:

- Timely investment in skill development and training at enhanced level.
- Enhancement of education and skill level of workers.

- Responsive training system.
- Need for effective partnership of all stake holders.

INDIAN EMPLOYMENT AND UNEMPLOYMENT SCENARIO

In India, due to the agrarian sector with seasonal operations, time disposition and availability for work have been the criteria for measuring employment. The accepted method of measuring employment is the usual status. Reliable estimates of employment/unemployment are generated through National Sample Surveys conducted once in 5 years by National Sample Survey Organization (NSSO). The concept recognizes time utilization only. Quality of work or income does not get reflected in the approach.

As per the results of the National Sample Survey conducted in 1999-2000, total work force as on 1.1.2000, as per usual status approach (considering both principal and subsidiary activities) was of the order of 406 million. About 7% of the total work force is employed in the formal or organized sector (all public sector establishments and all non-agricultural establishments in private sector with 10 or more workers) while remaining 93% work in the informal or unorganized sector. The size of the organized sector employment is estimated through the Employment Market Information Programme of DGE&T, Ministry of Labour. The capacity of the organized sector to absorb additional accretion to the labour force, taking into account the current accent on modernization and automation, is limited. In other words, an overwhelming proportion of the increase in the labour force will have to be adjusted in the unorganized sector. About 369 million workers are placed today in unorganized/informal sector in India; agriculture workers account for the majority of this work force. Growth rate of employment is less than the growth rate of the labour force indicating an increase in the unemployment rate. Self-employment and casual labour continued to play a pivotal role in rehabilitation of the unemployed.

RECOMMENDATIONS OF PLANNING COMMISSION

Considering the problems of employment and unemployment situation in the country, Planning Commission set up a task force under the chairmanship of Dr MS Ahluwalia to go into the details of the employment generation taking place in the economy and suggest measures for creation of 100 million jobs (10 million per year) in a period of 10 years. The task force has recommended intervention in five major areas as under:

- Accelerating the rate of growth of GDP, with a particular emphasis on sectors likely to ensure the spread of income to the lower income segments of the labour force.
- Pursuing appropriate sectoral policies in individual sector, which are particularly important for employment generation.
- Implementing focused special programmes for creating additional employment of enhancing income generation from existing activities aimed at helping vulnerable groups that may not be sufficiently benefited by the more general growth promoting policies.

- Pursuing suitable policies for education and skill development, which would upgrade the quality of the labour force and make it capable of supporting a growth process which generates high quality jobs.
- Ensuring that the policy and legal environment governing the labour market encourages labour absorption, especially in the organized sector.

The special group has also suggested restructuring in the following sectors in favour of labour intensive activity for generating additional gainful job opportunities for the Tenth Plan.

a. Agriculture and allied sectors.
b. Greening the country through Agro Forestry.
c. Energy plantation for biomass power generation.
d. Rural sectors and small and medium enterprises (SMEs).
e. Education and literacy.
f. Employment through ICT development.
g. Health, family and child welfare.

But along with the employment generation, self-employment or entrepreneurship will be crucial for bringing about a holistic development in a country like India.

WHAT IS ENTREPRENEURSHIP?

Entrepreneurship can be defined as (*AH Cole*)—"a purposeful activity of an individual or a group of associated individuals, undertaken to initiate, maintain or organize a profit oriented business unit for the production or distribution of economic goods and services".

ROLE OF GOVERNMENT IN ENTREPRENEURSHIP DEVELOPMENT

Government has been implementing various programmes which support women to take up new ventures and start self-employment, which has been categorized under four heads.

Empowering Strategies

Indira Mahila Yojana (IMY), Mahila Samriddhi Yojana (MSY), The Rural Women's Development and Empowerment Project (RWDEP) now called as Swa-Shakti Project, Development of Women and Children in Rural Areas (DWCRA).

Employment and Income Generation

Training of rural youth for self-employment (TRYSEM), Swayamsidha, Swalamban, Support for Training and Employment Programme (STEP), Norwegian Agency for International Development (NORAD), Socio-economic Programme (SEP), Condensed Courses of Education and Vocational Training (CCEVT), Swarnjayanti Gram Swarozgar Yojna (SGSY), Women's Vocational Training Programme (WVTP), Swarna Jayanti Shahari Rozgar Yojna (SJSRY), Urban Self-employment Programme (USEP), Development of Women and Children in Urban Areas (DWCUA), Jawahar Rozgar Yojna (JRY), Trade Related Entrepreneurship Assistance and Development (TREAD). Efforts are being made to merge STEP with other three programmes, i.e. NORAD, SEP and CCEVT, thus bringing out an umbrella scheme of "Training and Employment for Women".

Welfare and Support Services

Hostels for working women (HWW), short stay homes (SSH), Swadhar, creches/day care centres for the children of working and ailing mothers.

Other Enabling Measures

Rashtriya Mahila Kosh (RMK), a national level mechanism to meet micro-credit needs of poor and assetless women in the informal sector. Also known as the National Credit Fund for Women (NCFW).

ROLE OF NGOs IN ENTREPRENEURSHIP DEVELOPMENT

The major NGOs in rural entrepreneurship development are:
- National Alliance of Young Entrepreneurs (NAYE)
- World Assembly of Small and Medium Entrepreneurs (WASME)
- Xavier Institute for Social Studies (XISS)
- Self-employment Women's Association (SEWA) of Ahmedabad
- Association of Women Entrepreneurs of Karnataka (AWAKE)
- Rural Development and Self-employment Training Institute (RUDSETIs) based in Karnataka.

Some of these NGOs work solely for women entrepreneurs like SEWA and AWAKE whereas others are common for both men and women.

Financial Support

There are a good number of financial institutions that support women to start any new enterprise. Some of them are:
- Rashtritya Mahila Kosh (RMK)
- National Agricultural Bank for Rural Development (NABARD)
- Small Industries Development Bank of India (SIDBI)
- Council for Advancement of People's Action and Rural Technology (CAPART)
- Access to credit through "Development Bank for Women Entrepreneurs" in small scale and tiny sectors
- Reserve Bank of India (RBI)

Entrepreneurial Training

Entrepreneurs can be trained to start an enterprise, if proper inputs in the form of training are given. Some of the specialized institutes for training are:
- National Institute of Small Industry Extension and Training (NISIET), Hyderabad.
- Indian Institute of Entrepreneurship (IIE), Guwahati.
- National Institute for Entrepreneurship and Small Business Development (NIESBUD), New Delhi.

Training programmes for women entrepreneurship are also organized by government organizations (both central and state), e.g. small industries service institutes, centre for entrepreneurship development, etc. as well as by public sector banks like NABARD.

AVENUES OF EMPLOYMENT/SELF-EMPLOYMENT IN AGRICULTURE AND ALLIED SECTOR

There are many avenues of employment/self-employment in agriculture and allied sectors. Ranging from researcher to consultant, breeder, extension worker, and also in the sales and marketing of agro products like pesticides, fertilizers, seeds, etc. Besides entrepreneurial opportunities are also plenty.

Below we look at some of the emerging employment/self-employment opportunities in agriculture and allied field.

Agriclinics and Agribusiness Centres

Every year about 11900 agriculture graduates pass out of agricultural universities of which only about 2000 get employed in public and private sectors. The remaining 9900 agriculture graduates add to the pool of under employed/unemployed agriculture graduates.

The scheme of agriclinic and agribusiness centres was launched on 9th April, 2002 as a follow-up of Finance Minister's budget speech for 2001. The objective of the scheme is to provide fee-based extension and other services to the farming community and also to create self-employment opportunities for agriculture graduates.

The agriculture graduates are provided training in agribusiness development for two months in over 67 institutions in public/private sector located throughout the country and coordinated by MANAGE. These institutions also provide handholding support to the trained graduates for a period of one year. The entire cost of training and handholding is being borne by the Government of India. Trained graduates are expected to set up agriclinic and agribusiness centres with the help of bank finance. The scheme is being implemented with the help of Small Farmers Agribusiness Consortium (SFAC), National Institute of Agriculture Extension Management (MANAGE) and National Bank for Agriculture and Rural Development (NABARD).

Food Technologies

In today's busy world, people do not have enough time to stay in the kitchen. With changing lifestyle, food habits and jobs profile the ready to cook, ready to serve and fully processed packaged food and beverages are becoming popular.

It is estimated that food processing industries is growing and generating new jobs to extent of 2.5 lakhs every year. Agro processing sector is further expected to grow faster and generate more employment in the near future. It is estimated that Indian food increases more than 5,00,000 crores by the end of the year 2005. The market of the value added specialized processed packaged food product will grow to Rs 2,30,000 at the end of year 2005.

Biotechnology

Biotechnology is a science that enables us to find the beneficial traits, in terms of added nutrition, increased flavour, or greater ability to fight pests or diseases, and incorporate them into various organisms.

Biotechnology is able to isolate a particular gene (or trait) in one organism, remove it, and then transfer it to another organism, where this same gene replicates itself, creating a stronger and more resilient strain of the same substance.

Various roles in biotechnology are:

Molecular biologist: Functions in the area of genetic engineering.

Plant tissue culture specialist: Functions in the area of in vitro regeneration and propagation of plantlets.

Plant geneticist: Works to improve plants by developing new cultivars (horticultural varieties).

Extension Education

Extension education is the process of teaching rural people how to live better by learning ways to improve their farm, home and community institutions' (J. Paul Leagans). But the task of developing an individual is not so easy. For this an extension educator has to be a teacher, guide, friend and philosopher to the villagers/rural poor.

Thus if one aspires to be an extension educator he must be possessing an attitude and aptitude essentially demanded by the profession (i.e. interest and ability to work for the villagers) in addition to having a sound knowledge and understanding of the subject.

Floriculture

Floriculture denotes cultivation of flowers, developing new varieties of commercial value, sale of flowers as raw commodities, processing, distribution, etc. for the local and international market. Floriculture is emerging as a blooming business not only in India but in other countries as well. The annual domestic demand for the flowers is growing at a rate of over 25% and around Rs 90,000 crore internationally.

Floriculture industry in India comprises flower trade, nursery plants and potted plants, seed and bulb production, micro-propagation and extraction of essential oils. India's share in international market of flowers is negligible.

Enormous genetic, diversity, varied agro-climatic conditions, versatile human resources offer India a unique scope for diversification into new avenues which were hitherto unexplored or under-explored. India seems to have a blooming future of floriculture as there is a shift in the trend towards tropical flowers and this can be gainfully exploited by India.

Opportunities include consultants, farm/estate managers, plantation experts, and plantation supervisors, project coordinator. Research and teaching are some other avenues. Recently, marketing of floriculture products for different ventures has also emerged as a potential segment of this field. One can also work as entrepreneur and offer employment to others.

Dairy

Dairying is always considered as a viable occupation by the farm women and farmers as it generates regular income round the year. However, it can emerge as a profitable venture if undertaken as a business, based on proven scientific knowledge, latest package of technology, training and proper planning.

Milk Production Units

These units rear the milch animals and produce milk and sell it to the cooperatives, vendors and other consumers at remunerative prices, e.g. dairy farms.

Milk Procuring and Preserving Units

These units do not manufacture any new product. They merely procure and process the milk in order to increase its shelf-life, e.g. small-scale milk plants, chilling centres and raw milk pouch filling, etc.

Milk and Milk Products Manufacturing Units

These units produce entirely new products based on milk as the main raw material.

Packaging Units

These units can be undertaken in collaboration with any milk preserving and milk products manufacturing units. These units design attractive and safe packages for different milk products.

Horticulture

Horticulture is the main stream of agriculture. The term "Horticulture" is derived from the Latin *hortus* (garden) and culture (cultivation), which means garden cultivation. Horticulture is the branch of agricultural plant sciences that deals with the production of fruits, vegetables, nuts and ornamentals. It is a major source of food and employment. Horticulture provides a wide variety of jobs for many categories of people, directly or indirectly.

Job Opportunities

- Scientist.
- Academician.
- Training organizer.
- District horticulture officer/district agriculture officer.
- Technical assistant/technical officer in agriculture universities, ICAR, DRDO, IARI and CSIR.
- Horticulture inspector/fruit and vegetable inspector/marketing inspector.
- Training assistant in Krishi Vigyan Kendra (KVK).
- Farm supervisor.
- Horticulturist/horticulture officer or supervisor (landscape) in industries, farm houses, hotels, golf courses and construction companies, etc.
- Agriculture development officer.
- Village level worker.
- Agriculture inspector.
- Marketing job also in pesticides and insecticides companies.

Entrepreneurship Areas in Horticulture

- Horticulture consultant
- Agriculture clinic
- Raising commercial nursery
- Seed producer
- Fruit/vegetable/flower grower
- Floral decorator/florist
- Horticulture services contractor
- Mushroom grower
- Seed dealer/merchant
- Proprietor-cold storage
- Processing work of horticulture production

Plant Breeder

Plant breeders can make a career in education and research in 31 agriculture universities in the country, 40 ICAR institutes; seed production agencies of the government (National Seed Corporation, State Seed Corporations, SFCI, etc.). International crop research institutes under CGIAR system also offers very high quality jobs to plant breeders.

Sericulture

Sericulture refers to the conscious mass-scale rearing of silk producing organisms to obtain silk. Mulberry sericulture involves the cultivation of mulberry to produce leaf rearing of silkworm to convert leaf to the cocoon, reeling of the cocoon to obtain silk yarn and weaving to convert the yarn to fabric. Job opportunities for sericulture graduates include reapers, weavers, exporters, traders, etc.

Agronomy

Agronomy provides a wide variety of jobs for many categories of people, directly or indirectly. A large number of jobs require knowledge and training in Agronomy. The level of training could be vocational or at the college level. The work may be based on production aspects, demonstration trials in the rural areas and procurement of produce; marketing of inputs, viz. pesticides, insecticides, fertilizers and seeds of various crops in the urban as well as in rural outlets.

Other important job opportunities include scientist, educationist, training organizer, marketing job in pesticides and insecticides companies, agronomist consultant, seed producer.

Agricultural Engineering

There is tremendous scope for qualified engineers having professional degrees in agricultural engineering. Agricultural engineers work in production, sales, management, research and development, or applied science in agriculture. A large number of agricultural engineers work in academia or for research and development.

The job opportunities in private sectors include tractor industries for sales, R&D and management; irrigation equipment companies for sales, R&D and maintenance; dairy and food industries for quality control, R&D, and maintenance of processing machineries; computer applications for software development; instrumentation for automation and control; consultants to many organizations; agriclinic, agribusiness; and NGOs.

The job opportunities in government sectors include field executives and engineers, training assistants and organizers in areas of mechanization of agriculture, irrigation, drainage, soil and water conservation engineering, command area development, watershed management, rural development; and also in SAUs, ICAR, krishi vigyan kendras (KVKs), universities, colleges and other organizations for teaching, research and development, extensions and other scientific and technical jobs.

Lac Cultivation

Trained youth may select it as career to start their own training centre at village level. They can also share their trained manpower with NGO and agencies, which is working for rural areas. By adopting it as career, mass migration of youth from villages can be stopped.

Agricultural Meteorology

Agricultural meteorologists can work for research and developmental activities in private and government agencies such as Central and State Agricultural Universities, Indian Council of Agricultural Research (ICAR), Indian Space Research Organization (ISRO), Space Application Centre (SAC), National Remote Sensing Agency (NRSA), Department of Science and Technology (DST), Food and Agriculture Organization (FAO). In private sector, agricultural meteorologists work as consultants to many organizations including NGOs involved in water shed management, command area and rural development programmes.

Tea

There are a variety of jobs one can specialize in a tea industry. All together it is known as tea management. Tea tasting is one of the highly specialized areas of work. Other areas are that of researchers, plantation managers, tea brokers, consultants, etc. Work in the tea industry includes plantation management, processing, packing, auctioning, branding, marketing and research. Tea brokers who have a background in planting, tasting and knowledge of market trends auction the tea and the marketing personnel market the final product.

This is not an exhaustive list. There could be many more avenues of employment/self-employment in agriculture and allied sectors.

Some other entrepreneurial areas in agriculture are as follows:

1. Agribusiness centres
2. Agro-eco tourism
3. Animal feed unit
4. Biofertilizer production and marketing
5. Clearing and forwarding agency
6. Contract farming

7. Crop protection centre
8. Cultivation of medicinal plants
9. Cyber extension
10. Dairy
11. Direct marketing/retail marketing
12. Establishment of fodder farm
13. Farm machinery unit
14. Feed mixing plant
15. Fisheries development
16. Floriculture marketing
17. Food processing
18. Herbal based mineral water
19. Herbal processing unit
20. Honey agribusiness
21. Insurance
22. Landscaping and nursery
23. Micro-irrigation systems
24. Mushroom cultivation
25. Organic production/food chain
26. Pesticides production and marketing
27. Pickle, papad units
28. Plant clinics
29. Post-harvest management
30. Poultry
31. Research and development
32. Seed processing and agribusiness
33. Soil testing laboratory
34. Thermo foam tray production
35. Tissue culture unit
36. Vegetable production and marketing
37. Vermicomposting

AVENUES OF EMPLOYMENT/SELF-EMPLOYMENT IN VETERINARY

Qualified veterinary doctors in urban areas normally set up private practice where they deal with domestic canine and feline pets. Veterinary doctors in government hospitals in cities may find themselves handling mainly domestic pets, but government postings can also be in rural and semi-rural areas where responsibilities extend to cattle, sheep, goats, horses and poultry, etc.

Those who join government service are also often required for extension programmes at the block level, to educate and encourage livestock farmers to build up the quality of their animal stock, and handle the control and eradication of any notifiable disease. They also advise on animal farm management and animal health problems.

The dairy sector employs a large number of veterinarians who work at ensuring increasing yields in milk production, and also the health and breeding of dairy cattle.

There are also increasing opportunities in cattle development programmes, for those interested in research. Cattle breeding farms and artificial insemination centres all over the country provide input and extension support for the scientific breeding programmes of the government.

Veterinarians are also employed in the R&D departments of pharmaceutical companies, where they would handle the production of vaccines or development of animal feeds and fertilizers.

Another area of work for veterinarians is in poultry farms, for maintaining the health of poultry birds and to develop strains with high egg productivity, as well as poultry for table consumption. This is an area where veterinarians with relatively small amounts of capital and experience can set up their own poultry farms.

There are also opportunities for veterinarians in the armed forces. The Army Remount Veterinary Corps, equivalent to the Army Medical Corps, take on trained veterinary doctors as direct recruits. They are entrusted with the care of all defence animals including horses, ponies, camels, mules, cattle and poultry, and sniffer dogs for bomb detection.

Breeding of race horses is another area of specialization for veterinarians. With millions being spent on the care of thoroughbred horses, veterinarians play a very important role in ensuring the complete diet, health care and physical fitness of horses in a stud farm.

With increasingly environment consciousness, veterinarians are also required for the care and protection of wild animals in captivity as well as in sanctuaries. Veterinarians are therefore, employed by zoological parks and wildlife sanctuaries where they would handle the health of the animals, and the captive breeding of wild animals, feared to be getting extinct. They would also control the spread of diseases among animals, and help in maintaining the ecological balance in the forest areas.

Postgraduates in veterinary sciences can also opt for teaching or research.

Entrepreneurship Development

Scope for entrepreneur development in diversified areas is on the rise. Canine and feline practice in cosmopolitan cities, establishment of dairy and poultry industries, milk and meat processing venture, establishment of livestock business and marketing, etc. are gaining momentum.

Some of the areas could be:

- Cattle development
- Fodder development
- Goat development
- Piggery development
- Duck and poultry development
- Pig unit

- Dog breeding
- Modern feed mixing plant

SNAP-SHOT OF VETERINARY PROFESSION

1. India has the largest livestock population of more than 500 million heads, which contribute 15% of the world population. The demand of veterinarian to take care of this huge livestock is on the rise.
2. Due to commercialization of veterinary industry and the liberalization of Indian government policies more and more international industries of food manufacturing, pharmaceutical, diagnostic and vaccine production, etc. have opened avenues for veterinary professionals.
3. Increasing awareness towards veterinary education by introducing various schemes, viz. national talent scholarship, junior and senior ICAR research fellowships, internship allowance at higher rate and pay package to veterinary professionals equivalent to professional in other fields.
4. Job prospects in comparison to other professional and technical degree programmes are better for veterinary graduates.
5. Scope for entrepreneur development in diversified areas is on the rise. Canine and feline practice in cosmopolitan cities, establishment of dairy and poultry industries, milk and meat processing venture, establishment of livestock business and marketing, etc. are gaining momentum.
6. Opportunities for higher education in foreign countries and demand for qualified professionals in developed countries is attracting Indian veterinarians.
7. Liberalization of loans through agencies like NABARD, Rural Cooperative Banks, and Nationalized Banks under the rural development programmes, establishment of poly clinics, and livestock sector for operationalization and monitoring of the above schemes are boosting the demands for veterinarians. Most veterinarians also opt for clinical work and find opportunities in research laboratories and organizations.

The government of India, through the state governments have implemented various successful self-employment opportunities.

Some agri and allied sector companies, where one may find employment are as follows:

1. A.P. Engineering
2. Agricom Brokers
3. Agro Impex
4. AgroEngine.com
5. American Springs and Pressing Works Limited
6. Amit Biotech
7. APCL International: Exporters of Indian spice, agroproducts and plywood, etc.
8. Aries Exports
9. Arise Exports Ltd.—Exporter of oilseeds.

10. Asian Herbex Limited—Premium quality spice oleoresins from India
11. AVT Biotechnology
12. B&V Agro Irrigation Company
13. Bafna Agro Industries Ltd—Leading producers of agro-based products in India
14. Bagrrys India Ltd.
15. Bhilai Fertilizers and Agro-Chemicals
16. Bicco Agro Products
17. Bicco Agro Products Pvt. Ltd.
18. Blossoms inc., New Delhi—Flowers delivery service
19. Brahmaputra Valley Fertilizer Corporation Ltd.
20. Broadcast Engineering Consultants India Ltd.
21. BSA International Exports
22. Calcutta Tissue Culture Products Pvt. Ltd.
23. Central Institute of Brackishwater Aquaculture
24. Chamy Co.: Exporter and Importer of agroproducts
25. Chillies of India
26. Cochin Malabar Estates and Industries Ltd.
27. Coconut Development Board: Ministry of Agriculture, Government of India
28. Coffee Board of India
29. Coromandel Fertilizers
30. Costa Co. Private Limited, Goa
31. D.A.B. Exports—Export spices, agro food products
32. D.D. International
33. Dayal Fertilizers
34. Deepak Fertilisers and Petrochemicals Corporation Limited
35. Delphis Corporation
36. Dhampur Invertos Ltd.—Manufacturer of sweeteners
37. DSCL
38. East Coast Seaweed Technologies
39. Ekta Trade Link Pvt. Ltd.
40. Ekta Tradelink (P) Ltd.—Exporter of basmati and non-basmati rice, spices, etc.
41. Euro Fruits—Exporters of fresh fruit and vegitables
42. Everest Instruments
43. Gangadhar Industries
44. GANM Impex
45. Global Flora Tech
46. Gromax International, New Delhi
47. Growell India—Poultry products
48. Gujarat State Fertilizers and Chemicals
49. Guybro Chemical
50. Himachal Pradesh State Forest Corporation Limited

51. Hymatic
52. India Food Exports (IFE)—Cashew exoprts
53. Indian Centre for Aquaculture and Fisheries Trade
54. Indian Farmers Fertiliser Co-operative Limited
55. Indian Fisherman, Chennai
56. Indo Gulf Corporation Ltd—A Aditya Birla Group Company
57. Institute for Micronutrient Technology
58. Jegson Hi-Tech Industries—Eco-friendly and environmentally safe products
59. John Engineering Works—Manufacturers and exporters of world class pulveriseres from India
60. K.S. Intertrade Corporation—International brokerage firm
61. Kamal & Sons
62. Karuturi Networks Limited
63. Kerala Agro Machinery Corporation Limited
64. Khaitan Chemicals and Fertilisers Ltd.
65. Kisan Brother Pvt. Ltd.
66. Kisan Brothers
67. Koodath Agro Exports—Exports Cocopeat and Cocopeat bales
68. Krishak Bharati Cooperative Limited
69. Kumar Krishi Mitra Bioproducts
70. Labland Biotech
71. Link Systems Pvt. Ltd.
72. Link Trade Impex Services—International commodities brokers
73. Lovson Exports Ltd.
74. Madras Fertilizers Ltd.
75. Malloys India—Diesel engines, diesel generating sets, engine spares and agricultural implements
76. Mangalore Chemicals
77. Manjilas Agro Foods Ltd.
78. Manjushree Plantations Ltd.—Producers of tea, coffee, cardamom, roses and seeds
79. Marson Biocare Private Limited
80. Matrix vet Pharma Limited
81. Meerut Agro Industries
82. Monsanto
83. Nagarjuna Fertilizers
84. National Fertilizers Ltd.
85. Neotech Enterprises—Manufacturer of corn cob grits for the first time in india
86. New Age Agritech Ltd.—Manufacturer of drip irrigation systems
87. Nimbkar Agricultural Research Institute
88. Organica Biotech
89. Oswal Chemicals & Fertilizers

90. P. Mittulaul Lalah & Sons—Curry Powder
91. P.M.Diesel
92. Padgilwar Agro Industries
93. Paradeep Phosphates Limited
94. Pittie Agro Ventures Limited
95. Premier World—Irrigation Equipment
96. Priya Chemicals
97. Priya Exports
98. Priya Exports—Exporters from South India.
99. Pudumjee Plant Laboratories Limited—Jatia Group.
100. Ranawat Group—Shivagrico Implements—Animal drawn tools and hand tools
101. Rashtriya Chemicals and Fertilizers Ltd. (RCF)
102. Samde Aromatic Private Limited
103. Sap Exim Ltd—Manufacturer and exporters of agricultural machinery and equipments
104. Satnam Overseas Ltd.—Exporters of basmati rice, pulses and agro products
105. Sesame Seed
106. Shivnath Rai Harnarain (India) Ltd.
107. Shreeji International—Exporter of agroproducts
108. Shyam Industries
109. Smart Exporters—provide a line of healthy and economical food for cattle
110. Spices Board of India
111. Splashing Meadows Pvt. Ltd. Calcutta
112. Sri Pumps
113. Sun Beam Machines
114. Swani Corporation—Exporters of spices, oil seeds and medicinal herbs
115. Talakshi Lalji and Co.—Tilak brand products
116. Taruna International
117. Tata Tetley—Tea exports
118. Tea Board India, Ministry of Commerce, India
119. The Marine Products Export Devolopment Authority
120. Tinco
121. Trikaya Agriculture—Snow peas and baby corn vegetable exporter
122. Vikas Group, Mumbai
123. VVD Group of Companies
124. Westcoast Aquaculture
125. WynGroup—An Indian agribusiness company
126. Zuari Chambal

CONCLUSION

A part of the unemployment problem emanates from the mismatch between the skill requirements of employment opportunities and the skill base of the job-seekers. Rapid expansion of education, particularly of higher education, has also contributed to the mismatch in the labour market. While shortages of middle level technical and supervisory skills are often experienced, graduates and post-graduates in arts, commerce and science constitute a large proportion of job-seekers. The mismatch is likely to become more acute in the process of rapid structural changes in the economy.

It is, therefore, necessary to re-orient the educational and training systems towards improving its capability to supply the requisite skills in the medium and long-term, and introduce greater flexibility in the training system so as to enable it to quickly respond to labour market changes in the short run. The system should also be in a position to impart suitable training to the large mass of workers engaged as self-employed and wage earners in the unorganized sector for upgradation of their skills, as an effective means for raising their productivity potential and income levels.

5

Development of Enterprise in Livestock Sector

Rupasi Tiwari, MC Sharma

Livestock sector plays a multi-faceted role in socio-economic development of rural households. Livestock rearing has significant positive impact on equity in terms of income and employment and poverty reduction in rural areas as distribution of livestock is more egalitarian as compared to land. In India, over 70% of the rural households own livestock and a majority of livestock owning households are small, marginal and landless farmers. Small animals like sheep, goats, pigs and poultry are largely kept by the poor households for commercial purposes due to their low initial investment and operational costs. In the recent decade, demand for various livestock-based products has increased significantly due to increase in per capita income, urbanization, taste and preference and increased awareness about food nutrition. Livestock sector is likely to emerge as an important facet for agricultural growth in the coming decades and is also considered as a potential sector for export earnings.

Development of animal husbandry is envisaged as an integral part of a sound system of diversified agriculture. Emphasis is laid on mixed farming, a system in which crop production and animal husbandry are dovetailed for efficient and economic utilisation of land, labour and capital. The integration of agriculture farming with animal husbandry is essential for the better utilisation of farm by-products, maintenance of soil fertility, fuller employment for agriculturists throughout the year and increase in rural incomes (Kumar, 2007; Sharma and Tiwari, 2007).

LIVESTOCK REARING PRACTICES IN INDIA

Livestock rearing in India is mainly practised as a backyard production system wherein the farmers rear a few livestock specially for meeting the household requirements and the excess milk is sold in local market or milk collecting units. Thus, by being as an important means of income and employment for these households livestock helps to alleviate poverty and smoothen income distribution. In addition, livestock asset can be easily converted into cash, and thus acts as cushion against shocks of crop failure particularly in the less favoured environments. Further it has been found that most of the livestock population is owned by the small and marginal farmers, who possess 71% of cattle, 63% of buffaloes, 66% of small ruminants, 70% of pigs and 74% of poultry (Table 5.1).

This implies that marginal and small holders derive a considerable proportion of their income from livestock. Evidences indicate that increase in income from livestock in rural areas reduce income inequality.

Table 5.1: Size and distribution of land and livestock holdings, 1991-92

| Class based on land holding size | Percent of household | Size of land holding (ha) | Size of livestock holdings (numbers/household) | | | | |
			Cattle	Buffalo	Sheep and goat	Pig	Poultry
Landless	21.80	0.0	0.15 (2.4)	0.08 (2.8)	0.20 (5.1)	0.01 (7.7)	0.49 (6.4)
<1.0 ha	48.30	0.35 (15.5)	1.35 (47.1)	0.44 (36.1)	0.81 (46.2)	0.04 (49.5)	1.90 (54.8)
1.0–2.0 ha	14.20	1.41 (18.6)	2.34 (24.0)	0.90 (26.7)	1.15 (19.3)	0.06 (20.4)	2.23 (19.0)
2.0–4.0 ha	9.70	2.69 (24.2)	2.38 (16.6)	1.23 (20.2)	1.31 (15.0)	0.06 (13.9)	2.47 (14.4)
4.0–10.0 ha	4.90	5.78 (26.4)	2.34 (8.3)	1.72 (14.4)	1.66 (9.7)	0.06 (7.1)	1.41 94.2)
>10.0 ha	1.10	15.44 (15.3)	2.09 (1.6)	2.66 (4.8)	3.75 (4.7)	0.04 (1.0)	1.74 (1.1)
All	100.0	1.08 (100)	1.39 (100)	0.59 (100)	0.85 (100)	0.04 (1.0)	1.65 (100)

( ) indicate the percentage across column

ANIMAL CENSUS AND ECONOMIC IMPORTANCE OF LIVESTOCK SECTOR

India possesses one of the largest livestock populations in the world which is at present estimated to be more than 484.9 million with the top position in cattle (178.8 million), Buffalo (101 million), goat (126 million) and sheep (62 million). Further the country has about 14% of the world cattle population and 57.30% of the world buffalo population. The country possesses 6% of sheep and 17% of world goat population. Further our country has larger number of breeds of cattle (30), buffalo (10), goat (20) and sheep (42). Of the total buffalo and cattle breeds of the world, approx 75% and 20% respectively are available in Asia and 15% and 5% in India. The poultry which was considered as a backyard venture in the early 60's has now been transformed into strong agro-based farming activity. India accounts for nearly 3% of the world poultry population. Further with an annual production of about 102 million tones of milk and 46.1 billion eggs, India ranks 1st and 2nd in world respectively, and is one of the top ten broiler producers in the world. Our country has achieved annual growth rates of 4–5%

for milk, meat and egg production during the last decade. The value of output from animal husbandry and dairying to agriculture over the years has increased and is about 26% of the agricultural GDP and approx 5.7% of the national GDP. This has increased gradually from 14% in 1980-81. On the other hand, the contribution of the agricultural sector to the gross domestic product decreased from 35% in 1980-81 to 26% in 1997-98. Further agriculture got 4% share of annual budget but growth rate is not increasing and animal husbandry sector is getting only 1% share but there is increase in annual growth rate. Animal husbandry sector contribute 5.7 to 8% growth rate as compared to the 1.7–2% growth in crop production per year. In fact the increasing growth rate of animal husbandry will help the agriculture sector to acquire 4% increase in growth as a whole to make nation developed country. Although the contribution of livestock to Ag GDP has been rising continuously, its contribution to rural employment is not so encouraging. In terms of principal activity livestock employs about 5% of the rural work force, its share has, however, declined to 1% at present. Low share in rural employment is because livestock rearing in India is taken up as a subsidiary to crop production and mostly practised as a supporting and backyard enterprise.

Table 5.2 is indicating the census data of 2003, however, in text present estimated census and production data has been depicted.

Table 5.2: Livestock population in India

Animals	World	India	% Share
Cattle (million)	1371.17	185.18	13.71
Buffalo (million)	170.66	97.79	57.30
Pig (million)	956.02	13.52	1.41
Sheep (million)	1024.04	61.47	6.00
Goat (million)	767.93	124.39	16.19
Poultry (billion)	16605	489	2.94
Horse and ponies (lacs)	–	7.51	–
Mules (lacs)	–	1.76	–
Donkey (lacs)	–	6.5	–
Camel (lacs)	–	6.32	–
Yak (thousands)	–	65	–
Mithun (lacs)	–	2.78	–

17th Livestock Census (2003, Department of Animal Husbandry, GOI)

There is a tremendous scope of promoting the backyard livestock keeping in India into commercial micro-enterprises through entrepreneurship development programmes and entrepreneur favourable government policies. Apart from rearing of livestock, the livestock-based industry has vast scope of generating additional income and employment through its various allied enterprises such as the commercial livestock rearing units, livestock input industry, livestock product processing units and organic livestock production units which can be harnessed for increasing employment and income in the rural areas.

COMMERCIALIZING THE LIVESTOCK ENTERPRISES

Livestock rearing is the major subsidiary occupation in most part of our country. But keeping in view its potentiality for generating employment and providing food security to the country it needs to be taken up as a main occupation. This can happen only when the rural people are motivated to practice commercial livestock rearing rather than the subsistence or semi-commercial type of animal rearing. For starting any livestock enterprise commercially on scientific lines, the rural youth can avail loan from banks. For obtaining bank loan, the farmers/ entrepreneurs can apply to the nearest branch of commercial, cooperative or regional rural banks in the prescribed application form, which is available in the branches of the financing banks. Necessary help or guidance can be obtained from the technical officer for preparation of the project report which is a prerequisite for sanction of loan. The bank approves the loan on the basis of the economic viability of the project submitted. There are various livestock enterprises, which can be practised on commercial scale and can be started with small investment.

Development of Commercial Dairy Farms

In starting dairy farm, it is essential to decide which animal to be taken for this purpose. Normally cow/buffalo is the choice for dairy enterprise. Both the animals are milch animals but they differ in many aspects in production. The cow can yield high amount of milk and can be very economical at high production level. They breed regularly, giving one calf at every 13–14 months interval. Buffalo breed is also suitable for a commercial dairy farm. There is a greater demand for buffalo milk in the country because of its higher fat contents and its suitability for making ghee and other milk products. Other plus point in buffalo is that they can utilize crop residues with better efficiency than cows, and are more resistant to diseases. However, buffalo largely mature late and have longer calving intervals (16–18 months). These animals also need additional cooling facilities, e.g. wallowing tank or showers/foggers with fan. Thus in a commercial farm, a combination of cow and buffalo could work better than growing cow or buffalo alone. Cross-bred cow and buffalo should be kept in separate row under one shed.

The minimum economic size of commercial dairy farm under Indian condition should contain a minimum 20 (10 cows and 10 buffaloes) especially for a suburban area. The economic viability of the unit will depend on the production performance of dairy animals and the rates of various items including feed, fodder and milk.

The following points in selection of milking cow and buffalo, land, labour, feed and fodder requirements should be considered for economic commercial dairy farming.

1. Production level of the half-bred, Holstein Friesian, Jersy, Red Dane, Brown Swiss crosses should range from 3500–5000 litres, with an overall average of 4000 litres in a standard lactation period of 300 days in case of cows and the daily milk production should be about 10/12 litres in case of buffalo.

2. Freshly calved cows and calved buffalo in the second and third lactation should be purchased, preferably, from Govt. farms or from well-established commercial dairy farms or breeding tract in the district of Haryana, Punjab or other region of availability at a price of 20,000/- and 25,000/- respectively. For higher milk production, well-recognized breeds like Murrah, Niliravi or Jafarbadi are the breeds for dairy purpose.

3. 70–75% of cows and 60–65% of buffalo should be in milk throughout the year.

4. The period between successive calving should be on an average of 14–15 months in case of cows and 15–16 months in case of buffalo.

5. A total of six acre of well fertile land with assured irrigation facilities is required for fodder production at a level of about 700 quintal/acre/year. In addition to it the 10950 sq.ft. land for the construction of dairy shed and ancillary structure. Out of which under shed, paddock, store and office, manure pit and paved road and open space covered 2366, 3104, 875, 600, 4005 sq ft., respectively with construction cost @ Rs 100/-, 50/-, 150/-, 50/- and 25/-, respectively.

6. All cows and buffaloes at the farm should be insured against mortality.

7. One skilled person will be required to look after cow/buffalo and their followers. Therefore, two persons will be required to take care of all the activities of 20 cows/buffaloes dairy unit, which also includes the harvesting of fodders. Additional labour required at times, should be provided by the farmers himself and his family. The labour could be hired locally @ Rs 30000/person/year.

8. Farm grown green fodder will be required @ 25–35 kg/cow or buffalo/day and production cost will be nearly Rs15/- per quintal including the rental value of the land. Dry fodder (mainly wheat straw) will be required @ 2 kg/animal/day and it will be purchased from the market during wheat harvesting season @ Rs 150/- per quintal. The concentrate mixture will be required on an average @ 4 kg/animal/day. It may be either home made or commercial concentrate with its price about Rs 700/- per kg.

9. Under machinery and equipments a tractor with trailer including its implements, a feed grinder, a chaff cutter with 5HP electric motor, ten milk cane of 40 litres capacity, two hand driven trolley/cart to concentrate dispenser and mist cooling system in milking cow and buffalo shed with approx. cost Rs 2.5, 0.25, 0.20 0.08, 0.02 and 0.15 lakh respectively.

10. There are some operations that have to be followed on a regular basis in the respective farms. It is to be adopted to minimize the loss of diseases. It is true that "Prevention is better than cure". Below mentioned practices will help to prevent the occurrence of diseases.

Dairy Management

Milking animals, utensils, barn and paddock should also be cleaned. Feeding of half ration before morning milking and half ration before evening milking; separation of sick animals, identification of estrus animals, colostrums feeding to calf at proper time, balance feeding, exercise of bull, timely insemination, proper and timely vaccination, deworming, treatment of sick animals, keeping farm records and other miscellaneous work are the day to day activities which are to be followed sincerely. Keeping farm records is a key operation in livestock rearing. Without proper records, one cannot know how the enterprise is going on. There are different types of records that are essential for the enterprise which includes cattle history and pedigree sheet, production and reproduction records, breeding/service register, feeding register, calving register, herd strength register, daily milk record register, expenditure record register, etc.

Record keeping is essential for evaluating the performance and for taking remedial actions to maximize profits. Thus, the essential farm records must be maintained at a dairy farm like date of birth, pedigree, inventory, livestock, growth rate monitoring, reproduction, daily milk production, health and veterinary, feeding, estimated values, periodic test of milk quality, business records, etc. If we maintain these records, we may analyze the important information like reducing cost, proper utilization of land and labour, comparing performance with standard values, proper feeding of herd, making decision about culling of animals and facilitate in making claims from insurance companies. As far as economics of small dairy unit concern, Walli et al (2005) suggested that a livestock owner may get near about Rs 10000 as net income/animal/year.

Economics of Small Dairy Unit (Rathore and Sharma, 2007)

Capital Investment (Rs)

1. Cost of animal (10 cows + 10 buffaloes)	:	4,50,000
2. Building construction cost	:	6,53,175
3. Cost of equipments	:	3,20,000
Total capital investment	:	14,23,175

Non-recurring/Fixed Expenditure (Rs)

1. Interest on capital investment @ 10%/annum	:	1,42,317
2. Depreciation on livestock @ 12.5%/annum	:	56,250
3. Depreciation on building @ 3%/annum	:	19,595
4. Depreciation on equipment @ 10% per annum	:	32,000
5. Insurance @ Rs 800/cow or buffalo/year	:	16,000
Total (Rs)	:	2,66,162

Recurring Expenditure (Rs)

1. Cost of farm grown green fodder	:	62,415
2. Cost of purchased dry fodder	:	24,966
3. Cost of concentrate mixture	:	2,33,016

4. Labour charges : 60,000
5. Animal health care and reproduction
   charges @ Rs 400/- per animal/year : 9,000
6. Miscellaneous expenses including repair,
   electric bill, phone bill, purchase of chain,
   rope, etc. Rs 700/- per animal/year : 15,750
   Total expenditure (Rs) : 4,05,147
   Grand total : 6,71,309

Income of Sale

1. Sale of cow milk ($12.5 \times 7 \times 365 \times 15$) : 4,79,063
2. Sale of buffalo milk ($10 \times 6 \times 365 \times 18$) : 3,94,200
3. Sale of manure @ Rs 500/- per animal/year : 11,400
4. Sale of 4 buffalo male calves at 10 months of age
   @ Rs 500/- per animal : 2,000
   Total sale proceed (Rs) : 8, 86,663
   Net income/year : 2, 15,354
   Net income/month : 17946
   Net income/animal/year : 9529 say 10000/-

Development of Commercial Sheep Farms

Keeping in view the ever-increasing population of our country there is tremendous pressure on our natural resources such as land and water. Especially in the light of the marginalization of agricultural land holding sheep rearing is a better option as compared to other livestock, more so, in the semi-arid and the arid zones of our country. The sheep produce wool and meat. In spite of the fact that the country is endowed with 11.5% of the world livestock population it contributes little over 2.26% (5.74 million tones) to the world total meat production of 245 million tones. Considering 70% of human population non-vegetarian, the annual per capita availability of meat is roughly 8 kg as against the recommended intake of 11 kg of the total meat production more than 70% come from cattle (old bullocks), buffalo and pigs and for that preference is limited to socio-religious factors. Therefore, burden lies on goat and sheep meat, and in the recent years the domestic market price for mutton have increased from Rs 50 per kg to Rs 100–120 per kg. Moreover expected huge increase in demand for meat in developing countries (by 100%) especially in East and South-east Asia in next 20 years presents an excellent opportunity for enhancing export of live goat/sheep and their meat from India. Therefore, there is immense potential for entrepreneurship development through commercial sheep rearing in our country.

Development of Commercial Goat Farms

Goat rearing is an important subsidiary occupation especially practiced by the small marginal and landless farmers since it requires small amount of investment. But this occupation has tremendous scope and potentiality of generating income if practiced commercially on a small or a large scale. The small and landless youth can start a small scale goat farm of 10 goats with a small initial investment of Rs 25,000 only and this unit will yield him a net income of Rs 15,000/year, i.e. Rs 1250 per month. For starting a large-scale goat farm of 100 goats 1000 sq. mt. of land will be required in addition to an initial investment of Rs 2.5 to 3 lakhs and this enterprise can yield him a net income of Rs 1.5 lakh/year, i.e. Rs 12,500/month. The rural youth can get practical training in commercial goat rearing from either at IVRI Izatnagar or Central Goat Research Institute, Makhdoom, Mathura.

Establishing Commercial Poultry Farms

Today India is the 2nd largest egg producer and one of the top ten broiler producers in the world. This has been achieved due to the commercialization of the poultry sector. But, in spite of the considerable growth in the egg production (2.5 to 30000 million during 1950 to 2000) and broiler production, the per capita availability of poultry products is considerably low; 42 eggs and 500 g meat/annum as against the requirement of 180 eggs and 10 kg meat per annum, which shows that there is great potentiality for the development of poultry sector in the country thereby presenting higher opportunities of entrepreneurship development in rural areas.

For development of entrepreneurship in poultry sector following points to be kept in mind.

  i. The agro-climatic conditions must be suitable for rearing birds in the area.
 ii. It should be ascertained that the applicant has knowledge/experience in raising poultry.
iii. Selected site should be away from main roads and free from water logging conditions.
 iv. The poultry shed should be adequate to accommodate the number of birds to be raised. The poultry house should be according to standard requirements and should give protection to birds from sun, rain, wind and predators.
  v. Suitable arrangements should be made for purchase of high quality one day old chicks or layers from reputed sellers at reasonable prices.
 vi. Sufficient clean water should be available for birds. It should also be ascertained that the poultry feed is available from close proximity at reasonable price.
vii. Proper veterinary services must be available near the farm for treating the birds. Birds should be vaccinated against poultry diseases.
viii. Firm arrangements must be made for marketing of eggs/broilers/culled birds.
 ix. Arrangements should be made for insurance of birds and the insurance policy should be made in favour of the bank. Layers @ Rs 4.23/bird, Broilers @ Rs 0.71/bird, building and equipments @ 0.40% of cost.
  x. Proper records of all purchases and sales should be maintained:

Rural youth can earn attractive profits if they start the enterprise commercially. Further the two enterprises layer and broiler farming can be started on small scale with low investment also. A broiler farm of 1000 birds can be started with a covered land size of 1000 sq. ft. and an initial investment of Rs 50,000 as fixed cost for shed and other equipment. Around Rs 50,000 will be required for the variable expenditure on chicks, feed and other miscellaneous expenses. The broiler birds are ready within 42 days with an average body weight of 1.5 to 1.8 kg and can yield a minimum profit of Rs 10,000 per batch of 1000 birds (@ Rs 40/kg market price and 1.5 kg live weight of bird) which amounts to around Rs 70,000 per year (if the entrepreneur puts 7 batches of 1000 birds in a year), i.e. a net profit of Rs 5800 per month. The profit from a batch of 1000 birds can increase to Rs 20,000 with the increase in live weight of birds to 1.8 kg/bird. Further profits can be earned if the market prices are higher.

Development of Piggery Farm

In India, pig rearing is mainly carried out by the socially and economically backward class of our society. Moreover, it is a subsidiary occupation for them and the pigs are reared unhygenically under scavenging system. The pig can play a very important role in increasing meat production and thereby to meet the protein hunger. They excel all other farm animals in respect of edible flesh The pig rearing gives high returns with a low investment, so the popular name "mortgage lifter" is often give to them. The major advantages of pig rearing over the other livestock enterprises are its short generation interval, big litter size (6–7 in case of indigenous breed, 8–12 in case of exotic breed, 5–9 in case of cross-bred pigs), can be fed on cheap feed and food by products, high food conversion efficiency, quicker increase in body weight, 1 kg body weight at birth become 80–100 kg only in 7–10 months of age. Before starting a piggery, a suitable site is required to be selected. As feed cost accounts for about 70% of the total expenditure, the pig farm should either be established near to metropolitan city, where left food from hotel/mess/hostel is available or near a village where cheap by product from agriculture are plenty. A good land without ditches at higher level should be arranged near road side. Water and electric supply must be arranged.

The animals should preferably be purchased with following characteristics.
1. Pure bred Large White, Middle White and Landrace (white)
2. Physically strong and healthy with good condition
3. Normal body temperature (101°F)
4. Female of exotic and cross-bred must have 7 and 6 pairs of teats and belong to dams with good litter size.
5. Male should have good libido and semen quality.
6. Female of regular oestrus cyclicity.

Daily routine jobs in piggery is to perform like cleaning of all pigsties, feeding and water trough, farm premises along with disposal of dung/urine, checking the herd for spotting out the sick animals, spotty of sows/gilts in heat, if in heat then necessary breeding is to be planned and carried out, isolation of near parturition sows/gilts into furrowing pens or suitable place so that she is not disturbed by other animal. Whereas periodical jobs are also necessary like weighing of stock, which help the farmers to know the gain per unit for given inputs. Cutting of needle teeth which will prevent infection of wound from fighting or causing injuries to the teat of mother, piglets should be castrated when they are 2–3 weeks of age, weaning of piglets at 8 weeks of age, deworming periodically, culling and disposal of piglets as and when needed and vaccination against infectious diseases.

Preventive Measures

Following vaccinations should be given.

Swine fever: Freeze dried lapinised swine fever vaccine should be given 1 ml s/c as repeat dose every year at the age of 2 months.

Foot and mouth disease: Polyvalent oil adjuvant vaccine is available with IVRI, Bangalore and local market also. 2.5 ml of vaccine should be given I/m at 10 weeks of age and should be repeated after every 6 months.

Haemorrhagic septicaemia: 2 ml of H.S. vaccine is first given after weaning and should be repeated after every one year.

Deworming: Internal parasites specifically ascariasis, if uncontrolled can bring great loss to a pig farmer. Broad-spectrum anthlmentics like albendazole, fenbendazole, mebendazole, thiabendazole, tetramizole can be mixed in half of feed offered to piglets kept starved in previous evening. The pigs may be again dewormed after every 3 months depending upon the parasitic load which can got checked from a nearby veterinary laboratory.

External parasites: Two types of mites affect pigs and cause mange. The sarcoptic mange mite barrows into skin where it feeds and multiplies. The demodectic mite infests the hair follicles and sebaceous glands. Spray with 0.5% malathion, 0.04% deltamethrin and cyper-methrin 0.02% or Kilex Carbaryl (50% WP) 1% solution can be used to control it. Injection of ivermectin 1 ml/ 33 kg body weight controls external and internal parasites and should be repeated after 10 days.

Housing Management

Good housing must provide optimal environmental conditions such as fresh air, exercise, sunlight and protection from inclement weather and predators.

Breeding Management

Exotic pigs attain puberty at about 200 days of age, whereas cross-bred and indigenous pigs reach puberty at 150 and 120 days respectively. As pigs are polyestrous, females come into heat regularly at 21 days interval. Gilts tend to have shorter heat period than sows. Within this cycle, heat period lasts up to 48 hours. Females in heat are characterized by grunting, rest-lessness, following of teaser, mounting other females in pen and swelling of vulva. The period of maximum fertility in female occurs during mid-oestrus, some hours before ovulation. As the shedding of ova produced by the sow takes place over a period of several hours, maximum fertilization can be obtained by mating sow twice after mid-oestrus. Service time in pigs ranges from 5 to 20 minutes and average volume of semen is 250 ml. Gilts should be bred for the first time after their third heat period, at about 8 months of age and 60-70 kg body weight in exotics and crossbreds.

Boars may be used for first time at 7-8 months of age and get matured at 15 months of age. A mature boar can serve 20-40 times/month but boar under 15 months of age should not be used for service more than 25 times per month. In summer months, boars should be used either in early morning or late evening hours.

Feeding Management

Pigs are omnivorous in their feeding habit and can consume lot variety of edible materials including, grains, grasses like berseem, lobia, etc. hotel wastes, poultry wastes, etc. Although in organized govt. farms concentrate ration comprising costly grains is fed but it is not economical. Success of a pig enterprise depends upon the feeding programme adapted as feed cost accounts for 70–80% of total recurring inputs of pig production. Common conventional diets contain about 30–60% cereal grains primarily maize. The overall scarce supply of grains coupled with intense competition from ever increasing human population, the scope of feeding cereal grains to livestock is gradually becoming difficult. Therefore some alternative cheap diet from agro-industrial by-products like rice bran, rice polish, molasses, milk by-products and other cheaper materials are detailed below:

1. **Rice or wheat shorts:** These are by-products of the milling. Inclusion of rice shorts can make pig feed economical in paddy belts. They can be used up to 60% of the total ration.

2. **Rice bran:** It consists of the outer layer of the rice kernel and contains a high percentage of fats and fibre. It should not be fed at all to piglets or at more than 30–50% of total ration to the fatteners. In case, it is the only feed available, pigs consuming it will grow slowly and soft fat in their carcass.

3. **Potatoes:** Potatoes are available in most part of India. It can be mixed with grain three parts to one. Potatoes can also be dried and made into flour and this can form up to 30% of the rations.

4. **Root crops:** Cassava/tapioca and its peelings are both suitable feeds for pigs. Four part of cassava root can replace one part of maize. Prussic acid levels in fresh roots can be eliminated by drying or boiling the roots. Sugar beets, carrots can also be fed in small amounts.

5. **Bakery waste:** Stale bread and other bakery wastes, if cheaply available can replace total ration, white bread contains 64% dry matter, 85% protein, 2% fat, 0.3% fibre.

6. **Molasses:** Molasses can be used as substitute for carbohydrates. The metabolizable energy is two-thirds that of maize but the high potassium level tends to produce scouring. Cane molasses should not be used more than 20% in growing pigs and up to 40% in finishing pigs.

7. **Garbage:** The composition and feeding value of garbage vary from place to place and depends upon the prosperity of the people. Garbage from the public eating place is more nutritious than house hold garbage. Garbage should be cooked to control microorganism and other parasites. Garbage

should be thoroughly searched for and glass pieces, spoons, plastic bags before feeding. It can replace the total concentrate ration. In an experiment conducted at IVRI, it was found that one kg of pork can be produced at a cost of Rs 5.06 by feeding mess waste.

8. **Dairy by-products:** In vicinity of dairy plants, butter milk or separated milk are cheaply available. These may be mixed in creep feed to levels varying from 10-30%. Piglets of a galactic mother and orphan piglets can be given.

9. **Fruits:** Bananas which are green or over-ripe can be fed to pigs as a source of energy. These can also be used up to 20–30% in grower/finisher ration. Papaya, pine apple, bran, fruit pulp, sugar cane, green copra can also be used as pig feed in areas of abundant availability.

10. **Slaughter house waste:** Blood meal, bone meal or meat meal may be available and can be mixed up to 10% of the ration.

11. **Poultry by-product meal:** In areas of country where poultry keeping has been adopted at large scale, waste products from dressing plants such as head, foot, and undeveloped eggs, intestines can be used at the rate of 8.5 to 16% of total ration.

Economics of Small Piggery Unit (2 Males + 10 Females) (Rathore and Sharma, 2007)

A. *Total input (Rs)*

1.	Cost of construction of two sheds	:	50,000
2.	Cost of 12 pigs	:	28,000
	(Large White Yorkshire or Landress 60 kg) @ Rs 40/kg live wt		
3.	Feed cost		
	- Feeding of adult animal average concentrate 2 kg/day @ 4/kg for one year	:	35,040
	- Cost of creep feed for piglet of first farrowing	:	2,000
	- Cost of grower feed 70 g (for 5 months @ 1.5 kg/day/Rs 4/kg)	:	63,000
	- Creep feed for 2nd farrowing	:	2,000
4.	Other expenses		
	- Labour charges annually	:	30,000
	- Vet. med. including vaccine	:	5,000
	Total expenditure	:	2,15,040
	Interest @ 6%/annum	:	12,542

B. *Total output (Rs)*

1.	Sale of 12 adult pigs of appx. 100 kg bwt.	:	48,000
2.	Sale of 70 growers of 1st farrowing of about 60 kg bwt	:	1,68,000
3.	Sale of 70 weaners @ Rs 100/- each	:	70,000
4.	Cost of manure	:	5,000
	Total receipt	:	2,91,000
	Net income	:	63, 418 say 63500/-

The profit will be increased in 2nd year onwards as number of breedable sows will be more giving birth to piglets.

Buffalo Calves Rearing for Meat Purpose

Buffalo calves rearing for meat purpose is a very attractive entrepreneurship for rural youth as those buffalo calves can be reared partially on grazing and partially on the left out feed of the lactating animals. Later on fattening diet can be given to get proper body weight and good quality of meat. For meat purpose, buffalo calves may be purchased from urban and peri-urban dairy on throw away prices at the age of 2–6 months. These calves should be castrated at 3–6 months of age for good growth of meat. For rearing of 10 buffalo calves, an economic estimation is given below:

The cost of 10 buffalo calves @ Rs 300/- each will be (Rs 3000/-). Rearing cost of these 10 buffalo calves for 24 months to gain 250–300 kg body weight including feed, fodder and medication, etc. will be Rs 39,000 (excluding fixed cost of shed and land). The total returns after 24 months will be Rs 1,00,000 @ Rs 40/kg rate of buffalo meat. Thus net profit will be 61,000 and per calf Rs 6,100 per month.

Commercial Dry Cattle/Buffalo Rearing Units

Those animals which are in their productive age but dry are mostly sold off or given to the villagers on contract by the commercial dairy farmers especially in the peri-urban and urban areas as these farmers rear only the milch animals to have a stable amount of milk production all round the year. The rural youth can use this as an opportunity and can set up dry buffalo/cattle rearing farms and can purchase/take on contract dry animals and at parturition can sell them at higher prices. The practice of giving dry animals on contract to villagers presently exists among the commercial dairy farmers in the urban area but this can be used as an opportunity by the rural youth and they can take up this enterprise in an organized manner commercially and can start such type of farms in the rural areas.

Commercial Cattle/Buffalo Calf Rearing Units

It has been found that in the commercial dairy farms the management of calves is very poor leading to a high calf mortality rate. This is leading to a heavy loss to the farmers as well as to the nation in form of loss of good quality germplasm. Therefore such units can be established by the rural/urban youth and they can purchase cow/buffalo calves from these farmers and rear them till parturition and then can sell them at attractive prices to the same dairy owners. Further, the male buffalo calves can be fattened/reared especially for meat purpose.

Integrated Livestock Farming

Apart from rearing of individual livestock species, a new type of farming is emerging very fast these days, which is called the integrated livestock farming. In this type of farming, two or three livestock species are reared together and each species supplements the other. In fact it can be said that this type of farming is symbiotic in nature. Various types of livestock integration are practiced in our country such as:

1. Pig-fish integration
2. Poultry-fish integration
3. Pig-poultry-fish integration
4. Pig-poultry-fish-duck integration
5. Vegetable-goat-fish integration
6. Dairy-fish-duck integration
7. Crop-animal integrated farming

In these types of livestock rearing, the waste products of one species are utilized by the other therein enhancing the productivity of both the species in terms of waste utilization and lower expenditure on feed. For example, in the case of pig-fish integration, the excreta of the pig is used for manuring the pond which give rise to various planktons and phytoplankton's which are eaten by the fish thereby reducing the expenditure on manuring of pond. Further, the dead fish can be utilized for making the ration of pigs. Also it has been found that an individual can get a fish production of 6000 kg per hectare through the integration of livestock with fish by spending only on the purchase of fish seeds. Further such type of integration help in the use of barren and unproductive lands and water bodies, thereby effectively utilizing the natural resources.

LIVESTOCK INPUT INDUSTRY FOR ENTREPRENEURSHIP GENERATION

Another major area for entrepreneurship development in livestock sector is the livestock input industry, which can provide support to various livestock enterprises and can be taken up commercially. Various forms of inputs are required for the livestock enterprises such as feed and fodder, medicines, breeding services, etc. and practising these enterprises commercially can generate good amount of income and employment for rural youth. Various livestock input enterprises, which can be taken up by youth in rural areas, are given below.

Commercial Feed and Fooder Production

Feed and fodder account for the major cost of livestock products and are the major components of the livestock industry. Keeping in view the growing shortage of feed and fodder in our country, promoting these enterprises on commercial scale can solve both the problems, i.e. removing unemployment and developing adequate feed resources for our livestock. This industry has various avenues, which can be harnessed by the rural youth for entrepreneurship development.

Establishment of Area Specific Mineral Mixture Unit

It is a well-established fact that area specific mineral mixture is more profitable to our livestock community for increase in milk production and body weight in young animals. It will be a very good venture to establish unit for product of area specific mineral mixture and by this unit one can earn a lot of profit by sale of this product. The technology can be purchased from IVRI and commercial production can be started.

Commercial Dry Fodder Enrichment Unit (Preparing Urea-treated Straw)

Further, dry fodder enrichment units can be set up, wherein the nutritional quality of the crop residues can be enhanced thereby raising the market value of the poor quality roughages. The urea enriched dry fodder can be prepared on commercial level and can be sold to the dairy farmers at the time of shortage of green fodder which can fetch attractive prices.

Commercial Hay/Silage Preparation

Silage is the product obtained by packing fresh fodder in a suitable container and allowing it to ferment under anaerobic conditions, without undergoing much loss of nutrients. Hay is another form of preserved green fodder, which is made by converting the green forage into dry form without affecting the quality of original material. During the flush season when fodder prices are low, these can be preserved in form of hay and silage. And during the lean period (especially summer) when there is heavy shortage of green fodder, the hay and silage can be sold to the dairy farmers at attractive prices, which can fetch additional returns to the commercial fodder growers.

Growing Fodder Crops Commercially round the Year

Another option is to grow high yielding fodder crops commercially round the year and supply it to the urban and periurban areas, wherein there is heavy demand for green fodder as most of the commercial dairy farms are situated in these areas and can fetch the rural entrepreneurs good price for their fodder.

Establishment of Cattle/Poultry Feed Unit

A rural youth can start the cattle/poultry feed unit with a small initial investment of Rs 2,00,000 including fixed and variable cost, wherein he can get a bank loan of Rs 1,67,500 and rest he has to invest himself. This unit will earn him a yearly profit of Rs 1,16,600, i.e. Rs 9717/month.

Commercial Breeding Units

For commercial livestock rearing, one of the essential components is the availability of good quality breed of livestock, viz. cattle, buffalo, goat, pig or poultry. Keeping in view the importance of the breeding services, such activity can be taken up commercially and various types of commercial enterprises can be started in rural areas. These are discussed below.

Livestock Breeding Farms

Another important input for the commercial livestock rearing is the availability of high yielding breeds of animals like cows Sahiwal, Red Sindhi, Tharparker, Gir, etc. and of buffaloes like Murrah, Nili, Ravi, etc. It has been found that the dairy farmers have to go to other places especially other states, viz. Haryana, Punjab and Gujrat to get good quality cows and buffaloes. Further, most of them who are not able to afford bringing animals from distant places, just purchase the animals from the local market. For smaller livestock species such as goat, sheep and pigs the farmers do not bother to make any efforts for procuring a good breed of animal.

This gap between demand and availability of good breed of livestock poses excellent opportunity in front of rural youth to establish livestock breeding farms in their areas and sell the young ones at good prices. Different types of livestock breeding farms can be established viz.

1. Cattle/buffalo breeding farms
2. Sheep/goat breeding farms
3. Pig breeding farms

But the major requirement is of getting appropriate scientific training in running a livestock-breeding farm. Opening up of poultry hatchery is also a proposition that can be taken up by educated rural youth.

Providing Private Doorstep Artificial Insemination (AI) Services

The rural youth can be employed effectively for providing doorstep AI services by providing them a short para-vet training on AI from the state government, Krishi Vigyan Kendras or other NGOs after which they can purchase the necessary equipments, viz. the moped, AI kit, liquid nitrogen (LN) container and provide doorstep services to the livestock owners thereby upgrading the non-descript stock on one hand and generating additional income on the other. The rural youth can start the mobile AI unit with an initial investment of Rs 45,500 for which they can get loan from banks. In fact this activity is very successful in China.

Establishing Commercial Livestock Service Centres

Commercial livestock service centres can be established by the unemployed rural youth in the villages wherein they can provide both the natural services as well as the artificial insemination services for the livestock. Such type of activity is being practiced in rural areas but the farmers do not maintain good breed of cow/buffalo bull and charge Rs 50 to 100/service. Whereas in urban areas with good quality bulls the charges are Rs 100 to 200/service and this type of enterprise can yield good return to the rural youth also (Rupasi and Sharma, 2007).

Commercial Livestock First Aid Clinics

Timely health care is an important input required for any commercial livestock enterprise. In urban areas, there are a number of private doctors and clinics available for livestock , but such facilities are not available in the rural areas. Further, the government health care machinery is not so efficient as to provide adequate health coverage to all the livestock population. Therefore, the types of livestock first aid clinics that can be established in the rural areas are:

- Allopathic treatment clinics
- Indigenous treatment clinics or alternate system of treatment
- Combined system of treatment

The rural youth can be provided 6 months or one year training in first aid treatment of the livestock, through state government, NGOs, KVKs, dairy cooperatives, which will have dual benefits. On one hand, it will generate employment for rural youth and on the other hand, it will help in boosting the commercial livestock enterprise in rural areas through timely health care measures. Also in rural areas, a number of indigenous treatments are practised for livestock . The rural youth can learn the effective and time-tested indigenous treatment from their elders and can practice them in their areas to earn a living.

ORGANIC LIVESTOCK PRODUCTION UNITS

In the past decade, there has been an increasing awareness about the use of organic products especially in developed countries. The demand for organic products has created new export opportunities for the developing world. The organic products are sold at impressive premiums often at prices 20% higher than the identical traditional products. Therefore, there exists tremendous opportunities of entrepreneurship development through organic livestock production in our country. The major characteristic of the organic food is that it is produced in a naturally defined ecosystem without the use of any artificial means. But production of organic food especially in developed countries is a tough task as there is a heavy use of chemicals such as fertilizer, pesticide and herbicides. India has an edge over the developed countries in this aspect as still in most parts of our country the agricultural production is chemical free and the farmers are very close to being organic. The only difference is that they are not aware about the standards and procedures so as to get their products certified as organic products. Therefore the major requirement is of making our farmers aware about the national standards for organic production developed by APEDA, Ministry of Commerce, GOI, so as to help them fetch higher price for their produce. Such an effort will in turn generate additional employment and income in the livestock sector.

Livestock Product Post-Harvest Processing Units

In India, the revenue from livestock sector is mostly generated by the raw livestock produce, i.e. milk, meat and eggs. Hardly a small percent is being processed and value added. Post-harvest processing helps in enhancing the shelf-life of livestock products, which are a highly perishable commodity and also helps in reducing contamination thereby enhancing the palatability and market value of the livestock products. The annual production of meat and poultry products in India is estimated to be almost 4 million tones per annum, whereas about 1 percent of meat produced is converted into value added products. There is a tremendous opportunity in the livestock sector for employment generation through livestock product processing and value addition. The rural youth can establish various type of livestock product processing and value addition units to earn a livelihood, viz.

1. Milk chilling, storage and packaging units
2. Meat freezing and packaging units
3. Milk pasteurization units

4. Commercial milk product (ghee, paneer, khoa, etc.) production
5. Commercial meat products value addition unit for preparing nuggets, soup powder, papad, sausage, pickle, crackles, patties, samosa, etc. from mutton, chicken, fish pork and eggs.
6. Processing unit for important organs of dead animals or slaughter house by products.

Processing Units for Important Organs of Dead Animals

In India, many million animals die every year and there is no proper processing place or unit in rural area where remaining body parts of dead animals (skin, hides, hair bristles, horn, hoof, intestine, bones, etc.) can be processed and can be converted into value added products. Processing techniques are easy and rural youth can get the training from IVRI or any veterinary college. Collection of various glands from slaughter animals are also very beneficial to prepare various kinds of hormones, enzymes, medicines. The processed organ or parts of dead animals are in great demand not in our country but abroad also. Although these practices are already in vogue in villages and slaughter houses but in crude form not scientifically.

LOAN FROM BANKS

Various banks are providing loan for livestock-based enterprises. Here two models, i.e. financing for dairy and poultry unit have been given. However, time to time, and bank to bank financing terms and conditions may vary.

Model Scheme for Financing a Diary Unit of 10 Cross-bred Cows (Singh, 2007)

Economics of 10 cross-bred cows unit

A. Capital cost	Amount in Rs
i. Cost of 10 CB cows giving average daily milk yield of 10 lit. in a lactation period of 280 days (i.e. 14 days per day at the time of purchase) @ Rs 10000 per cow including transportation cost	1,00,000/-
ii. Cow shed @ 60 sq. ft/cow and Rs 60/sq ft.	36,000/-
iii. Calf cum heifer pens @ 25 sq ft/calf and Rs 60/sq ft	15,000/-
iv. Store cum heifer pen (200 sq ft @ Rs 100/sq ft)	20,000/-
v. Equipments @ Rs 200/animal	2,000/-
vi. Chaff cutter	5,000/-
vii. Insurance cost @ 4.5% of cost of animal for 1 year	4,500/-
viii. Concentrate feed for three months @ 3 kg/cow/day and @ Rs 5/kg	13,500/-
ix. Miscellaneous	4,000/-
B. Total scheme cost	**2,00,000/-**
Less margin @ 15%	30,000/-
Bank's finance	1,70,000/-

C. Annual lactation days and dry days

Considering 280 days as lactation period followed by 120 days of dry period (Details given at milk flow chart depicted at the end for 2 cows cycle).

Days	1st Year	2nd Year	3rd Year	4th Year	5th Year
Lactation days	2150	2600	2600	2550	2400
Dry days	550	1000	1000	1050	1200

D. Feeding cost during lactation period (LP) and dry period (DP) per cow per day

Items	LP Rs	DP Rs
a. Green fodder @ 25 kg during lactation 20 kg during dry period (@ Rs 40/q)	10	08
b. Dry fodder @ 10 kg (@ Rs 100/q	10	10
c. Contentrate feeds @ 3 kg and 1 kg during LP and DP resp. (@ Rs 5/kg)	15	05
Total	**35**	**23**

Financing for Poultry Units

i. The site should be dry, without water logging, well drained and properly accessible. It should be 500 meters away from the existing farm.
ii. Distance between brooder shed, grower shed and layer shed should be 100 ft from each other.
iii. Distance between two layers sheds should be 70 ft.
iv. The shed should have East West orientation.
v. Height of shed should 16 to 22 ft with a maximum width of 35 ft and a length of 100 to 400 ft.
vi. Feed mixing unit should be minimum 300 ft away from sheds.
vii. Floor space Norms   Sheds (sq. ft.)

		Layers		Broilers	
S. No.	Civil structure	Deep litter system	Cage system	Deep litter system	Cage system
1.	Brooder shed (0–8 weeks)	0.5	0.40	–	–
2.	Grower shed (9–20 weeks)	1.0	0.70	–	–
3.	Layer shed (21–72 weeks)	2.0	0.80	–	–
4.	Broiler shed (0–8 weeks)	–	–	1.00	0.60

viii. Feed and feed requirement

		Age in		Requirement (in kg)	
S. No.	Type of bird	weeks	Type of feed	Deep litter system	Cage system
1.	Layer (chicks)	0–8	Chick mash	2.0	2.0
2.	Layers (growers)	9–20	Grower mash	6.0	5.0
3.	Layers (adults)	21–72	Layer mash	40–42	37–39
4.	Broilers	0–4	Starter mash	3.75–4.00	–
5.	Broilers	5–8	Finish mash	3.75–4.00	–

ix. Vaccination schedule for layers and broilers as suggested by poultry experts should be strictly followed. All vaccinations should be completed before 15 to 16 weeks of age.

x. The birds should be insured. The premium rates of insurance of birds, equipment and building, etc. is:

Birds	**Building and equipment**
Layers @ Rs 4.23/bird	@ 0.40% of cost
Broilers @ Rs 0.71/bird	

xi. The total flock is brought in batches depending on the availability of sheds. Interval between introductions of batches should be 12 weeks.

xii. The economic size is 50000 birds for a layer unit in traditional area. For broilers, the unit size can be determined primarily based on the market potential in the area.

All the initiatives discussed above need massive financial support both from government and banks. The financial institutions should look at agriculture as a viable commercial activity rather than a traditional one and thus play a major role in changing the face of rural economy. It is all the more essential in the present day that all the institutions connected with agriculture and rural development should work with the spirit of partnership to give boost to the rural economy as per the policy initiatives of the government (Singh, 2007).

INSURANCE SCHEMES FOR LIVESTOCK SECTOR

Insurance of livestock is highly essential as animals suffer from many natural and unnatural calamities and animal may die due to various ailments at any time and age. There are certain diseases like FMD, HS, anthrax, leptospirosis, brucellosis, TB, paratuberculosis, chemical plant toxicity or poisoning, burn, electrocution, drowning of the animals in flood, death due to enemity, etc. So it is essential to farmers/livestock owners to protect themselves from these losses. They may insure their animals with any insurance company, viz.

1. National Insurance Co. Ltd.
2. The New India Assurance Co. Ltd.
3. Oriental Insurance Co. Ltd.
4. United India Insurance Co. Ltd.

The premium of the insurance of all the four companies are same. If farmers/ livestock owners are taking loan from any bank it become compulsory to get insured the animal otherwise also insurance always protect livestock owners from the losses of various causative agents (Bhasin, 2007).

CONCLUSION

Animal husbandry is the backbone of Indian agriculture and it is having potential to increase percent annual growth rate and GDP, for making livestock sector potential enterprise. A suitable infrastructure technical support is must.

There are 5 thumb needs to develop livestock industry, viz.

1. Proper breeding and reproduction policy at national level
2. Proper nutrition for all the seasons and adverse condition also. It can be decided on regional level by developing feed and fodder banks.
3. Proper management, i.e. proper housing and hygienic conditions.
4. Proper health management, viz. preventive and therapeutic.
5. Proper marketing awareness for livestock owners and trained them for result oriented techniques for value addition products.

Government of India should also provide subsidy to animal sector as well as frame such policies which develop the interest of farmers in livestock sector. Support of technocrat is highly needed to train the rural masses so that they can apply the latest technical knowledge for developing proper enterprise in this sector.

6

Need for Entrepreneurship in Agriculture Sector

JP Sharma, Rashmi Singh

From the 1960s onwards, India has had a population growth of around 23% per decade resulting with current population of more than 1.2 billion. Ours is the second country in the world after China to cross this mark. Half of the population in India is under 25 years of age and the percentage of literates to the Indian 1population is around 76%. This is an immense task ahead to provide meaningful employment to those ever-growing population. Also, the national employment pattern has undergone considerable change over the years. The agro-sector has witnessed a slide in employment from 64 to 54%, whereas opportunities in manufacturing and service sectors have gone up from 15 to 18% and 20 to 27%, respectively, which is a clear indication of the employment future of the country.

According to the 'Global Employment Trends for Youth 2004' report of the International Labour Organisation (ILO), Geneva, a large number of (42 million) unemployed in India comprises the youth. Days have gone when a higher secondary qualification or a graduate could fetch a job. There are over 99.54 lakh students enroll in higher education in India at present. India produces 36 lakhs graduates every year. The 1400 engineering colleges alone in the country produce 4.5 lakhs graduate annually. However, to create and provide jobs to such a large population will not be easier either for the government or the private sector. Therefore, the need of the hour is to encourage job creator rather than job seekers through entrepreneurship. Inculcation of entrepreneurial spirit among youth can resolve this enormous problem on the one hand and bring about speedier development of rural areas on the other side.

For a country like India where unemployment is a major problem, entrepreneurship can prove to be a gainful employment opportunity for our educated youth. Entrepreneurship is a strategy which is creating prospects through training, monitoring and providing other kinds of support system. Entrepreneurship is not inborn but can be developed through appropriate education, skills development and guidance.

Despite the serious need to create opportunities for the unemployed, entrepreneurship is one sector which has not been given the right focus as yet. Even the few institutes imparting entrepreneurship education are more focussed on producing managers than entrepreneurs. Some institutes offer short-term courses of 3 days to 4 weeks duration training and research programmes. But the scale on which entrepreneurial behaviour is needed to be enhanced among youth of present times, such courses fall short of expectations and effectiveness. Awareness generation, entrepreneurial skills inculcation and survival mechanism to cope with ambiguous market fluctuations is the need of the hour for making dent in the burgeoning problem of employment and rural farm distress situations.

Today agriculture in general is not in good health. National commission on farmer report, 'Jai Kisan—A National Policy for Farmers', states agriculture needs an all-round boost by providing farmers the necessary credit and marketing back up. Only this can save them from starvation and suicide conditions. Warning that there was "no time to relax", the report says if agriculture was neglected, the country could revert back to the times of "ship to mouth" existence, depending on imports to meet food requirements. "If agriculture goes wrong, nothing else will have a chance to go right. If, conversely, agriculture goes right, the vision of a hunger and poverty-free India can become a reality, sooner than the time-frame set under the UN Millennium Development Goals".

Dr MS Swaminathan, Chairman National Commission on Farmers suggested one of the solutions to the present crisis was the creation of more jobs in the non-farm sector, with a massive rural non-farm livelihood initiative on the pattern of the township and village enterprises of China. He gave a call to take about 20 million people from farm to non-farm sector by 2010 by integrating small farmers agribusiness centres, food parks, etc. into rural non-farm livelihood initiative to provide employment in rural areas.

This chapter highlights basic issues having bearing on country's employment scenario, needed interventions and possible outcomes through entrepreneurial efforts.

UNEMPLOYMENT SCENARIO

Unemployment is one of the basic problems the world is faced with. Estimates of the total number of people unemployed or under-employed in India vary from 50 to 100 million. Unemployment is the key link in the food security issue in the society these days. Unless a person is employed, he or she may not have the purchasing power to buy enough food for his or her family, though the food supplies may be abundant in the society and the market. The employment growth rate is lower than the growth of the labour force rate and also, the division between these two has grown over the period. The employment growth rate being less than 1% during the major part of the last decade, accordingly growth of employment decreased from 2.82% in 1972-73 to 1.15% in 1987-88. It was only 1% during the 1996-97 and continuously decreasing.

Jobless growth is joyless growth as termed by Dr MS Swaminathan. The most worrisome issue is the near jobless growth of many sectors in the economy, arising mainly from the increased capital intensity of many sectors, including the unorganized sectors. Further, the share of organized sector in the total employment is less than 10% and has decreased over time, pointing out the imperatives of employment generation in the informal sector. Our education system also has not resulted into employable human resources. According to an estimate given by NSSO, around 118 million youths are unemployed who are in the age group of 15–20 years. Out of these, more than 60% are educated.

Many economists believe that the way to solve the unemployment problem in general, is through higher economic growth, but this is not universally true as growth can be 'jobless' and being propelled by the use of capital-intensive technologies that enhance productivity growth. Industrialisation, mechanization and more use of innovative technologies requires less people to do the same job. For example, the robotics have changed the way car frames were earlier welded by workers. Today automatic robots are performing the same job much faster and with high level of precisive productivity. The direct labour deployment in hi-tech industry is decreasing. Mechanised conveyer system has reduced the need for labour. The effect of mechanisation on employment is more visible in agriculture sector, be it ploughing, sowing, weeding, irrigation, harvesting, transportation, every activity is performed mechanically drastically reducing employment potential in this sectors which directly or indirectly support two-thirds population of our country.

In developing countries like ours, only labour intensive techniques will absorb more workers and the variety of skills that the labour force possesses can be utilized. In our case, a large proportion of unemployed are young and many due to poverty, have dropped out of schools and are doing petty farm jobs instead of having a proper long-term employment. Many do not have any 'employable' skills. But there are also thousands of educated youth who are finding it difficult to find jobs because they lack job oriented skills. The skills like critical thinking, effective team playing, multi-tasking, multilingual and positive customer orientation are demanded by industries and other multinationals rather than just rote learning and rigid attitude (Fig. 6.1).

SHRINKING AGRICULTURAL FIELDS

Population growth, rapid urbanisation and industrialisation have resulted in decline in average size of holding and per capita land availability. If we see the population figures, it was 361 m in 1950-51, 439 m in 1960-61, 548 m in 1970-71, 683 m in 1980-81, 846 m in 1990-91, 1000 m in 1999-2000 and by 2020 India's population is like to be about 1300 m. Comparing that to food grain production as depicted in Table 6.1, we can conclude that it will be difficult in the years to come to properly feed out total population. The rate of food grain production is not increasing the way we are witnessing growth in nation's population.

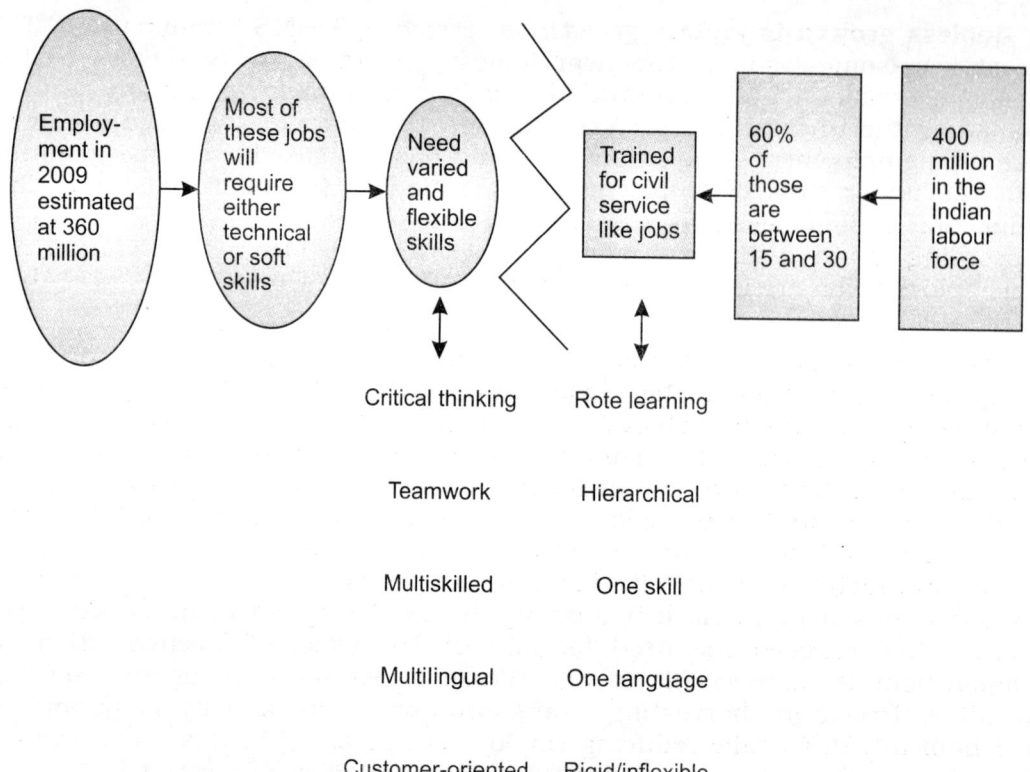

Critical thinking   Rote learning

Teamwork   Hierarchical

Multiskilled   One skill

Multilingual   One language

Customer-oriented   Rigid/inflexible

Source: Planning Commission (2000)

Fig. 6.1: Various skills required in multinational organisations

Table 6.1: Decadal growth in population and food grain production

Year	Population (millions)	Food grain production (million tonnes)
1950-51	361	50
1960-61	439	82
1970-71	548	108
1980-81	683	130
1990-91	846	176
1999-2000	1000	206

Source: Fertilizer Statistics (2000)

The number of small holders, encompassing small (1 to 1.99 ha), marginal (0.5 to 0.99 ha) and sub-marginal (less than 0.5 ha) increased from 49.1 m holders in 1971 to 83.4 m farm holders in 1991. The average size of land holding in India which was 2.28 ha in 1970-71 reduced to 1.55 ha in 1990-91 due to steady increase in number of families and almost no expansion of agriculture land. It has policy implications towards farm efficiency as an inverse relationship of productivity and farm size group has been found. It may also be noticed that land-man ratio has declined from 0.400 ha in 1971 to 0.258 ha in 1991 for all farm size groups and therefore, the pressure on land to attain household food security is further intensifying (Table 6.2).

Table 6.2: Distribution of operational holdings by farm size—All India

Farm size	Number of operational holdings (million)		Net cropped area (m ha)		Size of operational holdings (ha)		Land-man ratio	
	1971	1991	1971	1991	1971	1991	1971	1991
Sub-marginal	23.2 (33)	42.7 (40)	5.4 (3)	9.8 (6)	0.23	0.23	0.046	0.046
Marginal	12.5 (18)	20.6 (19)	9.1 (6)	15.0 (9)	0.73	0.73	0.140	1.124
Small	13.4 (19)	20.1 (19)	19.3 (12)	28.8 (18)	1.44	1.43	0.240	0.217
Medium	10.7 (15)	13.8 (13)	30.0 (19)	38.4 (23)	2.81	2.76	0.426	0.373
Large	10.7 (15)	9.2 (9)	98.3 (60)	73.4 (44)	9.18	7.95	1.257	0.994
All farms	70.5 (100)	106.6 (100)	162.1 (100)	165.5 (100)	2.28	1.55	0.400	0.258

Source: Agricultural Census 1970-71 to 1990-91, GOI
Figures in parenthesis indicate the percentage share in total corresponding to all farms.

There is continuous fragmentation of land due to ownership multiplication and division of joint families into smaller nuclear families; resulting in low per capita availability of land. The land to man ratio in our country is becoming very narrow. The employment situation in rural areas is rather more alarming in view of the shrinking agricultural land area. Due to low land-man ratio, more and more farmers and their children are finding themselves out of work. Increasing influence of education has also created a higher need for jobs amongst the rural masses. After finishing their education, rural youth also line up in front of employment exchange for seeking jobs. Although they have an option of starting their own enterprise but this option is usually ignored by them and they join the long queue of job seekers in front of offices. Sometimes they have to accept those jobs also which are not in accordance with their qualifications and experience. Thus unemployment and underemployment both are in existence. A large number of studies have clearly brought to light that the rural youth are serious victims of frustration, cynicism, goallessness, normlessness and misanthropy largely due to lack of employment opportunities. Their energy is not channelised in a positive direction. The situation has led to alarming increase in the rate of migration from rural areas to cities. If it continues uncontained, only a few years from now, it will not only create chaos in cities and towns, but it would also destroy the socio-cultural-fabric of rural India. Hence, even if agricultural productivity of India improves, a lot needs to be done in other aspects also for attaining economic prosperity and proper development of the rural India.

Many years ago, Mahatma Gandhi wrote in "Harizan" issue dated 29th August, 1936, "If the village perishes, India will perish too. India will be no more India. Her own mission in the world will get lost." He gave much emphasis on village industries and visualised village as a self-contained, independent and fully functional unit of Indian society. Fulfillment of his vision and much of the problems which have arisen because of lack of gainful employment opportunities in rural areas, can be tackled effectively if village industries are developed and agriculture moves from being just a way of life, i.e. culture to become a dynamic entity, i.e. agribusiness. Growth of village industries based on agriculture in rural areas has also been given priority by the government and policy makers in latest plans.

AGRICULTURE TO AGRIBUSINESS

Well-developed inter-linkages between agriculture and rural industry will be an effective mechanism of promoting rural transformation. While on one hand, farmers get just few rupees in the exchange of their produce; it is multinationals who are grabbing the major chunk of profits after selling it to the ultimate users. Whether it is potatoes, tomatoes and other perishable commodities, farmers are forced to sell their produce for very less amount while the ultimate consumer pays huge amount in case it is processed and packaged after grading the same produce. The cases of farmers of Ratnagiri district in Maharashtra and potato farmers of Farukhabad district in UP, illustrate this very situation where they suffered huge post-harvest losses and were forced to sell their produce at a throw away price. This is not a single case but true for all the perishable commodities which are produced in plenty during crop season but due to non-availability of storage and processing facilities locally, producers are not getting their due share. The big industrial houses having processing facilities and middlemen are making unbelievable profits. Take the case of potato chips. A farmer gets only Re 1 to 1.50 for one kg potato during potato harvest season or sometimes even less than this but beautifully packed potato chips are sold as high as Rs 300 per kg to the ultimate consumer. Similarly there are some regions where tomato production is very high and local demand is not enough to consume the produce and the farmers do not get remunerative price in absence of processing facility at the doorstep. So the same tomato purchased from the farmers at the rate of 1–2 rupees per kg is sold at the rate of 70–80 rupees per kg after making tomato ketchup. Here both the producer (farmer) and the consumer are at a loss and middlemen are making high profits. Hence, there is a great need to develop rural industries in villages itself based on agricultural products so as to reduce post-harvest losses and provide good returns to the farmers. It can be done and is highly in demand because of changing food consumption pattern and sufficient demand for value added products. The need is to prepare our people to go for such kind of economic activity.

NEED FOR ENTREPRENEURSHIP DEVELOPMENT

One of the major tasks before the developing countries is the building of human assets which is as important a pre-requisite of economic prosperity, as is the growth of physical and financial assets. In fact human resources can bring about transformations if they are able and efficient. Several empirical studies have shown that the entrepreneurs as the human capital have made a large contribution to economic development than non-human capital. Increase in population, which is considered a liability can also contribute positively towards overall national development if entrepreneurial qualities are inculcated among the masses. An attempt to develop entrepreneurial activity among persons may create a situation where people become capable of optimal utilization of the limited and scattered resources.

In fact there are four basic requirements for development to take place. These are financial, technical and infrastructural support along with matching human resource (Fig. 6.2).

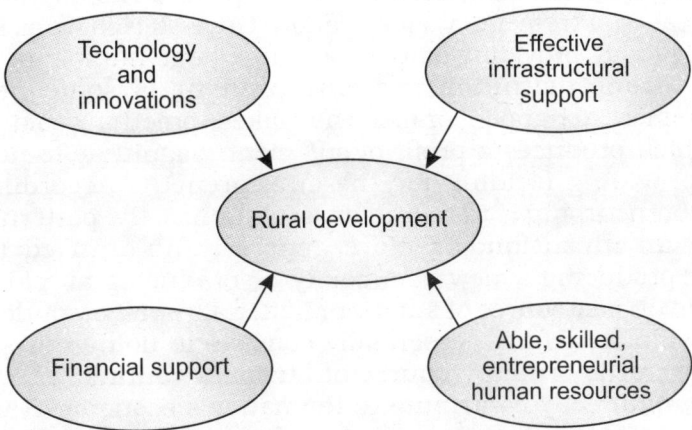

Fig. 6.2: Various components of rural development

Somehow our policy and planning emphasized only on first three and ignored the fourth one, i.e. human resource which is the most important. If a person is motivated, has a high need for achievement; he or she can mobilise other factors of development for the environment, but once this basic factor is missing all other facilities be it financial or technical, it will go waste or blatantly un-utilised or under-utilised.

WHERE DOES THIS LEAD?

Then what is the solution or the needed way out? We cannot always look up to the Government, the trade or the industry for employment. On the other hand, land availability cannot be increased, rather it is going to decline due to population growth and rapid urbanisation and industrialisation. Fortunately, now there are several opportunities in agriculture where the farmers can generate more income and employment per unit of time and land. This is possible through diversification and commercialization of agriculture one hand and exploitation of entrepreneurial opportunities in rural non-farm sector.

Here is where the entrepreneurs come to fill this vacuum. These are people who see potential gaps and perform value added jobs. These are people with a vision and see an opportunity for value addition and thereby getting that extra money, even by taking the risk associated with the job. Economic development will result in development of rural regions. The entrepreneurship concept is as old as the existence of human being. Even in Greek Mythology, the image of Hermes fits into the description of entrepreneur. The mythological story describes Hermes to have discovered a tortoise, from which he made an immense fortune by constructing its shell into a musical instrument. This was a simple technological invention, an indicative of the entrepreneurial behaviour. The entrepreneur with his vision finds out new opportunities and thereby creates wealth for himself and for others in the society. Many of today's industrial houses employing thousand of people, were once started by entrepreneurs, who had the vision and the courage to take risks associated with the opportunities. Role models emerging amongst us like Dhirubhai Ambani, Suichiro Honda, Narayanamurthy of Infosys are cases of tremendous inspiration. Once started off as small ventures have grown big today providing employment to a large number of people.

According to one definition, an entrepreneur is someone who makes something commercial happen, or one who makes something sold which benefits others and which produces a profit of sufficient magnitude to justify the risks inherent in providing funding for the entrepreneur. According to another version, entrepreneurship is to reform or revolutionize the pattern of production by exploring an invention, or more generally an untried technological possibility for producing a new commodity or producing an old one in a new way by opening up new source of supply or materials or a new outlet for products. Entrepreneurship as defined, essentially consists in doing things that are not generally done in the ordinary course of business routine.

Entrepreneurs directly contribute to the nation's economy. It is known from the history, that the Greek civilization grew from 900 BC to 100 BC, due to the entrepreneurs, and in Spain the growth took place from 1692 to 1710 due to the same spirit. England also witnessed the growth in the triggering of the industrial revolution around 1770 AD. In case of United States, the onset of World War I, triggered corporate growth mainly by entrepreneurs. During the II World war, again the American industry witnessed the growth of companies, mainly due to new entrepreneurs.

Japan is known for its business giants, like Sony, Honda, Yamaha, Mitsubishi, etc. But it is also worth noting Japan's small industry strengths, which is the first abode of an entrepreneur.

IMPERATIVE PATH

There is a need to develop entrepreneurship among the farmers in particular and rural masses in general. To convert a farm into an enterprise or business, the identity of the person managing it must change from a farmer to that of farm business operator or an entrepreneur. Any advancement in technology can never bring fruitful achievement until farmers become entrepreneurs. Agricultural advancement inspires farmers to be entrepreneurial, away from their conventional and hereditary vocational system. There is a great need to make our farmers entrepreneurial and this is an achievable proposition since the characteristics of entrepreneurs are not inherited but can be developed through systematic motivational training.

Entrepreneurship among farmers may be developed through systematic awareness spread programmes and training interventions. Awareness about available technologies, opportunities, resource support system and about market potential has to be systematically spread among the rural masses especially, the farming community. Then comes the second step of motivation development. Prior to it, an environment of awareness and need has to be prepared. This awareness and motivation has to be developed not only in the farmers but also in the field level extension workers. Once they become aware about entrepreneurship and convinced about its need in agriculture, they will be able to provide some thrust towards commercializing agriculture, as they are the one who are implementing government sponsored schemes. Entrepreneurship development programme (EDP) for agriculture has to go via the existing system itself. EDP aims to develop entrepreneurship through motivation development, providing support services and sustaining the efforts for the first time entrepreneurs.

Krishi Vigyan Kendras are nodal institutions, which are now making their presence felt in every district. Entrepreneurship development programme should be included in the mandate of KVKs. The staff of KVKs should be trained in entrepreneurship development in agriculture so that it reaches the ultimate users, i.e. the farmers who can then avail of the opportunities already existing in the system.

Experts feel that the spirit of entrepreneurship should be inculcated in students at the school level since by the time they undertake their graduation and post-graduation education they become too job centric. The Central Board of Secondary Education (CBSE) has recently introduced a two-year course on entrepreneurship at the senior school level as an elective subject. The curriculum will focus on developing entrepreneurial skills, values, motivation, understanding of patents, copyrights and trademarks and would provide inputs on managerial skills. Apart from the government sector, the B-schools and private sector should contribute to initiate more programmes in entrepreneurship, especially in rural areas. Some State Agricultural Universities have already included entrepreneurship development in their course curriculum but it needs to be made broad based. Vocational training can be given to school graduates and drop outs at various urban and rural centres using IT and this would prepare them better for getting jobs in the future. Training in manufacturing activities reserved for the small-scale sector should also be included and emphasized to enable the young to be self-employed. Young women should be given different types of training for income generation from home also.

Scientists should give emphasis on development of technologies which can be adopted by farmers rather than going on increasing the body of knowledge of science. It is not to deny the research efforts in basic sciences but applied aspects are more pragmatic and practical in present scenario. They must give priority to applied science in preference to basic science. Presently, outcome of majority of researchers is in the form of body of knowledge. If the consumer is willing to take up the knowledge, the application part is lacking. Scientists should develop adaptable technological packages. For example, lot of research has been done in the field of mushroom, floriculture or vermiculture but hardly any package in the form of project proposal is available for farmers. This package should be adaptable on farmer's fields. If a farmer is having a piece of land and money to invest even then there is hardly any package available to guide him to set up a viable enterprise. Farmers are developing interest in new technologies but these are not available in package form which can be adopted.

Many of the states like UP, MP, Bihar, Gujarat, Maharashtra, etc. have centers for entrepreneurship development or institutes of entrepreneurship development at state level. They are already providing entrepreneurship development training in rural non-farm sector for self-employment. They need to widen their area and effectively carry out entrepreneurship development activities in agriculture which is almost virgin and most potential area for entrepreneurship development in our country.

MICRO-ENTERPRISES TO BE PROMOTED

Micro-enterprises in rural areas based on agriculture and related non-farm activities can generate employment for rural youth in the villages itself; thus reducing the pulling factors for migration to nearby towns. Micro-enterprises can serve four major objectives of poverty reduction; employment generation, empowerment and enterprise development as an end in itself. Regardless of the stage of economic development among the Asia-Pacific countries, small and medium enterprises (SMEs) are generally considered as major sources of employment generation. They dominate the non-agricultural sector not only in the number of enterprises but also in the numbers employed. Promotion of such enterprises, therefore, is generally regarded as part of an employment-intensive industrialization strategy. They need to be promoted in agriculture sector as well.

Small and medium-sized enterprises are contributing to employment growth at a higher rate than larger firms. In the EU, economy about 99.9% of the enterprises are SMEs of which 93% are micro-enterprises. The private sector and in particular SMEs form the backbone of a market economy and for the transition economies in the long-term might provide most of the employment (as is the case in the EU countries). A world bank sector policy paper shows that their labour intensity is 4–10 times higher for small enterprises. Benefits of SMEs are well evident now, the only need is to apply it to agribusiness development.

MICRO-CREDIT AND SELF-HELP GROUP

Rural areas are characterized by the poor resource base and lack of capital and investment. Micro-credit support would stop this resource crunch and strengthen the development of micro-enterprises both the farm-based ones and non-farm-based enterprises. Micro-credit, in the sense of small loans to the poor, has its roots in the ancient India. But our neighbour Bangladesh's Grameen

Bank has well established that micro-credit is the way out for rural enterprises to take shape and fluorish.

Group action at farmers level by forming self-help groups in rural areas will enable farmers to overcome the common problems experienced by all in terms of marketing and delivery of services. The imperative issues facing micro-enterprises sustenance and smooth functioning can be addressed to a large extent by promoting self-help groups in rural areas. It provides the farmers greater bargaining power at micro-and macro-levels of our system. Their interests are kept into accounts at policy levels. The SHGs have excellent opportunities to work together to initiate small business or extend various essential services.

There is an immediate need to identify new opportunities, which should be based on the demand for the output both in local and outside markets. This calls for a network of SHGs, who can share information among themselves. They can also set up a common information service centre to learn about the demand-supply situations for their produce and modify their plans accordingly to optimize profits. Also there is need to train the members of SHGs regularly. The training should emphasize on managerial aspects of the business, in addition to technical skills.

SHGs can also initiate several development activities such as improvement in hygiene, sanitation, public utilities, kindergarten, primary school, adult education, child health care and immunization, family planning, safe drinking water and management of local bodies and public institutions. Indeed, these indirect benefits highly empower the local people to monitor public services and utilities provided by the government. With the local people demanding punctual services, staff working in the Panchayat institutions will have to be accountable by assuming their responsibilities. The enlightened community can participate in Gram Sabha meetings and pressurize the Gram Panchayat to improve their services. This will ensure transparency in public affairs. This indeed is the sustainable development managed by the people themselves.

ENABLING POLICIES

Facilitating the flow of information on jobs and markets for products, e.g. through publications and through the establishment of NGOs and other organizations that can provide such services. Local economic development programmes need to be inclusive, and ensure that the urban poor benefit from them. Then equally important is the issue of providing practical job training. The ability of the poor to benefit from growth requires good basic education and can be enhanced through job training programmes. Cities can organize job training programmes and workshops in collaboration with the private sector and central government to enhance the skills of the labour force.

Facilitating childcare to enable women to work, governments can initiate simple and cost-effective programmes with the help of NGOs and community-based organizations (CBOs). These child-care programmes can be supported with modest subsidies. Cities must ensure basic hygiene and safety through advisory services and minimal regulations. Community day-care centres started in Latin America are an example for such programmes.

Supporting the sectors that have higher employment generation capacity. For example, the construction sector (including housing and infrastructure) accounts for between 40 and 70% of gross fixed capital formation in developing countries. It also tends to be labour intensive. Therefore, both national and city level policies should be designed to eliminate factors that may impede development of the construction sector. Lack of financing mechanisms for both developers and homebuyers and undeveloped land markets can easily impede development of construction activity. Labour-intensive construction methods, like self-help housing, can also be supported. Government support of formal housing construction programmes, as well as self-help housing (which is more labour intensive), would boost employment and investment. Cities can also take a role in the creation of short-term employment, e.g. through public works programmes. Such programmes typically address urban infrastructure deficiencies through small works investments. Although the jobs created are only short-term, such programmes provide temporary supplements to income and promote small-scale entrepreneurs.

CONCLUSION

Way from agriculture to agribusiness and rural entrepreneurship development will stop migration to cities. Increasing population in cities can also be stopped and rural people will get employment in rural areas itself. Hence, this will help in maintaining villages as dynamic entities while reducing the chaotic conditions in cities and put a stop to ever increasing boundaries of townships. This will also help in shifting the economic power to rural areas and will be really a step towards decentralization of power. Rural manpower will be utilised by rural industries. Rural income can be increased which will pave the way for real development to occur in rural areas. Exploitation of farmers by traders and middlemen can thus be avoided. Agro enterprise can help in achieving. A balanced growth and development which will be eco friendly. Misuse and over-exploitation of natural resources will be minimized. Transportation costs as well as post-harvest losses of perishable commodities can be reduced if agro-industries are in rural areas. Nowadays, most of the processing of agricultural products is being done in cities which means farmers have to bear the cost of transportation. This is another thing which makes farmers frustrated. If agro-industries are developed in villages, a cycle can be developed whereby "agricultural products" can be utilised by these industries and also some enterprises can produce products which can be utilised in farming.

Enterprises in rural areas will improve their infrastructure and will have a boosting effect on other aspects like transports, roads, availability of products, economy, etc. Thus, it will result in overall development of these areas. Employment opportunities in rural areas will be able to utilize the energies of rural youth and thereby lessen the social evils and mischief in the villages. Hence, it will pave the way for developing a healthy society in rural areas. Thus, micro-enterprise promotion by providing training inputs to farmers, infrastructural support and micro-credit availability will make a dent in the vicious cycle of poverty, unemployment and scarcity in rural areas. It will help in fostering rural development and will help the majority of our population to have secure livelihood.

7

Entrepreneurship Development in Agriculture and Horticulture

Debashish Sengupta

India is a country with diverse agro-climatic conditions. Almost 70% of the population lives in the rural area and they are mostly dependent upon agriculture for their livelihood. The development of the nation largely depends upon the development of the rural population. Mahatma Gandhi (1926) had once said— *India's way is not Europe's. India is not Calcutta and Bombay. India lives in her several hundreds of villages.* The green revolution came as a boon at a time when India was struggling to achieve self-reliance in food grain production. This was realized to a large extent but the conditions of the farmers did not improve drastically. The reason was that the green revolution largely concentrated on the cereals. Agriculture in India is understood to be synonym to cultivation of cereals and pulses. The real picture and the scope of this sector are not properly understood even to the people who are engaged in this sector. In our country, the agricultural sector provides livelihood to around 650 million people, representing roughly 58.4% of the country's workforce. Its more than obvious that the development of the nation as a whole is not possible without the development of the people involved in this sector. Majority of the country's workforce is engaged in agriculture and their development will be key if we wish to charter an exponential growth curve for ourselves.

MAIN PROBLEMS IN THIS SECTOR

We are the second largest populated nation of the world, have very favourable agro-climatic conditions and more than half of the working nation is involved in the agriculture sector; still the terms and conditions are dictated to us by the American and the European countries. The reason for this anomaly is the lopsided development of this sector. Majority of the farmers are small or marginal farmers. The awareness level among the farmers regarding the scope of this sector as well as how they can prevent their exploitation at the hands of the unscrupulous intermediaries for marketing of their produce is a huge underbelly.

After about four decades, we have realized that the sustainable growth and rural empowerment was possible through concentrating on other commercial crops as well and one of the booming sectors is **horticulture**. India's horticulture

73

production currently nearing 150 million tonnes a year has not only bought prosperity to the small and marginal farmers but also provided food and nutritional security to the nation. Ranked as second largest producer of fruits and vegetables in the world, horticulture in India has emerged as an important sector for diversification in agriculture.

Sole dependence on cultivation of cereal, pulses and some cash crops like cotton, sugarcane and tobacco cannot redefine the picture. There is an increasing need for entrepreneurship development in agriculture, horticulture, animal husbandry and allied sector to truly empower our people and pave way for sustainable growth.

AGRIPRENEURSHIP (AGRI-ENTREPRENEURSHIP): THE RAY OF HOPE

The people involved in agriculture are slowly realizing that they cannot afford to look at the government for each and every thing. Self-reliance is key. Besides, with the changing global agricultural scene in light of WTO round of talks, over-dependence on traditional format of farming and on traditional crops will not be enough. Entrepreneurship in agriculture sector or agripreneurship is the order of the day. There are tremendous opportunities in the agriculture and allied sector for promotion of agripreneurship. The allied sectors like sericulture, dairy farming, bee-keeping, mushroom cultivation, fisheries, etc. have a lot of potential for agripreneurial development. Horticulture, which encompasses olericulture, pomology and floriculture in itself, provides lots of scope for entrepreneurial ventures. Besides, the farmers should also identify the related cottage industries like tomato sauce and squash making units, fruit jam making units, mentha oil making units, jaggery units, etc. This will lead to regional as well as individual growth. Such entrepreneurial ventures can increase the disposable income of the farmers largely and can make them more financially independent.

The following can be prospective agripreneurs:

- Progressive farmers.
- Unemployed agriculture graduates.
- Retired persons settled in their native regions.
- Women cooperatives.
- Self-help groups.

Possible Areas of Agripreneurial Development

Contrary to popular belief, there are large number of areas of agripreneurial development. Some of the possible areas where agripreneurship can be undertaken are as follows:

1. **Herbal processing unit:** It involves setting-up of mentha oil extraction units, herbal products manufacturing like neem soaps, oils, etc.

2. **Honey agribusiness:** Bee-keeping and honey production provides a vast unexplored opportunity to the budding entrepreneurs. Honey extraction units like in Jeolikote, Nainital are a model example.

3. **Plant clinics:** Diagnosis and effective treatment of crop pests, diseases, microbial attacks and weeds is a major problem faced by farmers. Agriculture graduates can position themselves as plant doctors and set-up plant clinics.

4. **Insurance:** Government is of-late rolling-out crop insurance schemes for the farmers. Possibility exists to facilitate such policies through enterprising agents.

5. **Mushroom cultivation:** Mushroom cultivation and marketing have a lot of potential and scope. Although the consumption pattern by large is still not developed to that extent, however, that's what needs to be done.

6. **Landscaping and nursery:** There has been a steady growth among the people in general regarding the green issues and consecutively a desire to make their surroundings greener. However, there is still a lot of gap between the demand and the supply especially with the aspect of accessibility. Nursery business provides an opportunity to many for filling-up this gap. Corporate and commercial landscaping sector is also growing and creative people can do wonders in it.

7. **Agribusiness centres:** Agri-trading centres, commercial agri-hubs, etc. are some of the prospective entrepreneurial areas to be tapped on a larger scale.

8. **Food processing:** Food processing industry in India offers on palate tremendous scope for expansion. Small to medium level entrepreneurs can set-up units like potato chips plant, finger-chips plant, tomato sauce plant, etc.

9. **Herbal-based mineral water:** Herbal is the word in vogue today. Thanks to the relentless campaign against chemical hazards. The discovery of higher degree of pesticides in drinks and some other similar incidents have reinforced the view to a large extent that herbal is safe. Moreover, when it comes to water herbally treated mineral water will definitely have many takers. However, the need is to have such units, which is only possible if budding entrepreneurs embrace the idea.

10. **Micro-irrigation systems:** Manufacturing and trading of micro-irrigation systems is possible on a small-scale too and hence vast opportunities.

11. **Agro-eco tourism:** Development of ornamental gardens, forest areas and agro-expos can facilitate the agro-eco tourism.

12. **Animal feed unit:** Animal feed is something, which has still a huge demand-supply imbalance more due to the unavailability of cheap animal feed. These units be set-up at a small scale; as it has also an existing demand.

13. **Biofertilizer production and marketing:** I remember once to have visited a person's place in Shantipuri near Pantnagar (Nainital, Uttarakhand). He was making cow-dung manures, neem manures in his house itself. He had dug-up pits and put cow dung in it. Then covered it with soil rich in earthworms. The manure would be ready after some months. He would then be packing it in polythene bags and giving it a brand name. Biofertilizer

production and marketing can be taken-up very easily with minimal investments.

14. **Clearing and forwarding agency:** Clearing and forwarding agents are an important link in marketing of agriculture goods. Enterprising people can become clearing and forwarding agents, distributors, etc.

15. **Contract farming:** Farming for landless people is not impossible. Agriculture graduates desirous of applying their learning into practical can opt for contract farming by taking farms land on lease.

16. **Crop protection centre:** Crop protection is a big issue in India especially due to the lack of proper initiatives from the government. Crop protection centres offering crop solutions under one roof can be a valid option.

17. **Cultivation of medicinal plants:** Cultivation of medicinal plants offers a good entrepreneurial opportunity for the people. The reason behind has been the growing fad of herbal medicines and the bent of the pharmaceutical companies towards manufacturing such medicines. For this, they will require raw material in the form of medicinal plants products. Such growers can fulfill this demand.

18. **Cyber extension:** ITC's e-chaupal has open floodgates in the sector of rural internet extension. Cyber presence in rural areas is almost negligible. However, contrary to the popular belief the interest and need can be generated among the farmers regarding the use on internet in knowing soil conditions, weather forecast, crop protection tips, etc. Cyber extension with a little bit of rural customized approach is definitely a good entrepreneurial option.

19. **Dairy:** Dr. Kurien showed through Anand Milk Union Limited that how lakhs of unorganized milk women can be converted into successful entrepreneurs. Dairy if taken-up in a more organized manner with effective local branding and with genuine quality assurance can generate a lot of income. Veterinary graduates can show path.

20. **Direct marketing/retail marketing:** Marketing of agriculture goods provides a vast arena for entrepreneurship in India.

21. **Farm machinery unit:** There is a serious need for customized farm machinery equipments. For instance in hills, the traditional farm machineries do not work because of the terrain. Here we need small, handy and sturdy farm machinery and equipments. Such units can be set-up by innovative agriculture engineering graduates.

22. **Fisheries development:** Fisheries provide good opportunities in both the domestic as well as the export sector. Entrepreneurial efforts in this direction can be highly useful.

23. **Floriculture marketing:** Floriculture is all set to become the next big thing in India. The growth in this sector will be phenomenal, if the efforts carry on as they have started now. Floriculture marketing offers huge opportunity

for entrepreneurial explorations. Florist shops, wholesale trading, electronic retailing and so on; the possibilities are unlimited. There have been many examples where entrepreneurial efforts in floriculture marketing have brought wonderful results. One such example is Ferns 'n'Petals. Ferns'n'Petals started as small florist shop in Greater Kailash area of New Delhi. With its entrepreneurial efforts and effective branding strategy, it went on to become the first branded online chain of corporate and marriage floral decorators. Its presence on internet made it even more versatile. Today it holds about 10% share in India's total floriculture trade. A phenomenal achievement, considering the journey from an ordinary florist to a big player at national level. Recently in an International Floriculture Conference held at Bangalore an entrepreneur demonstrated his online flower-retailing portal named Phoolwal.com.

24. **Organic production/food chain:** Food processing industry is rolling big bucks in India already. Organic food is all set to come and takeover the market like a whirlwind. The pioneers will be the biggest gainers. Organic food in very simple terms will be naturally or organically processed foodstuffs. This is very much a part of our ethnic culture. So making entrepreneurial forays in these fields will require explorations at local level.

25. **Poultry:** Egg and meat consumption have shown a steady rise over the years. This provides a very good opportunity for the budding entrepreneurs to take up poultry business. Poultry farming provides reasonable diversification.

Some Other Agri-entrepreneurial (Agripreneurial) Areas

- Pesticides production and marketing
- Post-harvest management
- Research and development
- Seed processing and agribusiness
- Soil testing laboratory
- Thermo foam tray production
- Tissue culture unit
- Vegetable production and marketing
- Vermicomposting
- Veterinary clinics
- Pickle, papad units

Agripreneurship Promotion and Development

Of late, the significance of agripreneurship is being realized more and more. This has seen efforts from the government as well as from the NGOs for the promotion and development of the same. The following data showing the state-wise success stories of the agripreneurs facilitated by the agriclinics and agribusiness centre schemes, is in itself a testimony of the new found focus (Table 7.1).

Table 7.1: Statewise success stories of agripreneurs

S.No.	Name of the state	No. of success stories
1.	Karnataka	130
2.	Rajasthan	104
3.	Maharashtra	72
4.	Andhra Pradesh	60
5.	Tamil Nadu	45
6.	Gujarat	41
7.	Orissa	28
8.	Uttar Pradesh	17
9.	Haryana	12
10.	Bihar	11
11.	Uttarakhand	11
12.	Madhya Pradesh	8
13.	West Bengal	6
14.	Punjab	4
15.	Jharkhand	3
16.	Kerala	3
17.	Assam	1
18.	Pondicherry	1
	Total	**557**

(*Data Source:* National Bank for Agricultural and Rural Development and National Institute of Agriculture Extension Management.)

Indian government and its allied agencies have come out with a range of promotional and developmental schemes for entrepreneurial, marketing and export growth with an objective to mobilize the people to engage more and more in entrepreneurship. Some of the schemes are as follows:

Schemes of National Horticulture Board (NHB)

National Horticulture Board contribution has been multi-dimensional, supporting the farmers and entrepreneur to face the challenge of the globalized markets with improved production, post-harvest management and value addition. Committed to the 'golden revolution' NHB has formulated broad-based entrepreneur-driven schemes to facilitate integrated development of the horticulture sector. Some of the NHB schemes, pattern assistance, etc. are as follows:

Development of Commercial Horticulture through Production and Post-harvest Management

The components are:

Production related: It includes high quality commercial horticulture crops, indigenous crops, aromatic plants, seed and nursery, biotechnology, tissue culture, bio-pesticides, organic foods, establishment of horticultural health clinics, consultancy services, bee-keeping.

Primary processing related: It includes grading/washing/sorting/drying/ packing centres, pre-cooling units, refrigerated van containers, special transport vehicles, retail outlets, auction platform, ripening curing chamber, market yard/ ropeways, radiation unit/dehydration unit, vapour heat treatment unit, primary processing of products, horticulture ancillary industry and crates/cartons/ aseptic packaging and nets.

The pattern of assistance is back-ended capital investment subsidy not exceeding 20% of the project cost with maximum limit of Rs 25 lakhs per project (Rs 30 lakh for north-east/tribal areas) for production, post-harvest management and primary processing of the horticulture produce. Project must be submitted in prescribed format to the NHB state office.

	Processing fees	
1.	Project with cost up to Rs 10 lakh	Exempted
2.	Project with cost above Rs 10 lakh	0.25% of the project cost
	and upto Rs 20 lakh	
3.	Project with cost above Rs 20 lakh	0.5% of the project cost

Capital Investment Subsidy for Construction/Modernization/Expansion of Cold Storage and Storage for Horticulture Produce

Components		
	Pattern of assistance	
	Back ended capital subsidy not exceeding 25% of the project cost with a maximum limit of Rs 50 lakh per project (Rs 60 lakhs for north-east areas) @ 33% of the project cost	
	How to apply	
	Project involving term loan may be submitted to banks/ NCDC for appraisal/sanction of loan. For self-financed project, LOI in prescribed format is required	
	Processing fees	
1. Cold storage	Project with cost up to Rs 10 lakh	Exempted
2. Controlled atmosphere (CA)/modified atmosphere (MA) storage	Project with cost above Rs 10 lakh and up to Rs 20 lakh	0.25% of the project cost
3. Onion storage	Project with cost above Rs 20 lakh	0.5% of the project cost

Some other schemes of NHB are grouped under the following—**technology development and transfer market information service for horticulture crops** and **horticulture promotion service**. In almost all these categories 100% assistance is provided. The eligible organizations are NGOs, association of growers, individuals, partnership/proprietary firms, companies, corporations, agricultural produce committees, agro-industry corporations, etc.

Agricultural and Processed Food Products Export Development Authority (APEDA)

APEDA set-up by the ministry of commerce and industry, government of India, is an endeavour to augment agro-exports and provides financial assistance to the exporters under various schemes for horticulture and general agriculture.

The various schemes of APEDA can be divided under 4 categories:

1. Scheme for market development
2. Scheme for infrastructure development
3. Scheme for quality development
4. Scheme for research and development

1. *Schemes for Market Development*	
Components	**Scale of assistance**
(A) Packaging development	
(i) Activity for development of packaging standards and design	APEDA's internal scheme for development work through involvement of institutions/organization in India and abroad with the cost sharing with exporters and/or organizations involved in the export promotion. Maximum amount in case of sharing with exporters/organization is Rs 5 lakh or 50% of the cost of development whichever is less or 100% in case of APEDA.
(ii) Assistance to exporters for the use of packaging material as per standards and specifications developed or adopted by APEDA.	30% subject to ceiling of Rs 1.50 lakh per beneficiary.
(iii) Assistance to exporters, producers, growers, service providers, co-operative organizations, etc. for purchase of "intermediate packaging material" for domestic transportation of produce.	50% of the cost of the material subject to ceiling of Rs 5 lakh.

Feasibility studies, surveys, consultancy and database upgradation	
(i) Development and dissemination of market information	100% to be implemented by APEDA
(ii) Assistance for conducting feasibility surveys and studies to exporters	50% of the total cost subject to ceiling of Rs 2 lakh per beneficiary
(iii) Assistance for conducting feasibility surveys and studies to semi-government and PSUs	50% of the project cost subject to a ceiling of Rs 10 lakh per beneficiary
Export promotion and market development	
(i) Supply of materials, samples, development of websites, events sponsored by APEDA	100% to be implemented by APEDA
(ii) Preparation of publicity and promotional material for APEDA	100% to be implemented by APEDA
(iii) Brand publicity through ads	40% of the cost subject to a ceiling of Rs 1 lakh per beneficiary
(iv) Export promotional activities	100% of the cost
2. *Schemes for Infrastructure Development*	
Part-I	
(i) Establishment of common infrastructural facilities by APEDA	100% grant in aid
Part-II	
(A) Assistance for purchase of specialized transport units	25% of the cost subject to a ceiling of Rs 2.5 lakh per beneficiary
(B) Assistance to exporters producers, growers, cooperative organizations and federations for horticulture and floriculture sector.	
(i) Mechanization of harvest operation	25% of the cost subject to a ceiling of Rs 5 lakh per beneficiary
(ii) Setting-up of sheds for storage, grading, etc.	25% of the cost of equipment subject to a ceiling of Rs 5 lakh per beneficiary
(iii) Setting-up of mechanized handling facilities	25% of the cost of equipment subject to a ceiling of Rs 10 lakh per beneficiary

(iv) Setting-up of pre-cooling facilities	25% of the cost of equipment subject to a ceiling of Rs 10 lakh per beneficiary
(v) Providing facilities for pre-shipment treatment	25% of the cost of equipment subject to a ceiling of Rs 10 lakh per beneficiary
(vi) Setting-up of integrated post-harvest system	25% of the cost subject to a ceiling of Rs 25 lakh per beneficiary
(vii) Setting-up of vapor heat treatment, electronic beam processing or radiation facilities	50% of the cost subject to a ceiling of Rs 25 lakh per beneficiary
(viii) Assistance for setting-up of environment control system	25% of the cost subject to a ceiling of Rs 25 lakh per beneficiary
(ix) Setting-up of specialized storage facilities	25% of the cost subject to a ceiling of Rs 10 lakh per beneficiary

3. Schemes for Quality Development

(i) Assistance to exporters, producers, trade associations, public institutions, etc. for setting, up/strengthening laboratories	50% of the cost subject to a ceiling of Rs 5 lakh per beneficiary
(ii) Assistance to exporters and producers for installing quality management, quality assurance and quality control system	50% of the cost subject to a ceiling of Rs 2 lakh per beneficiary for each system
(iii) Activities related to standardization and quality control	100% internal scheme of APEDA
(iv) Upgradation and reorganization of labs for export testing	For upgradation up to 50% of cost for private labs and up to 100% of the cost for central/state govt. and university laboratories to a maximum of 50 lakhs
(v) a. Samples which involve testing for pesticide and heavy metals	50% of cost of or Rs 5,000 per sample whichever is lower
b. Samples which involve testing for antibiotics, hormones, etc.	50% of cost of or Rs 10,000 per sample whichever is lower

Organizational building and HRD

(i) Assistance for up gradation of technical and managerial personnel	(i) 50% of the cost for approved training programme subject to Rs 50,000 per beneficiary (ii) 100% of organized by APEDA

(ii)	Assistance for organizing seminars/group activities including study tour within the country	50% of the cost of seminar workshop, etc. subject to a ceiling of Rs 1 lakh for national seminar and Rs 2 lakh for international seminars.
(iii)	Seminars organized by APEDA	100% if organized by APEDA
(iv)	Assistance programme for study tour sponsored or organized by APEDA abroad	50% of the total cost of travel and distribution of study material

4. *Scheme for Research and Development*

(i)	Assistance to support research development for export efforts trough R&D organizations in govt sector	100% APEDA's internal scheme
(ii)	Assistance to support relevant research and development for export enhancement trough R&D organizations in co-operative/ private sector	Up to 50% of the total cost of the project subject to a ceiling of Rs 10 lakhs

SYNERGY FOR INTEGRATED DEVELOPMENT

The efforts of the **central government and its allied agencies** will have synergistic impact when it has the co-operation of: **(a) State Governments, (b) Mandi Parishads, (c) Farmer's/Grower's Associations** and **(d) Private Companies**. Some of the examples discussed below will showcase the integrated efforts required at a larger level.

Example of State Government's Efforts

Karnataka enjoys a prominent position on the horticulture map of India. Horticulture has become an important land-based activity in the state during the last two decades. It is perhaps the only state in India, which has a minister for horticulture. At present, the area under horticulture crops in Karnataka is about 17.9 lakh ha, with annual production of about 128 lakh tonnes.

S. No.	Crops	Area (in lakh ha)	Production (in lakh tonnes)
1.	Fruits	3.15	54.50
2.	Vegetables	2.59	54.56
3.	Plantations (spices and coconuts)	11.24	26.00
4.	Flowers	0.21	1.24
	Total	**17.19**	**128.00**

Thrust Areas

1. Production and distribution of quality planting materials including tissue culture.
2. Disseminating advanced horticultural technology.
3. Organizing credit support to growers to grow more horticultural crops.
4. Organizing marketing, processing and export facilities for horticulture produce.

Example of Mandi Parishad's Efforts

Uttar Pradesh Krishi Utpadan Mandi Adhiniyam was enacted in 1964 to regulate and organize the marketing of agriculture produce with an objective to provide a level playing field for the traders and fair remunerative price to the farmers along with availability of quality produce to the consumers. Mandi Parishad's assets and reserves are Rs 42.87 crores and Rs 159.84 crores, respectively. The Mandi Parishad has embarked upon a modernization drive with prime thrust on horticultural development. Some of the steps planned are:

- Computerization and networking of mandis, divisional offices and headquarter by the year 2007.
- To provide quality agri-inputs to farmers, Krishak Sewa Kendras have been established in 4 mandis on a pilot basis.
- Proposal for commissioning of specialized mandis like a modern fruit and vegetable market in Lucknow (Apna Bazar) and flower auction centre at Noida.
- Establishment of cold chain systems.

Example of Farmer/Grower Association's Efforts

South India Floriculture Association was formed in 1995 as Cut Flowers Growers Association and it started with 20 hectares by 7 members. Today it represents over 38 growers comprising an area of over 150 ha. It has established export markets in Europe, Japan, Australia, Singapore, Middle-east, New Zealand and Malaysia.

Achievements

1. Instrumental in establishment of cold storage facilities by APEDA at Bangalore airport.
2. Establishment of adequate and reliable air fright transport facilities.
3. Partnered with APEDA and government of Karnataka in setting-up of International Flower Auction, Bangalore (IFAB) of International standards.

Example of Private Company's Efforts

In this we take the example of a German company to be treated as a role model for Indian companies of how investment in horticulture can benefit them as well as bring sustainable development in the rural areas. NBV UGA is German's leading sales organization for cut flowers, potted plants, fruits and vegetables (Fig. 7.1).

The total turnover in 2001 amounted to over 602 million Euros. More than 3000 German, European and International growers supply the NBV UGA and

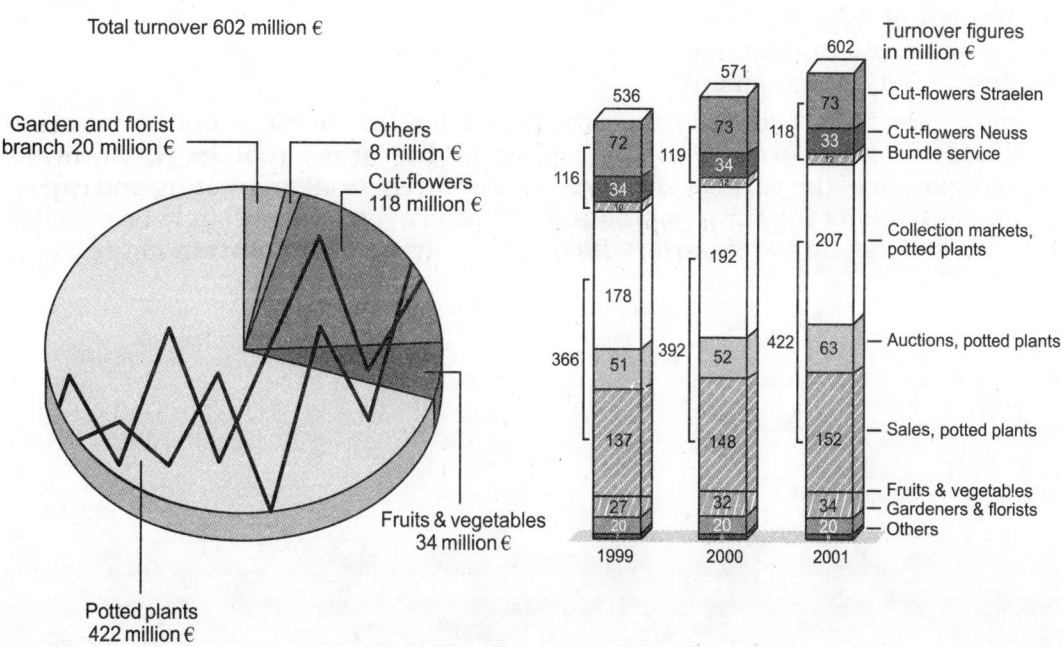

Fig. 7.1: A German company's effort

guarantee a comprehensive offer of flowers, plants, fruits and vegetables to the auctions, the mediation services, and to the sales and collection markets. Its customers include more than 25000 wholesalers and retailers. NBV UGA has over 1200 employees.

UNDP'S ENTREPRENEURIAL PROMOTION INITIATIVES IN UTTARANCHAL

UNDP is the UN's largest source of grant assistance for development. UNDP assists governments and civil society organizations in developing economic and social policies to address the causes of poverty. *It works for the full realization of the right to development—a paradigm that places people at the centre of all development activities* (Source: www.undp.org.in). The thrust of UNDP interventions in the state is aimed sustainable human development; on all critical issues in areas such as employment in the small scale and informal sector, women in agriculture, technology for urban renewal and community development. UNDP support programmes are aimed at capacity development for strengthening decentralisation, sustainable livelihoods, empowerment of women, and the safeguarding and regeneration of natural resources. Some of its entrepreneurial promotion initiatives in Uttaranchal are:

1. Setting-up of cane and bamboo technology centre
2. Sector based interventions in village and small industries—Khadi and Village Industries Commission (KVIC)
3. Mission for application of technology in urban renewal and engineering (MATURE)
4. Women in agriculture
5. Small grants programme
6. Community development

Agripreneurship promises a bright future for the development of the rural sector and empowerment of the people at the grass root level. However, dissemination of the various schemes for entrepreneurial, marketing and export promotion among the rural population will be crucial. This will only be possible by such synergistic endeavours, which can catalyze the **Revolution** in the truest sense.

8

Strategies for Entrepreneurship: Poultry Farming

Simmi Tomar, K Dhama, M Mahendran, JM Kataria

The Indian poultry sector, in the recent past, has become a major contributor to the national economy largely due to the revolutionary and scientific approaches in avian health care management and superior breeding policies, giving rise to promising and highly profitable poultry enterprise. Today, India ranks globally at 4th and 5th in egg and meat production, respectively. Being one of the most vibrant, dynamic and ever expanding sectors with tremendous potential, there is wide scope for its exploitation in the country. Even though there is significant upsurge in the commercialized poultry sector, the involvement of small-scale farmers residing in the rural areas has not improved as desired. About 70% of the total population resides in rural areas which is vast and at present, the poultry production is more concentrated around urban and periurban areas. For full utilization of the potential that the poultry sector bears, there should be strong, concordant and sincere efforts from the part of administration, veterinarians and scientific community so as to enable the rural people, especially the youth and women, to indulge in economic poultry rearing. A drive towards creating an awareness of the benefits of poultry rearing can help in alleviating the unemployment problems due to population explosion, malnutrition and financial insecurity which are all common to a rural society. Also the energy of unemployed youth in the rural villages could be directed in the right perspectives by adapting poultry farming as a useful source of income. Women can also play a major role in improving basic health care of backyard poultry that does not require much manpower. Poultry farming can be a very important occupation for majority of the landless families and suitable measures adapted to upgrade the backyard poultry and promote small to medium scale poultry farming would provide a good source of self-employment and livelihood security and in the long run have the potential to drastically transform the economy of the rural India.

Even though poultry rearing brings in good returns, lack of proper and scientific poultry management can cause significant losses, the major culprits being infectious diseases that prompt the farmers, who are not well supported by the knowledge regarding immunoprophylaxis, disease monitoring, biosecurity and hygienic practices, to restrain from poultry farming. The advancement in the field of science and technology has made it possible to identify and control the disease causing agents at the earliest and thereby preventing serious losses. Before jumping into the poultry farming business, care should be taken to educate the rural people about the prerequisites of poultry farming and disease prevention strategies to achieve better productivity and economic returns. In this context, the utilization of advanced techniques and facilities should be made available to the rural poultry farmers by the government through agencies involved in disease diagnosis and management, which will instill in them the much needed confidence to undertake poultry farming as an economically viable livelihood.

ADVANTAGES OF ADOPTING POULTRY FARMING

Among the several developmental schemes adopted in the livestock sector, poultry rearing has shown to have the highest growth rate with backyard poultry farming getting slowly transformed into commercial poultry units. The importance of the choice of poultry farming as successful and economically viable solution for alleviating poverty and unemployment in rural areas arises from the fact that it can bring in good profit through poultry products which are in great demand in the country such as India where the per capita consumption of meat and egg is far below the required standards. The per capita consumption of eggs in the country is only 36 eggs and poultry meat is 850 grams against a recommended consumption of 180 eggs and 10.8 kg poultry meat per person per annum by the Nutritional Advisory Committee (NAC) (Table 8.1). So there is wide scope to meet out this nutritional requirement through upgrading poultry farming. The urban people consume about two-thirds (65–70%) of the total eggs and poultry meat, though the urban areas have only 30% human population. While, the rural people consume only 7 eggs/head/year, and there is also insignificant consumption of poultry meat by the villagers, though the rural areas have 70% human population in the country. Total meat production in India is 6.5 million tons, and poultry has 3rd rank in total meat production with nearly 25% contribution. Broiler meat contributes nearly 70% of total poultry meat production, the rest 30% is derived from culled layers/breeding stock, cockerels and desi fowl, so presently the desi fowl is contributing very less towards the meat production. Also, the rural poultry production contributes only 20% of total egg production, which should be increased as per the demand and the tremendous potential and the huge exploitable scope of the rural

Table 8.1: The amount of nutrients provided by 100 g of poultry meat, eggs and other selected foods

Food item	Energy (k cal)	Protein (g)	Calcium (mg)	Iron (mg)	Vitamin A (μg)
Egg (fresh)	158	12.1	56	2.1	156
Poultry meat	139	19.0	15	1.5	0
Maize	353	9.3	10	2.5	0
Rice	361	6.5	4	0.5	0
Sorghum	345	10.7	26	4.5	0
Plantain	135	1.2	8	1.3	390

(*Source:* FAO)

poultry farming. Chickens in traditional village poultry systems provide good and cheap source of animal protein in the form of meat and eggs. The value-added products based on poultry meat and eggs are gaining much popularity among the urban consumers, which is another potential source of additional profit for the rural poultry farmers. Apart from this, by-products such as poultry manure can be used as an effective fertilizer in agro-farming, which adds to the profitability of poultry farming. The poultry sector requires minimal investment and starts giving results in a very short time period. Rural poultry production is recognized as a major generator of livelihood security in rural regions of most of the developing countries as they are considered as livestock that can be owned by very poor households with limited land resources. Thus the potential for growth of the sector is huge particularly in rural India, where 70% of the people reside. Government reports clearly show that the poultry sector has the potential to grow at 20% per annum over the next 10 years. Poultry, in fact, has registered the maximum growth rate among all the sectors of agriculture, the annual contribution of the poultry sector to the Gross National Product being Rs 7,810 crores.

THE RURAL POULTRY PRODUCTION SCENARIO

Poultry is generally managed in a backyard system of rearing by the village people. Village chickens are often essential elements of poor households because of their low labour and investment requirements. Although the output of traditional village chickens is low due to chick mortality, reduced weight gain and less number of eggs per hen per year, it is obtained with minimal input in terms of housing, disease control, management and supplementary feeding. The backyard poultry rearing in rural areas is particularly based on scavenging, feeding of grains (wheat and barley) or giving household refuses. This adds to the profitability as the majority of the cost involved in poultry rearing is due to the feed, which may account for 60% of the total cost incurred as in case of commercial poultry units. Any cost-effective strategy that increases the productivity of these birds can, therefore, assist in poverty alleviation and the improvement of food security (Table 8.2).

Table 8.2: Features of rural poultry production

Breed and flock size	Local indigenous type, <50 birds.
Housing	Specific poultry houses are rarely built.
Feed resource	Scavenging, feeding with home grains, household refuses.
Health programme	No regular health programmes/disease control measures in place.
Markets	Marketing channels or links are weak.
Infrastructure	Underdeveloped infrastructure.
Product storage and processing	No refrigeration, the sales of live birds and eggs are only means.
Technology/information	Local knowledge, with moderate or no extension services.

Supported by several developmental schemes of the government, the rural farmers are attempting to adopt the poultry farming as a business by starting rearing 500-2000 chicks or even on larger scale, but the lack of the proper knowledge on poultry nutrition, diseases and their management along with improper support of professionals especially the poultry health care specialists has many a times forced the farmer to leave this profitable business. The potentials, major constraints and possible solutions for improved poultry health care, management and production have to be identified in advance. In conjunction to promoting the backyard poultry farming, appropriate strategies need to be implemented to encourage the rural people of the country to develop entrepreneurship via adopting poultry rearing in the form of small to medium or even large scale poultry farms or enterprises. Given the integrated nature of most farming systems, a holistic interdisciplinary approach should be followed to promote the rural poultry production in a profitable manner.

STRATEGIES FOR PROMOTING SUCCESSFUL POULTRY FARMING IN RURAL AREAS

Successful poultry farming requires a good knowledge of poultry husbandry practices, viz. good management principles and procedures, awareness of the nutritional requirements of the birds, biosecurity, immunoprophylaxis, disease monitoring, and hygienic and disinfection principles. Poultry farmers should also be acquainted with the economic poultry feed resources, they should be oriented and encouraged through education and training programmes, interactive health camps, promotional subsidies and professional interactions. There should be a drive to strengthen the veterinary services, diagnostic facilities, disease surveillance and monitoring programmes, research and diagnostic activities (scientific and technological advancements), feed availability and the marketing facilities. Poultry diseases, the major concern in the backyard system of rearing and adapting the rural poultry farming as an enterprises/business, can be avoided to some extent by knowing their causes, clinical signs and lesions, modes of transmission, detection, prevention and control measures. At present the poultry farming in rural areas is confined to marginal farmers who are not well versed with the basic knowledge of poultry farming. Therefore, care should be taken that the rural people get familiarize with the prerequisites of poultry farming, before venturing into this profitable business, to achieve better productivity and economic returns. For farmers, to gain confidence in poultry rearing and mass popularization of poultry business, it is therefore essential to provide them the sound knowledge of poultry husbandry and the needful poultry health care and management support through well planned training and extension programmes.

MANAGEMENT PRINCIPLES FOR RURAL POULTRY FARMING

The incidence of diseases in indigenous flocks depends upon the management practices, prevailing environment, nutritional status and health coverage followed by the farmers. The real problem starts at the beginning of brooding or rearing of poultry, where the issues of disease morbidity and mortality in chicks and sanitation and hygiene are the universal problems in rural area, and which get aggravated by unawareness towards the basic principles of poultry farming.

Appropriate and systematic management practices should be followed to reduce the disease incidences in poultry and subsequently the economic losses. Successful management of poultry diseases is the most important factor that determines the economic returns from this industry. The health cover programmes should be implemented and well planned in advance and executed in time without allowing an alarming situation to arise for this purpose. Useful tips for rural poultry farmers include the awareness about the following disease management practices.

Poultry House Management

Proper environment is a necessity for healthy living of the flocks. The farmers should adopt indigenous and traditional farm management principles depending upon the resources available at their disposal, for the successful rearing of poultry. The poultry houses should have sufficient space to accommodate the birds with proper ventilation and clean water facilities. This helps in reducing the environmental stress to the poultry. There should also be an efficient drainage system. Location of the poultry house must be appropriate with respect to other poultry production area, road facilities and direction of farm. Practice all in all out (one age group per farm) breeding management.

Source of Chicks

Follow business with suppliers who practise good biosecurity standards. For staring a poultry farm, the rural farmers should take chicks or other poultry from reputed hatchery or disease free certified sources. Indigenous or improved indigenous poultry flocks with better immunocompetency and suitablility of survival should be reared. It has been observed that the indigenous birds face maximum casualties during early stage of life. Therefore, for layer poultry farming, it is advisable to rear the chicks in a nursery following complete vaccination programme, before releasing to the rural farmers as it is difficult to vaccinate all the rural birds under village conditions.

Nutrition

Vitamins and mineral supplements are to be provided to the birds to avoid deficiency diseases and to make them immunologically competent. Availability of economic poultry feed resources should be known.

Hygiene and Disinfection

The poultry houses, feed and water troughs, etc. should be cleaned regularly to check the disease spread. Prompt removal and proper disposal of dead birds and contaminated materials by incineration or burial methods should be followed so that they are not approached by the scavenging animals and birds. This can check the spread of diseases.

Diagnosis, Prophylaxis and Treatment

The flocks should be tested regularly for important poultry diseases and should be exposed to regular vaccination programmes. With the present disease scenario in indigenous poultry flocks, the birds should be protected against economically important diseases like MD, ND, IBD, fowl pox, etc. Routine treatment should be provided against bacterial infections and parasitic diseases. If needed, antibiotic susceptibility should be evaluated in case of bacterial diseases so as to avoid the development of drug-resistance bacteria and prevent the economical losses timely.

Biosecurity: The First Line of Defense

Biosecurity refers to the methods adopted to secure a disease free environment by preventing the exposure of the birds/flock to transmissible infectious diseases, parasites, and pests. It is a term that embodies all of the measures that should be taken to prevent viruses, bacteria, fungi, protozoa, parasites, insects, rodents, and wild birds from entering or surviving and infecting or endangering the well-being of the poultry flock. The rural environment is a vast reservoir of infectious agents, which have easy access to birds. A disease is the outcome of the interaction between the host (bird), environment and pathogens and this has to be interrupted to check the influx of the pathogen and the disease in a flock. In rural conditions, the birds are mostly maintained as semi-intensive or scavenging backyard flocks and kept in sheds during night. Hence the birds are exposed to disease causing agents that may quickly spread among the entire flocks in the area. Moreover, the improved varieties of chicken from urban areas, which are highly sensitive to diseases, often remain as the carriers of different emerging diseases and have been found to be a potential source of transmitting different diseases in indigenous flocks. The biosecurity practices may help the researchers and local veterinarians to control, contain and eradicate certain diseases from the country, which may help improve trade of poultry products.

Key Principles of Biosecurity

Isolation

It is the confinement of birds within a controlled environment. A properly built fence keeps the poultry flocks in and all other free flying or wild birds out. Mechanical transmission of disease agents by carriers can thus be prevented. Care should be taken to avoid introduction of birds of unknown disease status into the flock and institute a suitable vector control programme.

Traffic Control

Disease spread between poultry premises almost always follows the movement of contaminated material, people and equipments. Separate the personnels working in infected sheds and healthy sheds. Limit the entry of visitors and restrict their direct contact with the flock. Control the human traffic judiciously. Fences and barriers are very effective ways to direct on-farm traffic and the traffic on to the farm.

Sanitation

It addresses the disinfection of materials and equipments entering or going out of the farm and the cleanliness of the farm and the personnel hygiene. A clean sanitized environment is a good insurance against disease outbreak and hence, a high standard of hygiene is required in the poultry farms. Plan periodic clean out, clean up and disinfection of houses and equipment thus limiting the spread of disease causing organisms. Add sanitizer in the drinking water provided to the flocks.

DISEASE PREVENTION AND CONTROL PROGRAMMES

Infectious diseases of poultry, responsible for causing huge losses, are considered to be the most important factor that impedes the development of rural poultry enterprises. Outbreaks of infectious diseases like Newcastle disease (ND), infectious bursal disease (IBD), litchi heart disease, egg drop syndrome (EDS), salmonellosis, colibacillosis, coccidiosis, etc. can lead to huge losses due to high mortality, reduced production performances and carcass condemnation. The velogenic form of Newcastle disease (Ranikhet disease) virus (NDV) frequently destroys most of the rural poultry flocks. Litchi heart disease caused by inclusion body hepatitis (IBH) virus has already been identified a cause of 'spiking mortality' in broiler flocks. Other economically important diseases include fowl pox, infectious bronchitis (IB), Marek's disease (MD), avian reovirus (ARV) manifestations, chicken infectious anaemia (CIA), egg drop syndrome-76, colisepticaemia, fowl cholera, infectious coryza, chronic respiratory disease (CRD) (mycoplasmosis) and aspergillosis. Mycotoxicosis caused by mycotoxins like aflatoxins present in mouldy feed also have serious detrimental effects on health and productivity of birds. IBD, CIA, ARV, MD, litchi heart disease and aflatoxicosis are the important immunosuppressive diseases, which predisposes poultry flocks to secondary infections leading to huge economic losses. Parasitic and nutritional deficiency diseases also plays role in decreased production output under the rural environment due to the lack of proper sanitation and hygiene practices and the balanced nutrition. Indigenous poultry flocks reared in free-range system are always susceptible to these diseases. These economically important diseases as well as diseases of zoonotic implications such as bird flu are spelling doom over the poultry keepers and discouraging them to undertake poultry farming as a successful enterprise. The economic loss as a result of poultry diseases is more important from the perspective of a landless rural poultry farmer and mortality of birds, especially in poor rural families, and can even lead to economic catastrophe that may exaggerate the socio-economic impact of poultry diseases.

For the effective control of the common viral diseases of poultry, it is essential to follow strict immunoprophylactic measures to prevent the occurrence of these diseases. Diseases such as ND, MD, IBD, EDS, fowl pox, etc. can be effectively controlled by vaccines procured from public or private sector biologicals. These diseases, which are the major constraint as far as the rural poultry producers are concerned, should be given priority at all stages. Strategic measures should be implemented for developing sustainable community-based ND control programmes with due importance. There is a need for more coordinated research on the most appropriate and cost-effective vaccine for controlling ND in rural poultry. The recent development and use of thermostable vaccine (ND-V4) in many developing countries has created fresh interest for the control of ND. The V4 vaccine is more cost-effective where oral administration can be used and this vaccine could be a future breakthrough for ND vaccination in village chickens. The thermostable vaccine can be used along with pelleted feed or coated on suitable food grains which can help to control diseases in birds. In the current scenario of various IBD virus strains circulating in the field and different vaccination practices being followed, particularly after the emergence of very virulent (vv)-IBDV in the country, a judicious vaccination programme for the prevention and control of this highly immunosuppressive disease is to be planned out. The indiscriminate use of hot vaccines (intermediate plus strains for vv-IBD virus) should be discouraged and they should be practiced only in those regions where vv-IBDV is a major problem. Regular monitoring of vaccinal responses including maternal antibody evaluation for IBDV is suggested, which is the need of the hour for designing judicious immunoprophylaxis strategies for IBD. Incidences of vertically transmitted diseases such as EDS-76, CIA, salmonellosis, mycoplasmosis, etc. can be minimized by procuring healthy chicks from certified hatcheries. When compared to the viral diseases, bacterial diseases including colibacillosis, salmonellosis, fowl cholera, fowl coryza, CRD, etc. can be prevented by good management practices as well as timely treatment with specific antibiotics. Many anti-coccidial agents are available that can be added in feed so as to prevent the incidence of coccidiosis, a protozoal disease which is responsible for high flock mortality resulting in severe economic loss. Anti-fungal agents are also available for treating and controlling the fungal diseases in poultry. Feed additives such as probiotics help in reducing the losses due to few of the infectious diseases. Nutritional deficiency diseases can be minimized to a great extent by providing balanced formulations supported with necessary mineral and vitamin supplements to the birds. Parasitic diseases can be avoided by following a regular prescribed de-worming schedule during poultry rearing.

The development of effective poultry health care and disease management programme requires reliable information on the epidemiology of diseases, which is lacking in village chicken production systems. Epidemiological studies in rural areas should be undertaken to understand the host-pathogen-environment interactions. Results from such studies could be used in developing suitable vaccination programmes, as well as selecting the most cost-effective vaccines. Disease surveillance is further limited by poor infrastructure, communication and networking, as well as inadequate diagnostic facilities. These limitations have resulted in under-reporting of disease outbreaks, as observed for ND and other diseases in many places of the country. At the village level, contacts between flocks of different households are the main sources of infection transmission. Similarly, other domestic fowls and wild birds form another source of infection, because the chickens roam freely in the villages. Apart from this, the people who are following poultry farming in the rural areas are not usually practicing the basic principles of biosecurity, sanitation, hygiene and disease management, which make their flock easily susceptible to various diseases, leading to the economic assault and finally they get discouraged and leave the poultry business.

Describing the epidemiology and economics of village poultry production, suggests the need to develop appropriate epidemiological techniques for rural poultry, because of the nature of the host-pathogen-environment interaction specifically in these areas. During disease outbreaks, it is essential to carry out early diagnosis and follow appropriate therapeutic (medication and treatment) measures along with proper disposal of carcass, good sanitation, hygiene and biosecurity practices. If necessary, suitable prophylactic measures should be followed immediately.

STRENGTHENING OF EXTENSION ACTIVITIES

Relevant information on poultry health care, nutrition and management, if appropriately delivered, will help the rural poultry owners to effectively prevent the diseases affecting their birds and follow suitable primary treatment measures. This has a direct and important bearing on the success involved in poultry rearing. Extension programmes should be encouraged and supported in national institutions, universities, non-government organizations, krishi vigyan kendras, etc. for promoting poultry rearing as a livelihood for rural people. More centres should be established by the animal husbandry departments for promotion of poultry production as a valuable alternative source of income and employment. It is the responsibility of the extension volunteers to infuse courage and confidence among the rural people. The important issues and know-how related to the poultry health care and management could be effectively disseminated by the extension worker keeping in mind the following strategies.

Education and Training

Community participation in disease control programmes is a key factor which is crucial for the development of sustainable and fruitful results. Farmer's education and training using extension messages through the media, i.e. television, radio, newspapers, posters, leaflets, etc. should be part of rural poultry upgradation programmes. Farmers participation should be encouraged in conferences, seminars, workshops, exhibitions, orientation programmes, etc. for inculcating good poultry rearing practices in them. Poverty, ignorance and illiteracy among the rural backyard poultry rearers and those adopting poultry farming as a business or a source of earning are the main hurdles in delivering the extension services. By designing appropriate knowledge dissemination methods, the relevant information on poultry health could be transferred from "knowledge centres" to the farmers. The poultry producers in rural areas should be given enough know-how regarding various aspects of poultry husbandry viz. poultry production and health care management; rearing and feeding practices, balanced feed formulations; knowledge of important diseases, their early detection, prevention and control measures (biosecurity, hygiene and disinfection, vaccination schedule and treatment practices); knowledge of major cross and desi breeds of poultry and their suitability to the agro-climatic conditions of the respective regions, etc. through organizing short-term training programmes with the help of information centres and research and development (R&D) organizations such as the Indian Veterinary Research Institute, Central Avian

Research Institute, Izatnagar (UP), Poultry Breeding Farm, Hessarghata, Bangalore, Project Directorate on Poultry, Hyderabad, agricultural universities/ veterinary colleges, poultry development schemes/corporations under the state animal husbandry departments, and private organizations. Through this attempt of imparting training, a profound knowledge on poultry farming would be passed on to the farmers via poultry management and health care experts so that the losses incurred due to unscientific rearing practices can be minimized.

Mass Popularization

Information and Communication Technologies

Use of electronic and print media (radio, television, newspapers, leaflets, manuals, books, internet, etc.) should be exploited appropriately to popularize and educate the rural masses about the good farm practices. Mass communication needs improvement by publishing more literature, popular articles, books, periodicals, journals, producing documentaries and launching websites on the advantages of poultry farming in creating self-employment and entrepreneurship development. Advances in information and communication technologies (ICTs) should be utilized to educate the rural farmers in an efficient way and at a mass scale. Computer based information and communication technologies is seen as a giant leap forward in people's ability to access the information they need, particularly where internet access is available. This could include improving existing extension services through the use of IT tools, opening new communication channels by which updated information can reach farmers about advances in poultry farm practices and the services provided by the authorities. There is a tremendous scope of ICTs application in rural areas, which can reduce the globe into a village thus addressing the issue of marginalization, and promoting mass education regarding successful poultry farming. It can help improve the economic status directly through e-commerce applications and indirectly through access to varied kind of poultry business information. Internet can empower people by inducing transparency and accountability in the system and also building a smooth interface with the Government. It is important to emphasize that the ICT solutions should be sensitive to the rural characteristics. The applications should be designed in such a way that it speaks the rural poor's language, reflect their culture and above all should address their needs and requirements.

Databases

Searchable databases with salient information for various diseases and their control, biosecurity principles, economic feed formulations and resources, poultry rearing and management with user-friendly interfaces, etc. are convenient ways in mass popularizing and promoting the poultry enterprise among the rural people. User friendly softwares, citing the disease and control methods with graphics and animations, audio delivery of information and choice of language should be designed to minimize the labour involved in extension activities. Establishment of poultry health and production information databases at district level will be a highly useful tool to the rural poultry producers of a particular region. For this purpose, reliable databases need to be established through regular disease surveillance programmes for the poultry disease occurrences (epidemiology) control of endemic, epidemic, emerging, re-emerging, economically important and transboundary diseases through the systems analysis approach so as to impart confidence to the rural poultry farmers. If possible, a disease forecasting system based on epidemiological/disease prevalence data may be evolved keeping in view the agro-climatic conditions and disease scenario in the area, which can help in planning efficient disease prevention and control strategies well in advance and thereby infusing in them enough confidence to adopt poultry farming. Data-bases can also be developed reflecting the economic returns of poultry business so that rural people can be encouraged for adopting poultry farming as a successful business enterprise.

Veterinary Health Services

Disease Surveillance and Monitoring

Poultry consultancy, disease diagnostic facilities and routine health coverage need to be strengthened and made available to the rural farmers. Complete veterinary cover should be provided to the poultry farmers. Testing of poultry flocks should be done regularly for the commonly occurring diseases like ND, IBD, MD, salmonellosis, mycoplasmosis, etc. using suitable diagnostic kits, at the farmer's door steps. Regular surveillance and monitoring of diseases in rural poultry flocks and routine health coverage could help achieve sustainability in rural poultry production with assured success. Scientific and technological advancements in the field of poultry disease diagnosis and control make feasible the early and confirmatory diagnosis of the disease causative agent and thus helps in timely planning and execution of suitable prevention and control strategies. These methodologies and facilities should be utilized widely for the beneficiaries, which will instill confidence in rural farmers to undertake poultry farming as a successful business.

Vaccination Campaign

Intensive vaccination programmes should be implemented for the prevention of economically important viral diseases and efforts need attention for the creation of disease free zones, for the eradication of deadly disease like Newcastle disease (ND) as has been achieved in the case of Rinderpest (RP) in animals. These practices may help the researchers and local veterinarians to control, contain and eradicate important diseases from the country, which may help the export of poultry products. The researchers may try to develop thermostable live vaccines against infectious avian diseases which can be useful in controlling diseases in rural areas with adverse environment and lack of facilities to maintain cold chain. There is need to develop combined vaccine and pelleted feed based vaccine for ease of administration. Facilities should be generated for maintaining the cold-chain for vaccine storage in rural areas.

Health Camps

Interactive health camps should be organized in order to make the rural people aware of the importance of personal hygiene and prevention of avian diseases that are transmissible to man, i.e. of zoonotic importance. For consumer awareness, the nutritional benefits of consuming poultry eggs, meat and value added products should be highlighted. Efforts should be made to remove some misconceptions about egg, viz. egg being considered a non-vegetarian food, produces more body heat on consumption, desi eggs are more nutritious than farm eggs and the cholesterol related health issues. Confidence need to be inspired in poultry farmers by providing a backbone of basic facilities and needful support.

Balanced Feed and Nutrition

Enhancement of feed production units and knowledge of common and locally available and cheap feed resources for meeting the nutritional requirements of the poultry flocks is essential for successful and profitable poultry rearing in rural areas. Balanced feed supplemented with vitamins and minerals should be ensured. Feed resources are a major input in poultry production systems, estimated to account for about 60% of total production cost in commercial poultry sector. So the backyard poultry is the alternative, which can strive on scavenging, kitchen wastes and local flora and fauna. But these flocks are affected with nutritional disorders and deficiency diseases very often. So partial supplementation of compound feed to eliminate the deficiencies and provide a balanced nutrition will give desired results.

Diversified Poultry Production System

Diversification involving rearing of bird species other than chicken, such as turkey, quail, guinea fowl and duck, has the potential to provide solution to meet national and international challenge in food production, nutritional security, employment generation and alleviation of poverty. Diversification should be promoted due to increase in demand of poultry and poultry products in world market, consumers always looking for products with a change. There is increase in the human population and changes in their lifestyles, with more people becoming non-vegetarian. Modernization, with the establishment of large number of fast food restaurants such as McDonald's, Pizza Huts, etc. are mostly poultry meat based in our country. This adds to the importance of endeavouring prospects in diversified poultry production.

Development of Marketing Facilities and Value-added Poultry Products

Rural poultry farmers should be guided in finding the market for their products. Strengthening of marketing and transportation facilities for poultry and its products needs a special attention. Cold storage facilities for poultry products in rural areas should be established. Assistance with feeding, housing and disease control measures between different marketing points is also needed. Marketing requires institutional and organizational support with intensification approaches to make the egg and poultry or its products locally available. Setting up of more number of small poultry processing units should be encouraged to cater the consumer's preference for value added products at an affordable price. Market surveys should be conducted to assess consumer's demand and preference for poultry products. Efficient and attractive packaging, competitive pricing, reliable service, strict quality assurance measures and widened retail outlets in rural and urban areas are needed. These approaches can very efficiently promote the consumption of poultry and its products in the country and also could help in increasing the export potential of the country for these commodities.

Interactions and Networking

The poultry health scientists, veterinarians, extension personnel, policy makers, officials and administrators should interact regularly with the farmers in rural areas on the essential farm practices and viability of possible modifications that should be implemented to address the proper survival of flocks with the optimum use of available resources. Feedbacks of the rural farmers should be taken up on priority for making improvements. Networking should be encouraged in village chicken production. There is a need for more national support to the existing network for rural poultry development programmes and understanding the socio-economic problems of the farmers. Closer and dynamic linkages with research and development (R&D) institutions for technical know-how and training support for rural people should be made. The network should endeavour to identify key or priority problems, the solution of which would benefit the rural farmers. Linkages with the nearby city/town's fast food outlets, restaurants, hotels and other institutional and retail markets should be boosted in rural areas.

Encouraging Women in Rural Poultry Production

It is a known fact that till recent years, man has been the sole bread winner in the family and women were known for their culinary skills and house keeping. But for the past few decades or so considerable advancement and parity in the field of education has given the impetus for gender equality. This scenario has made possible for the feminine gender to become more confident and to undertake challenges that were once forbidden. This change has been reflected more in urban societies when compared to rural population which is still lagging behind far and are unable to recognize the importance of utilization of 'women power' to generate additional income and stability to the family. On this pretext, the aim should be to find out suitable ways and means for the rural women to provide monetary support to her family. The poultry rearing as a backyard system has proved easier for women to manage successfully by themselves. This can be an excellent source of income that can contribute much to the income of the family and requires less time and energy expenditure, which will be suited for women. Apart from her day to day household works, this will create an opportunity to use her time and energy sagaciously. As the backyard poultry rearing systems do not require much infrastructural facilities and the capital required is less when compared to other small scale enterprises, it could be seen as a viable source for generating additional income in rural families. A flock of 50-100 birds in a rearing system will give enough supportive income to the family. The problem of undernourishment basically seen in rural population will be answered, as the poultry is an excellent and cheap source of animal protein.

Several assumptions are made about the involvement of women in rural poultry projects: helping women to increase rural poultry production, increases women's income and thus empowering them; an increase in food production as a result of increased rural poultry production increases equitable distribution of food in the household; village chickens are easily managed within homesteads, and are therefore appropriate development projects for women; women are more resourceful in managing village chickens, and therefore their involvement in development programmes increases production efficiency. Through the instruments of self-help groups and village development committees initiated by local NGOs, a large number of women drawn from the backward communities have been able to find more respectability both within household and in the community, with increased access to financial resources. Interface with the outside world has brought about a significant enhancement in the awareness and confidence levels of the womenfolk in many areas, and a large number of women are now engaged in livelihood activities. Women can play a good role in improving basic health care of birds, if only they are properly trained for the purpose. The enhancement of knowledge and work force among women can help to a great extent cherish our envisaged dreams of becoming a 'truly developed' nation.

Research and Development (R&D) Strategies

In order to make an impact through rural poultry as an income generating activity, research and development efforts are required to develop suitable genotypes and to provide appropriate low cost health cover for sustaining their production potential. Integrated and coordinated approach should be made for promoting scientific outlook and research on poultry production and performances. Efforts must be made to upgrade poultry breeds. Special disease resistance breeds and breeds suitable to different agro-climatic conditions of the country should be developed and improved genetically, so that this valuable source of income remains available to the farmer, especially the small and marginal farmers. Effective strategies for eradication of fatal diseases like Newcastle disease and other economically important diseases should be devised. Combined vaccines, pelleted vaccines and *in-ovo* vaccination methods should be devised to avoid stress, labour and cost. Designer eggs utilizing modern scientific advances for producing cholesterolless eggs and other similar poultry products favouring better health needs promotion. Utilization of poultry eggs as transmission vehicles for immunogens need to be explored, which when administered to humans, especially children, could render them immune to a particular disease. Special funds should be provided to encourage both public and private sector research institutions to undertake result-oriented and time-bound projects for promoting poultry farming. Feeding of unconventional feed resources that have been tested on a small scale should be developed further to increase the scavenging feed resource base. Appropriate farm structures, including housing, feeders, waterers, nests and cages for transportation should be developed and strengthened. Since the poultry sector has great potential for poverty alleviation utmost importance should be given for future research in this field by establishing R&D centres in different areas.

Breed Improvement Programmes

Disease resistant breeds and breeds with good climatic tolerance are needed to improve the poultry farming in rural areas. Certain indigenous poultry breeds such as Naked Neck, Frizzle fowl and Tini are well adapted to the tropical climatic zones as they have better heat dissipation abilities. The genes of these indigenous breeds responsible for this heat tolerance ability can be introgressed into the germplasm of the meat and egg type breeds which could lead to the evolution of high performance heat resistant flocks that could well suite to the rural regions of the country. The breeding programmes should also aim to develop disease resistant varieties of poultry. Genetic strategies have already provided with breeds that are resistant to Marek's disease by selection of B^{21} allele which is responsible for the reduced susceptibility to this particular disease. As the major histo-compatibility (MHC) gene plays an important role in resistance to many diseases, the future studies should be directed to elucidate the underlying mechanism and thereby providing disease resistant breed varieties to the poultry farmers in rural areas.

Encouraging Entrepreneurship and Promoting Skills

Specific funds and subsidies should be allotted through government organizations for infrastructural facilities and promoting rural poultry farming. It should also be ensured that the rural people interested in poultry farming should get loans from banks on low interest rates and the channel for getting loans should be made easy. More awards should be instituted by the government and private organizations for researchers as well as successful poultry farmers in order to initiate, undertake and promote research and innovations in the field of utility and contribution towards poultry promotional and mobilizing activities. Small scale farmer oriented groups should be encouraged to adopt poultry farming as a successful and profitable large scale enterprise. Women and youth power should be mobilized in the right directions for adopting poultry business as a successful enterprise. Pro-poor policy is the need of hour to uplift the socio-economic conditions of the rural farmers.

For any enterprise to flourish, it needs to develop sound managerial and marketing skills in the entrepreneur. This coupled with a strong practical sense or approach is most essential in germinating a fruitful enterprise. For developing a successful poultry enterprise, whether it is small scale or large scale, it needs profound knowledge among the entrepreneurs, regarding the flock management and disease control measures. Apart from these, the major constraint and the weak link in poultry production being the marketing sector, it has also to be addressed in the right perspective. Escalating input cost due to unscientific rearing practices has virtually thrown out many from poultry business even though compared to other enterprises poultry farming requires less infrastructural facilities and capital investment. All this points to the lack of managerial and business skills, especially among the rural people. So it is high time to take this matter into account and steps should be taken to impart training for the future entrepreneurs to inculcate in them these skills in addition to the technical know-how of successful poultry rearing. The lack of these 'soft skills' if supplemented could very well establish the highly lucrative poultry business which could in the long run help the nation to surge ahead.

Development of High-tech Model Villages

As a future plan there should be strong recommendations for the development of high-tech model villages, which are self-sufficient in all aspects. This could help in improving the general living standards of the people residing in rural areas of the country.

Advantages of Promoting Poultry Farming in Rural Areas

- Provides subsidiary employment and helps alleviating unemployment and job scarcity.
- As a source of regular income provides financial security and dwindles down poverty.
- Inspires self-confidence and self-sufficiency in rural people.
- Reduces malnutrition and ensures nutritional security.
- Management does not require much manpower—ladies and children can be involved easily.
- Poultry farming needs minimal use of land and capital.
- By-products such as poultry manure have excellent value in organic agro-farming, which would fetch higher return to villagers.
- Job opportunities can be created through consultancy services.
- Overall improvement in rural economy.
- Sustained growth of poultry sector could be achieved.
- Increased poultry production will strengthen the national economy.

CONCLUSION

Poultry farming has tremendous potential, which has not been exploited to its full capability in rural areas. Rural poultry is an important element in diversifying agricultural production and increasing household food security. Chickens provide readily harvestable animal protein to rural households. Poultry, like other short-cycle animal stock, is a crucial element in the struggle for sustained food production and poverty alleviation. In India, even though, the commercial poultry production is increasing rapidly, no significant efforts have been made for developing backyard poultry and poultry farming practices for small farmers, which still contributes much towards the poultry production in the country. If effective measures are implemented to improve the production performance with minimum monetary input this can form the basis for transforming the rural poultry sector from subsistence to a more economically productive base. Pro-poor policy is needed to uplift the socio-economic conditions of the rural/ tribal farmers of the country. For them, the rearing of poultry is a viable alternative for alleviating poverty by providing self-employment opportunities and economic security. The current scenario of 'population explosion' has limited the number of job opportunities in both government and private sectors. By utilizing the prospects of successful poultry farming this problem can be sidelined to a great extent and also the energy of unemployed youth and women in the rural villages could be directed into right channels. Thus, educating and supporting the rural farmers for development of poultry enterprises can to a great extent instill in them greater economic stability. In order to encourage poultry production by rural people, emphasis is required to develop indigenous poultry flocks, which can thrive well under rural conditions having adverse environment, in small units as backyard, family and small to large scale poultry farming system. It is also essential to provide timely and appropriate low cost health cover to the rural poultry and to identify cheap and locally available feed resources for sustaining their production potential in a profitable manner. Taking stock of the situation it is the responsibility of the administration to set up plans for the future that can help improve the awareness about poultry rearing and disease prevention and control measures. This can be achieved by promotional campaigns on scientific and economic rearing of poultry with the help of mass media and by providing subsidies for infrastructure facilities. The farmers should be given enough know-how regarding the disease management aspects by rendering training programmes with the help of information centres and professional organizations so that the losses incurred due to unscientific rearing practices can be minimized. Therefore, the poultry health scientists, extension personnel, planners, policy makers and officials should interact regularly to have information on the production potential, health management requirements and other problems and feedbacks of rural poultry rearers, and execute the modification of the practice, if necessary, which may help in success and sustainability of rural poultry production.

A strong resolve towards educating the rural farmers and to transform the energy of rural youth and jobless women to help them gain financial security is the need of the hour and all efforts from the governmental organization should be properly channelized to obtain the desired results. This in turn can ingrain in them the confidence to surge ahead in the coming decade, which can drastically transform the economy of the rural India. For this, the traditional rural poultry farming practices should be supported with the backbone of a precise knowledge on poultry health care and management along with appropriate follow-up of extension policies and activities. The rural poultry farming, in country like India where 70% of the population is rural, if promoted in the positive directions through an integrated approach can have significant impact in generating small, medium to large enterprises in rural areas; help in achieving livelihood security, alleviating malnutrition, poverty and unemployment; and shall improve in the long run the socio-economic status of the rural families as well as the Indian economy and thus the sustained growth of poultry sector could also be achieved. Therefore, efforts need to be made for public awareness about the "virtues of poultry business" and its "products" by blending science, spirituality, wisdom and mass popularity so that the poultry farming should gain popularity not only in traditional rural families but also in highly educated and scientific society.

9

Piggery Enterprise: A Case Study

R Prasad, C Singh, RA Rawat

In 1951, the country's population was 361 million. It crossed 600 million mark in 1976 and 1000 million or one billion by the end of 2000. During, initial 25 years, the population grew by 240 million and subsequently between 1976-2000, it increased by 400 million. Continuing, at this speed, the country would be having 16000 million faces in 2025 who will be faced a severe problem of employment, nutrition and health care. The case of child labours under 16 years and migration of mass rural youths to urban areas for seeking employment are the burning evidence of ill effects of rising population graph in our country.

There is a good scope of agro/livestock based enterprises, e.g. seed production, nursery raising, fruit preservation, mushroom cultivation, milk product processing, layer, broiler and piggery farming, etc. in villages itself for unemployed rural youths. Piggery enterprise is one which require least expenditure to establish as compared to other enterprises and hold tremendous production potential in generating employment opportunity in rural areas. Therefore, efforts should be made to promote and accelerate the piggery enterprise on industrial mode to meet the objectives of employment generation, support to economically weaker section, prevention of rural youths migration and enhancing the availability of animal protein per capita. Some of the salient features of pig/pig farming are:

- Piggery enterprise is contributing about 5.90% of the total revenue from livestock production. Pigs are the most efficient feed converting and litter bearing animal, having a short generation interval, high prolificacy, faster growth rate and higher dressing percentage as compared to other meat producing animal species.

- Pig farming complement well with mixed farming system to sustain the crop production. Pigs are the fertilizer factory which convert/recycle the farm/domestic waste into valuable plant nutrients for agriculture. It is estimated that a herd of 15–20 pigs can produce one ton of ammonium sulphate annually.

- India has achieved self-sufficiency in cereal production in recent years. But the availability of animal protein per capita per day to an average Indian is only 7.6 g against the world average of 24.70 g. To bridge this wide gap between requirement and availability of animal protein the milk, mutton, chevon or chicken, etc. cannot fulfill, together the demand of fast growing population without pork production. Thus, piggery development may play an important role in solving the problem of animal protein, which is comparatively cheaper and reachable to an average house hold.

- Pig population increased with an annual compound growth rate of 6.27% from 3.70 million to 16 million between 1945 and 1998, which constitute 1.48% of world pig population (FAO, 1998). Uttar Pradesh had the largest pig population (2.90 million), followed by Assam (1.40 million), Bihar (1.10 million) and West Bengal (0.96 million). It reflects the future scope of piggery development in Uttar Pradesh.

- The pig population in Uttar Pradesh indicate that the majority of the pigs reared in rural areas are local (>85%) and very less (<15%) are improved, which is one of the major cause of low productivity of rural pigs. Although, the annual growth rate of improved breed (8.74%) is accelerating as compared to local breed (2.60%) which is a good indicator of replacing the poor productive, non-descript breed (Table 9.1).

Table 9.1: Changing trends in pig population in UP

Years	Indigenous pigs	Cross-bred/exotic pigs	Total
1988	2192871 (88.35%)	289287 (11.65%)	2482158
1993	2477459 (85.62 %)	416052 (14.88%)	2893511
Annual growth rate (%)	2.60	8.74	3.31

Figures in brackets indicate the percentage of total pig population

Source: Livestock Census 1988 and 1993, Government of Uttar Pradesh, Lucknow.

- Pigs are generally reared by socially and economically weaker section or tribal people in a traditional way on almost zero investment (mainly on scavenging) with local, poor productivity or non-descript breed and without input of modern technology. As a result, the production and productivity of pig farming is low.

- Pigs provide a regular source of income to a large number of farmers. It provides good quality pork containing 15–20% protein with all essential amino acids and important B group of vitamins. Besides meat, pigs provide valuable by-products viz skin, hair, fats, hoofs, blood, bones, meat scraps, intestine and bladders, endocrine glands, collagen, etc. of important.

- Thus, pig farming can play an important role in creation of employment opportunity and upliftment of socio-economic status of weaker section in rural areas. Piggery enterprise require lesser funds to set up a small unit, give quick return on investment and convert rapidly the inedible feed into pork and valuable by-products, aid soil fertility and supplement other enterprises. Keeping in view, Krishi Vigyan Kendras (KVKs), viz. Gonda, Allahabad and Chitrakoot have come forward to set up the piggery unit at their centre with Large White Yorkshire (LWY) breed to disseminate this breed and technology at farmers field in rural areas.

Introduction of LWY Breed at Farmers Field

The project "Integrated Piggery Development" was sanctioned and financially assisted by Ministry of Agriculture, New Delhi, during January 2000 to KVK Gonda, Allahabad and Chitrakoot. The technical know how guidance was provided by IVRI, Izatnagar, Bareilly. A piggery unit was set up with 1+5 LWY breed. A total number of 724 piglets were produced from 2000 to 2005 as centre and yearwise details given in Table 9.2. The interested rural youths were selected and trained properly on various aspect of breeding, feeding and management of pigs. After a well orientation, 124 rural youths were provided LWY Piglets @ 1:4 to establish the unit at their own field in different batches and years. Besides, the culled and weaned piglets were also sold them to rear for slaughtering purpose. As a result, 124 small units have been established up to 2005 under close monitoring of KVKs. The centre and yearwise set up of piggery units at farmers field is given in Table 9.3.

Table 9.2: LWY piglets produced by different KVKs during 2000 to 2005

Years	KVK Gonda		KVK Allahabad		KVK Chitrakoot		Total
	Female	Male	Female	Male	Female	Male	
2001	58	41	–	–	11	09	119
2002	59	73	01	01	11	04	149
2003	50	47	39	26	14	08	184
2004	26	24	27	23	10	09	119
2005	19	12	31	29	22	40	153
Total	**212**	**197**	**98**	**79**	**68**	**70**	**724**

Table 9.3: Year and districtwise set up of piggery units at farmers field

Year	Gonda	Allahabad	Chitrakoot	Total
2001	8	–	4	12
2002	18	–	–	18
2003	24	16	10	50
2004	11	7	4	22
2005	7	5	10	22
Total	**68**	**28**	**28**	**124**

Feeding Management

Pigs were allowed for scavenging or grazing (5–6 hrs daily) in surrounding areas of the house, pasture and garbage. During scavenging time, pigs ingested different feed materials like leafy vegetables, arum, grasses, root of different plants and standing crops, viz. sugarcane, potato, berseem, jowar, bajra, vegetables, etc.

In addition to grazing, the animals were offered various feed materials like cooked rice with rice police or gruel, wheat/rice bran, cereal/pulse shortenings in uncertain amount and improper ratio. Besides these, kitchen waste, vegetables and leafy soft fodders were also given as per availability. No mineral mixture and protein substitute like oil cakes were given because farmers could not afford for these costly ingredients.

Housing Management

Majority of the farmers constructed piggery shed of asbestos/thatched roof, brick/wooden wall but cemented floor. There were well sanitation and ventilation in almost all the sheds. They cleaned the pigsty and bathe the animals daily. The pigs wallowed in pond, canal or retained tube well water to keep the body cool. Majority of the pig owners provided bedding materials of paddy straw, gunny bags for their piglets. The sheds were constructed near the house and the old ladies and children of the family took care of reared pigs.

Breeding Management

The piggery owner reported that the gilts were bred at an average age of 10.5 months and male pig were used at first time at an average of 10.8 months. As a routine practice, the male and female pigs were sent together for grazing, therefore, farmers did not take care for heat detection and insemination of animals. Hence control breeding was not followed.

Management of Piglets and Pregnant

Majority of pig owners cleaned the mucus from mouth, nostril and body of newly born piglets and provided comfortable bedding materials. The piglets were fed colostrums from the suckling sows. However, very rare farmers clipped the needle teeth. Instead of starter ration, farmers offered only rice gruel to piglets in addition to mother milk. Majority of the farmers did not provide iron pills, minerals and vitamin supplements to piglets. Vaccination, weaning and castration (male piglets reared for slaughter) were also not followed. However, the pregnant gilts/sows in advance stage were specially cared for providing good quality feed and comfortable accommodation. The remaining was reared as their usual practice.

Marketing Management

In district Allahabad and Chitrakoot, farmers were bound to sell their pigs to local consumer, because there is no such market. As a result, farmers did not get remunerative return and faced a problem of vigorous bargaining to sell their pigs. However in district Gonda, there was no such problem because, the district is well connected by railways and highways to North Eastern Hill (NEH) Region. These states are mostly dominated by Christians and have good demand of pork.

RESULTS AND DISCUSSION

The data pertaining to various production potential traits, viz. age of puberty, body weight gained at puberty, age at first farrowing, gestation period, litter size, mortality of piglets, farrowing intervals and slaughter weight at 12 months age were collected from entire 124 small units set up at farmers field. Consequently, these observations were also collected from the farmers in same areas, rearing the indigenous pigs for comparative study.

Performance of LWY Breed at Farmers Field

The age at puberty in LWY gilts ranged from 210 to 260 days with a mean value of 235 ± 5.85 days. It tooks longer duration as compared to the observations of Babu et al (2004) and Sein (1985) as 167.70 ± 3.41 and 179.70 days, respectively. The body weight gained at puberty of LWY gilts was recorded as 75 ± 2.70 kg and ranged from 64 to 90 kg. Comparatively, the body weight in present study is lower than the findings of Babu et al (2004) and Sain (1985). The average age at first farrowing was 401 ± 4.50 days, which is comparatively higher than the reported values of other authors (Table 9.4).

Table 9.4: Reproductive and productive performance of LWY pigs at farmers field

	Particulars	Gonda	Allahabad	Chitrakoot	Mean
1.	Age of puberty (days)	229	230	246	235 ± 5.85
2.	Body weight at puberty (kg)	75.0	72.5	77.5	75.0 ± 2.70
3.	Age at first farrowing (days)	345	470	388	401.33 ± 4.50
4.	Litter size (number)	10	7	8	8.33 ± 0.65
5.	Pre-weaned piglet mortality (%)	17.5	20.0	23.0	20.16
6.	Farrowing intervals (days)	205	194	244	214.33 ± 4.70
7.	Slaughter weight at 12 month age (kg)	80	60	70	70.0 ± 2.75
8.	Net profit (Rs./pig)	997.00	1112.00	918.00	976.66

The higher age and low body weight gained at puberty and further higher age at first farrowing were mostly due to imbalanced nutrition. Farmers gave maximum emphasis on scavenging with minimum on supplementary feeds. They did not provide protein (oil cakes), vitamins and mineral supplements. As a result, piglets did not attain desired body weight at specified age and took longer duration at puberty vis-a-vis to farrow at first time.

The average gestation period of LWY gilts/sows was 114 ± 0.25 days which is almost similar as per the observation of Babu et al (2004) for LWY breed. The average number of piglets born per gilts/sows was 8.30 ± 0.65 and ranged from 7 to 10. Similar range in litter size (7.09 to 10.10) was reported by Singh et al (1989) for LWY breed.

In present study, the pre-weaned piglet mortality was higher (20.16%). The major mortality were due to severe cold in winter, genetical/congenital defects or by crushing beneath the mother.

The mean farrowing interval in sow was observed to be 180 ± 3.20 days. Similar farrowing interval was reported by Babu et al (2004). Comparatively, shorter farrowing interval was reported by other authors as 166.40 to 56.30 days in LWY breeds. The longer interval in present study was mainly due to imbalance nutrition and to some extent by not following the weaning practice by the farmers.

The extra male piglets were reared for slaughter purpose which attained a body weight of 70 ± 2.50 kg in 12 months and gave a net profit of Rs 976 per pig. However, Kumar et al (2004) reported higher income of Rs 1444 per annum per pig of same breed. The lower body weight at slaughter age was mainly due to imbalance nutrition and culled/defective piglets reared for pork purpose. The lower profit received by the owners was due to non-availability of organized market facilities.

Although, there were no any outbreak of swine fever, foot and mouth disease or other contagious diseases seen or reported from any district, without adopting the vaccination schedule, even though, it must be followed.

Comparative Performance of LWY vs. Local Breed

The comparative economic traits recorded for both the breeds are given in Table 9.5. The average age of gilts, when first came in heat, were 10.80 ± 1.52 and 7.70 ± 1.05 months, body weight at puberty were 50 ± 2.59 and 75 ± 2.70 kg, age at first farrowing were 15.2 ± 1.98 and 13.24 ± 0.97 months and farrowing intervals were 7.76 ± 1.69 and 7.02 ± 1.65 months for local and LWY breed, respectively. Similarly, the average birth weight of piglets were 0.55 ± 0.02 and 0.87 ± 0.03 kg, body weight at slaughter age were 55 ± 1.85 and 70 ± 2.50 kg and net profit/pig/year were Rs 550 and 976 in indigenous and LWY breed, respectively. Study revealed that under identical condition of feeding and management practices, LWY has shown quite higher prolificacy, faster growth rate and other economic traits as compared to existing local one. Hence, LWY breed could be successfully raised and multiplied at farmer's field.

Table 9.5: Comparative economic traits of indigenous and LWY breed

Particulars	Indigenous breed	LWY breed
Age at puberty (months)	10.80 ± 1.52	7.70 ± 1.05
Body weight at puberty (kg)	50.00 ± 2.59	75.00 ± 2.50
Age at first farrowing (months)	15.20 ± 1.98	13.24 ± 0.97
Litter size (numbers)	5.90 ± 0.35	8.33 ± 0.65
Farrowing intervals (months)	7.76 ± 1.69	7.02 ± 1.65
Birth weight of piglets (kg)	0.55 ± 0.02	0.87 ± 0.03
Body weight at 12 months (kg)	55.00 ± 1.85	70.00 ± 2.50
Net profit/pig (Rs.)	550.00	976.00

Constraints and Feedback

The LWY breed had shown quite encouraging performance at farmers field and at productivity level like good quality pork, high feed conversion efficiency and large litter size. Even then to popularize the piggery enterprise at large scale, there are few limitations which needs urgent remedial measures, as given under:

- Lack of organized market facilities to sell the surplus pork.
- Costly feed/feed ingredients/supplements.
- Non-availability of improved/desired breed.
- Very high pre-weaned piglets mortality.
- Lack of technical knowledge.
- Social/religious taboos.

In case piggery enterprise as employment generating enterprise among the rural youths, following points should be given due considerations:

Availability of Market Facilities

Government should make industrial pork production strategy on the pattern of operation flood and encourage entrepreneurs to venture in this sector. State department of animal husbandry and private agencies should come up for establishing pork processing units/bacon factories. Self-help group and Cooperatives should be constituted at village level. The consumption of pork and pork products should be popularized by hygienic production, quality control and suitable processing technique in local market as well as possibilities for export market should be explored. The products should be well labeled and given trademark as dairy products. The valuable by-products should also be properly utilized for industrial purposes. This will encourage the piggery enterprise and ultimately the farmers will get better return and be saved from exploitation by middle man.

Availability of Economical Ration

It is an important input of piggery farming, since, it alone account 65–75% expenditure. Therefore, efforts should be made to formulate the more economical ration, using local available ingredients and resources. Area specific mineral mixture should be developed as per different agro-climatic zones. A general composition of creep, grower and finisher rations are given in Table 9.6. Few alternate sources of ingredients to make the ration economical based on cheap availability, unfit for human consumption, cereal and pulse shortenings, etc. are suggested below:

- Maize can be replaced by broken wheat, rice, barley, sogrhum, jowar, bajra or kodo; groundnut cake by other oil cakes like linseed, sunflower, sesamum or coconut; wheat bran by good quality rice bran and fish meal by slaughter house waste meat meal, meat scrapings, skim milk powder, etc. as per availability.
- Waste of hotel, hostel, kitchen, bakery, etc. (properly boiled to avoid any diseases); molasses, potato/sweet potato/tapioca + cereals (3:1) may be fed up to 40% of total ration to growers and adults to save the feed.

Table 9.6: Composition of creep, grower and finisher rations

Ingredients (%)	Creep ration (from 15 days, up to 2 kg body wt)	Grower ration (up to 35 kg body wt)		Finisher ration (above 35 kg body wt)	
		Cereal based	Non-cereal based	Cereal based	Non-cereal based
Maize	60	35	–	40	–
G. N Cake	10	10	10	11	11
Wheat bran	10	47	47	47	47
Rice polish	–	–	35	–	40
Fish meal	6	6	6	–	–
Min. Mixt.	1.50	1.50	1.50	1.50	1.50
Common salt	0.50	0.50	0.50	0.50	0.50

Add supplevit-M @ 250 g or problend @ 200 g per 100 kg feed

- Green leafy vegetables, succulent soft cereal and leguminous fodder waste fruits and their remaining, soft seasonal edible weeds, leaves of fodder trees may be fed *ad lib* to adults. These are the cheapest source of minerals and vitamins.
- Regular scavenging may also reduce the feeding cost to a great extent but depends upon the situation of grazing resources.

Availability of Improved Breeds

Farmers should be made available the improved breed or cross-bred between of exotic and indigenous breed rather than pure exotic breed. Therefore, the most specific and appropriate exotic breed for different agro-ecological situations should be identified for better growth, adoption and disease resistance. Besides, the State Department of Animal Husbandry and Veterinary Services should make available the vaccines (swine fewer, FMD, etc.) and essential drugs at their centre situated in rural areas.

Piglet Mortality

It was reported that about 20% piglets died before weaning. The major causes of mortality were congenital/genetical defects, under weight, large litter size and severe cold during winter. About 4–5% piglets are born with some genetical/ congenital defects and are not expected to survive. As congenital defect is not curable but balance feeding to pregnant can provide healthy piglets. However, in case of large litter, few piglets may be shifted to a foster mother, which farrowed within 48 hours. If foster mother is not available, warm cow milk may be given in small quantities, 5–6 times a day up to 3 weeks. The mortality due to severe cold (15 Dec. to last Jan.) may be checked by control breeding, considering the gestation period of 114 days, i.e. during 4th week of August to 1st week of October.

Technical Knowledge

As observed, farmers require systematic exposure of scientific technology related to various aspect of pig farming and also desire to develop proficiency in its efficient use. Study revealed that majority of the farmers did not follow the important practices like prevention during cold and hot weather, feeding of surplus piglets via foster mother or cow milk, disinfection of novel card, clipping of needle teeth, feeding of iron pills, vitamins and mineral supplements (piglets), weaning, vaccination, castration, deworming, care during farrowing, lactation and breeding, etc. mainly due to lack of awareness. Therefore, it is essential to provide and upgrade the technical knowledge of the farmers about important practices. Thus can be done by organizing long duration vocational trainings, visits of demonstration units, scientists visit to farmers fields, scientist-farmers interactions, animal health veterinary camp and making availability of folders, pamphlets, booklets, leaflets in simple language, making films, etc. to acquisite the knowledge and utilize into practice for the success of piggery farming. Few farmers from different zones may be selected, trained properly and used as satellite farmers for dissemination of technology.

Religious/Social Taboos

Pigs are not reared by Muslim people. Even in Hindus, pig rearing is restricted mostly up to schedule caste and schedule tribes. But now the scenario is changing many people from Hindu communities are coming up and engaging themselves into pig farming and also not hesitating in consuming pork. Intake of pork or pork products are also increasing tremendously among the working and middle class in metropolitan cities. So the religious/social taboos are not a big constraint and will vanish gradually in future.

CONCLUSIONS

In our country, there is a large scale migration of rural youths of different regions to urban areas for seeking employment. To prevent this migration, it is absolutely necessary to create self-employment opportunities in their own villages/areas itself. Piggery enterprise is one of the effective tools in bringing out the socio-economic change and generating employment opportunities. The study revealed that the adopted pig farmers under project were highly satisfied and convinced with the high feed conversion efficiency, superior pork quality, large litter size and production potential of Large White Yorkshire (LWY) an exotic breed. Simultaneously, they are facing, few major limitations, like lack of organized market facilities for surplus pork or pork products, non-availability of desired/improved breed, costly feed/feed ingredients/supplements and lack of technical skill in scientific management of improved breed make the piggery farming an unremunerative enterprise. Thus, the success in overcoming these obstacles, therefore, offers every encouraging incentive in making the piggery farming more profitable and adoptable enterprise. Obviously, this will increase the production potential of their pig and will help in improving the standard of living.

10

Entrepreneurship Development: A Success Story of Hiware Bazaar Village of Maharashtra

Shahaji Phand, Rupasi Tiwari

Livestock sector is a powerful tool for sustenance of millions of poor worldwide, who otherwise become a victim of monsoon vagaries due to crop failure. This particular sector has immense potential for entrepreneurship development, which will ultimately address the issue of widespread unemployment. Though the veterinary sciences have been blessed with a powerful tool but mere awareness and availability will not suffice the purpose. The ultimate end user, i.e. the farmers should be in position to take advantage of this situation. Therefore, the basic issues should be addressed first which are in the way of entrepreneurship development in livestock sector.

Entrepreneurship development in agriculture and livestock sector mainly depends on three major critical inputs, i.e. land, water and capital. The ongoing government policies on farm credit have solved the problem of capital to some extent through various nationalized banks and grassroot level government institutions like cooperative societies. Secondly, the land without water availability for irrigation and fodder growing mainly jeopardizes the entrepreneurship development in this sector, so the major constraint in development of entrepreneurship is water availability. The state like Maharashtra, where only 16% of land have assured irrigation facilities, the rest of land is rainfed. Due to changing climatic conditions as a result of global warming, vagaries of monsoon have shown widespread impact on farming systems including livestock. Frequent drought condition leads farmer to sell his animal to butchers. In such situation there is urgent need to solve these basic problems.

NATURAL RESOURCES MANAGEMENT

FAO has defined it as the management and conservation of the natural resource base, and the orientation of technological and institutional change in such a manner as to ensure the attainment and continued satisfaction of human needs for present and future generations. Such sustainable development conserves land, water, plant and animal genetic resources and is environmentally non-degrading, technically appropriate, economically viable and socially acceptable.

Village economy and its development are based on its natural resource and their successful management by the village community for production. Natural resource management therefore has to be the key pin for an effective strategy for rural development in general and entrepreneurship development in particular. Livestock has been seen always as a subsidiary of agriculture rather than as a separate entity, therefore failure in one will always affect the other. If this symbiotic relationship between these two sectors has to succeed, there is necessity of a holistic approach the development, which should address the basic issues such as strategy to overcome frequent draught through watershed development; and thereby agriculture and livestock development. Development of infrastructure for marketing and processing of livestock products at village level through cooperative societies, which will ultimately result in development and diversification of entrepreneurship in livestock sector.

In 1985 with this holistic approach, the Government of Maharashtra came forward with its new programme called *Adarsh Gaon Yojana* (AGY) (Ideal village scheme), which was based on natural resource management by the village community. The programme was undertaken in 300 villages across 300 blocks in Maharashtra to provide safe drinking water, employment, green fodder, education and health so that a village may achieve self-sustenance by development of entrepreneurship in agriculture and livestock sector.

Hiware Bazaar village in Ahmednagar district of Maharashtra is one of them, where the Government of Maharashtra has implemented this programme through *Grampanchayat*. The implementation of the programme was based on the following "Panchasutra" (the five principles):

• Donation of labour (Shramdan)
• Ban on grazing (Kurhad Bandi)
• Ban on tree cutting (Charai Bandi)
• Ban on liquor (Nasha Bandi)
• Family planning (Kutumb Niyojan).

The criteria for selection of village under this programme is that, village should be located in a drought prone area and should have shortage of drinking water as their major problem. The villagers should have to take an oath to follow above five principles. The 'AGY' aims at encouraging the villages to become self-sufficient and self-reliant by following the five principles and involving them in the watershed development programme with the assistance of NGOs and government departments.

The present study was carried out at Hiware Bazar village of Ahmednagar District of Maharashtra to find out the impact of AGY where, Government of Maharashtra implemented *AGY* since 15 August 1994 and under the scheme this village has been awarded 'Ideal village' (*Adarsh Gaon*) status in 1998. A research design used for the study was 'before-after' with control. Data was collected through personal interview and secondary sources. A total 117 respondents were selected randomly for the study consisting 54 each from Hiware Bazaar (Experimental village) and Jamgaon (Control village), which consisted 51 landholder and 3 landless respondents in each village. In addition, the data were collected from 7 government officials such as Block Development Officer, Village Development Officer, Livestock Development Officer, Medical Officer,

Water and Soil Conservation Officer related to the concern villages. Data from secondary sources were collected from Grampanchyat office and NGO ('Yashwant Krishi Gram and Watershed Development Trust') involved in the implementation of AGY regarding the people's participation in creating various community assets in the village, various activities for natural resource management, watershed development and soil conservation measures (Table 10.1).

Table 10.1: Salient features of the village Hiware Bazaar (2002)

Physical features		Social situation	
Total geographical area	976.84 ha	Total population	1245
Cultivatable land	795.23 ha	No. of males	620
Forest land	70.03 ha	No. of females	625
Pasture land (public)	6.75 ha	No. of farm families	205
Pasture land (private)	62.00 ha	No. of land less families	11
Gaothan	4.46 ha	No. of milch animals	560
Irrigated land	795.23 ha	No. of farm use animals	120

HISTORY OF HIWARE BAZAAR

This is the story of a village, which rose like phoenix from ashes. It was not cursed by anything, but their own deeds which lead them to years of sufferings and hardships. Roots of their sufferings were in neglect of "Mother Nature", which lead to persistent drought. Drought caused poverty, alcoholism and several addictions, which took over the village completely. Families were destroyed. Many people migrated to all direction for survival. Homes lost homeliness and village its identity. Suffering continued for 2–3 decades amidst curse of drought, until a young committed son of the village determined to change the things for good.

Implementation of *Adarsh Gaon Yojana* brought unity and peace in village, faith and services took place of evils of alcoholism. Poverty and suffering came to end, families were rebuilt and prosperity pervaded everywhere. A village once crippled by several political and social evils, once again became independent. Villagers got enlightened with new vision. Their tears gave way to happiness. The villagers, who are witnessed of this great transformation, say that, this is miracle, but it was a real transformation and this is the story of that transformation.

This village happens to fall in Nagar block of Ahmednagar district of Maharashtra and the name of village is 'Hiware Bazaar'. It has a history of being a part of empire of king Shivaji 400 years ago. Merchants used to flock to the village for marketing. The things started changing for worse with the advent of British. Destruction of forests started for meeting the needs of marketers. Trees were felled and used for fuel. The trend continued unabated during the British regime and turned the green landscape of 'Hiware Bazaar' into bleak and bare. Independence did not stop this destruction and ultimately lead to reduction in the rainfall of the area. Soil became bare and got eroded over the time. It became unproductive. It gradually led to drought like situation. Then came the drought of 1972. It created havoc in Maharashtra. 'Hiware Bazaar' was among the worst hit. Wells dried, fields became cropless. Women had to search for water in all the directions. There was no food and no work, life and living became difficult. 'Hiware Bazaar' turned out to be incapable of supporting its people (Fig. 10.1). People went to Mumbai-Pune-Ahmednagar to earn their daily meals (Warghade, 2003).

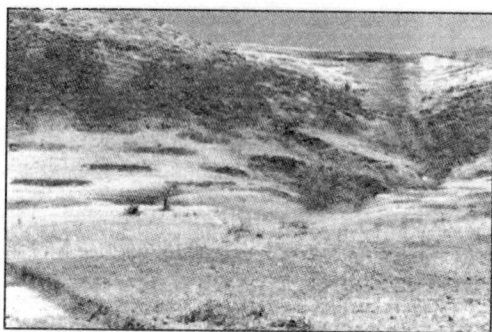 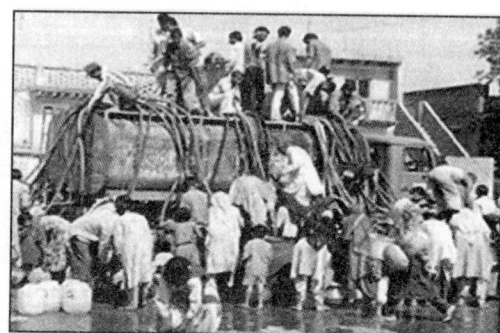

Fig. 10.1: Hiware Bazaar (Before 1989)

Poverty and sorrows of life frustrated the people. They found no way to overcome it, which resulted into several addictions to forget their sorrows. In this way scourge of alcoholism entered in 'Hiware Bazaar'. Eventually alcoholism took over the village completely. Yet things came to an all time low when, in 1982, there was a murder case in the village.

There was no co-operation to Government employees working in the village. Residents claim that, the village was marked as a punishment village, where employees of the civil service were transferred if they had offended higher-ups or had disciplinary action taken against them. It weakened *Panchayat Raj* System and became obstruction to any kind of development activity. The law and order situation had deteriorated so much that, the police did not venture into the village unless they were armed and numbered. The village topped the blacklist in police department.

NEW LEADERSHIP: NEW DIRECTION

In 1989, Mr Popatrao Pawar, a young committed son of the village was in fact an unnatural choice as Head of *Grampanchayat*. He was inspired by the well-known social activist Anna Hazare and decided to devote himself to social work. He reviewed village situation and with the cooperation of some youth of village he started intervening in various village problems. In 1990 there was extreme scarcity of drinking water and there were only two hand-pumps in the village which also were not in working condition. Women had to fetch water from 2–3 km away but no one was caring. Mr Pawar personally went several times to *Panchayat Samiti* (Block) office and solved the problem of water by repairing the hand-pumps.

NATURAL RESOURCE MANAGEMENT THROUGH VOLUNTARY LABOUR

Mr. Pawar had gathered youth of the village and discussed on the various issue of the village problems. He strongly believes that any development actions need to be performed with the villager's participation right from its selection, planning and execution. He advised youth, that, "We should not depend on government or any such other help for our development. If we keep on waiting on such hope then, it will take years together to come out of this poverty. We have to bring out our own development". Youth were impressed by his thoughts and decided 'Natural resource management through voluntary labour' as means of their transformation. They decided that at least one member of every family will work for village development in a week.

It has been proved by several experiences that the local peoples' participation in any kind of development process or creation of community assets (such as creating of village road, social forestry, watershed development and management) is very crucial factor for its success as well as sustainability (Fig. 10.2). As pointed by Pushpalatha, KBC (2001) that, in the recent past, aquaculture development programmes have failed due to the absence of participation of local communities.

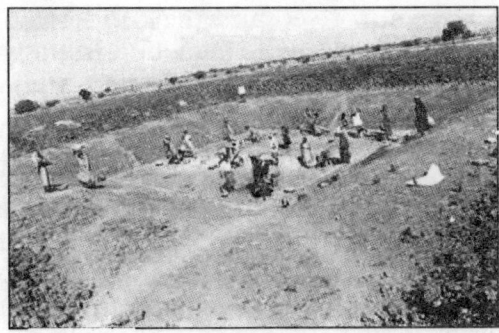 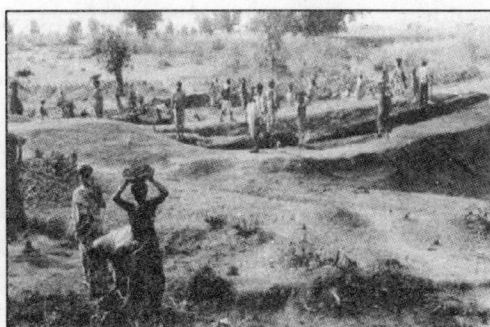

Fig. 10.2: Watershed development through voluntary labour

IMPACT OF NATURAL RESOURCE MANAGEMENT AND WATERSHED DEVELOPMENT

Agriculture is the means of livelihood of about 90–95% of people of Indian villages and water availability for irrigation is the crucial factor in the development of villages particularly in drought prone areas. 'Hiware Bazaar' was not different, which is surrounded by the small hillock from three sides. Though it received average rainfall of about 250 mm yet, overgrazing and deforestation had created barren hillsides incapable of retaining water. Consequently, the little rain that the village received would runoff soon after the rainfall, before it could recharge the local water table in any significant way. The village had not a single source of water for irrigation nearby due to its typical topography. But water availability for irrigation was the ultimate answer for the widespread poverty in village. Mr. Pawar called *Gramsabha* and explained about watershed development. In 1993, they took the first step for watershed development with the co-operation of forest department and about 40,000 continuous counter trenches (CCT) were created on the slope of 70 hectares of hillock through labour donation. Trees were planted on the sides of trenches after the first rainfall in June. Meanwhile cattle's grazing was strictly banned on that area. As a result about 300 tones of grass were produced in first year, which was not only fed adequately to all its cattle, but was also in abundant and some fodder was sold to neighbouring villages to meet their needs. Farmers had made a transition towards stall-feeding their cattle to reduce overgrazing and raise milk yields. Henceforth, the *Gramsabha* decided that only a headload of fodder per family per day could be collected from these hills, and that the *Panchayat* for this privilege would charge nominal user fees of Rs 100 per family per year. These funds would later be used for different village welfare programmes. No outsiders were allowed to have access to these grasslands.

Thus, collected amount of Rs 30,000 was used for village development. Rainwater was not drained out but, it got percolated through land due to CCT and recharged aquifer which drained into the wells and tube-wells. Even the wells and tube-wells which became dried earlier got flooded with full water. Previously water in the village got depleted after 1–2 months at the end of monsoon. But now it remained for about 3–4 month. The irrigated land which was only 15–20 hectares rose to 70 hectares due to their first effort of watershed development (Warghade, S. 2003). People were surprised and they understood the importance of watershed development. The success of this small initiative was sufficient to inspire and recharge the community.

IMPLEMENTATION OF ADARSH GAON YOJANA

During the period in which the State of Maharashtra was celebrating the Golden Jubilee of its existence, the state government announced the *Adarsh Gaon Yojana*, which was based on well-known rural transformation model of "Ralegan Siddhi" under the leadership of Anna Hazare. Perhaps the 'Ralegan Siddhi' model of Anna Hazare is the most notable, which is based on people's participation in natural resource management. The *Adarsh Gaon Yojana* was undertaken to provide safe drinking water, employment, green fodder production, education and health so that a village may achieve self-sustenance.

Mr. Pawar recognized the need of *Adarsh Gaon Yojana* to cope up with the situation and accordingly, in *Gramsabha*, in it's meeting on 15th August 1994 accepted the challenges and the opportunities presented by this scheme, and decided to implement it whole heartedly. For this purpose, the *Gramsabha* formally established the 'Yashwant Krishi Gram and Watershed Development Trust'. (Rao 2000) reported that institution-building and leadership formation is necessary for ensuring effective participation of people on a sustained basis. He explained the importance of *Panchsutra* in *Gramsabha* again and again and sought approval of all its components. Then he submitted the necessary documents for the nomination of village in AGY to Shri Anna Hazare, who was the chairman of *Adarsh Gaon Samiti*.

After 4 years of planned efforts to development of watershed structure and natural resource management villagers were able to solve the basic problem of water availability (Figs 10.3 and 10.4), which resulted into revitalization of the agriculture and livestock sector. He gave loan to farmers to get loan from various government

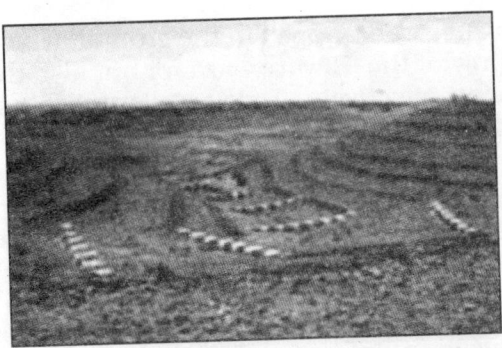
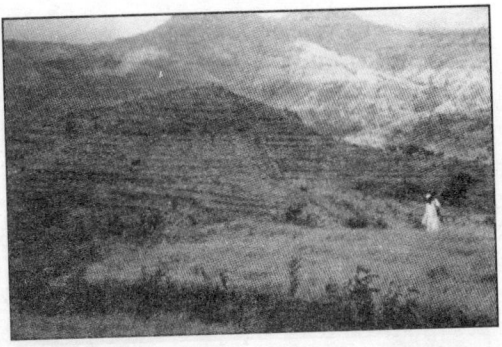

Fig. 10.3: Natural resource management

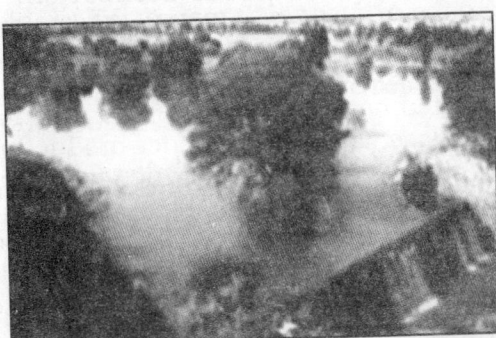
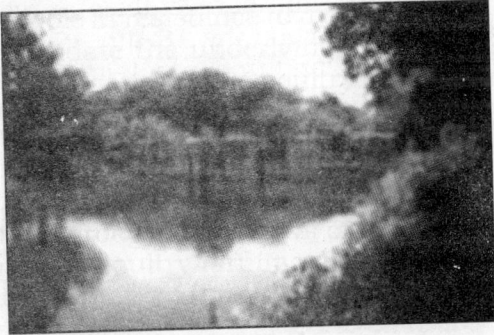

Fig. 10.4: Water everywhere

schemes to start the dairy farming, goat farming, digging of wells and tried to change their way of subsistence. In 1998 'Hiware Bazaar' was rewarded as *Adarsh Gaon* (Ideal village) by the Government of Maharashtra. After selection of village in the 'Adarsh Gaon' group it started receiving the finance under the AGY for watershed development and various other development activities in the village. The panchayat researched and developed a database of the different government schemes that, they could use to improve their agricultural or water development programmes. Using this information, they sought the services of various government experts to plan their watershed development. Officers and residents together surveyed the lands in and around 'Hiware Bazaar' to determine the sites for tanks and bunds. Based on this knowledge, they structured five years duration plan of water harvesting in four stages through their NGO, i.e. 'Yashwant Krishi Gram and Watershed Development Trust'. In the first stage, work was undertaken on the government land of the village, second on the *Gram Panchayat* land, third on the private and fallow land of the village and massive tree plantation programme was undertaken in final stage. They created several water storage structures in the village within a span of 3 years, such as continuous counter trenches (CCT) on the 180 hectares of land, earthen structures-2, cement bunds-4, storage tank-7, percolation tank-2, van tale-2, loose boulders-120, repairing of *Nala* bunds-11, and tree plantation on 206 hectares of land and also along the 6 km roadside. Thus today about 9 lakh trees are growing on the village land, adding the beauty in the greenery of village (Phand, S. 2005).

In this way each and every drop of rainwater was trapped in the ground, which resulted into increase in water-table not only of the 'Hiware Bazaar', but also the nearer villages. It also checked soil erosion effectively. Today wells and other water storage structures remain flooded with plenty of water throughout the year.

ENTREPRENEURSHIP DEVELOPMENT

As an impact of watershed development, 795.23 ha of the total geographical area of 976.44 ha became cultivable. Previously only 250 hectares land was under the protective irrigation, which today spread over to the entire cultivable land. As the water become available for irrigation, people started farming with full speed. Today, village is having 318 wells full of water. Villagers started to grow vegetables, fodder, flowers, fruits along with the cereals and pulses. They sell about 680 tons of vegetables everyday in the Ahmednagar market. Vegetables raised their income by 18 times and pulses about 23 times per year. Earlier there was no land under fruit crops in the village, but now about 10 hectares of land is under the fruit crops, which has created new income generation avenue in the village. Regarding the livestock enterprises, land under fodder production increased by 9.5 times (Phand, S. 2005) and total fodder production in the village reached up to 3,000 to 5,000 tones per year with 25 times growth (Warghade, S. 2003). As the fodder production increased, about 70% of villagers started commercial dairy farming, and number of milch animals (crossbreds and buffaloes) increased by 7 times (Fig. 10.5). Earlier there was no cross-bred

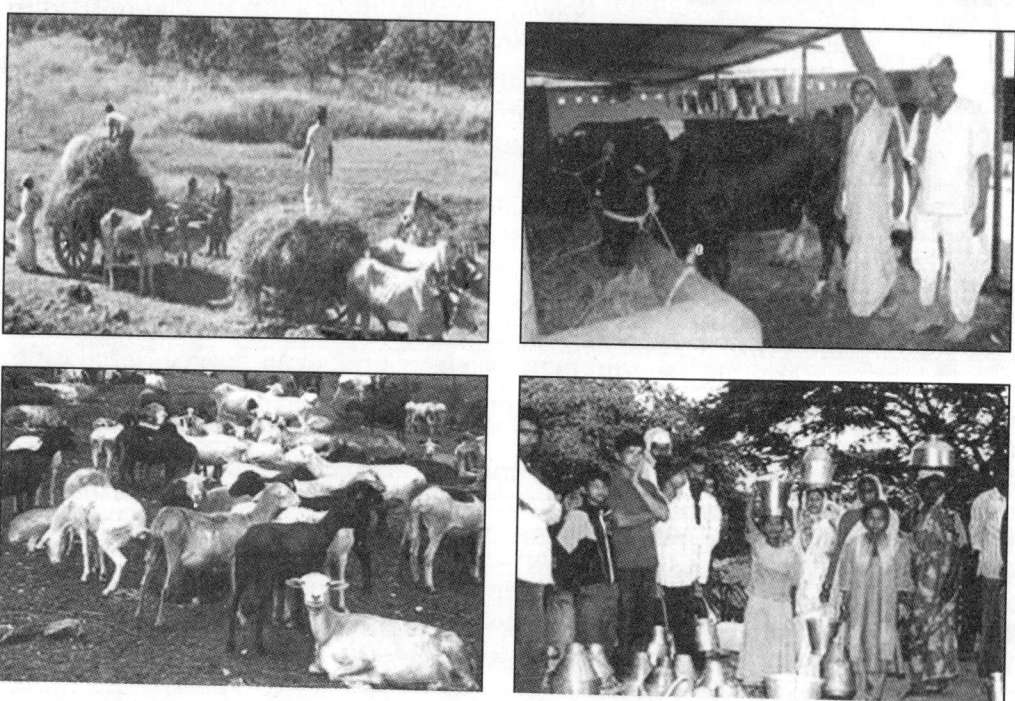

Fig. 10.5: Entrepreneurship development in livestock sector

in the village, now among milch animals 80% of milk production come from cross-breds. Previously milk production of respondent's family was only 1.5 liter per day, which now rose to 15 liter per day. Village has two co-operative dairies, where they sell their milk. The per capita income before AGY was merely Rs 1004, which is increased by 16 times and reached to Rs 16701. The people of 'Hiware Bazaar' have spent their increased incomes on improving the quality of life in their village (Phand, S. 2005). As the agriculture and dairy farming flourished in the village, villagers were busy throughout the year and not a single person remained unemployed. Rather the village is facing problem of labor, so they started "Community Farming" to solve it. During harvest and planting seasons, people work on single farms together. This social practice ensures that the village can simultaneously harvest large tracts of land.

Thus, the curse of drought and poverty of about two decades came to an end. All families have enough food grains and income to meet their day today needs. The living standard of villagers improved substantially, prosperity pervaded in each and every household. In the economic survey of 1992, out of 180 families, 168 families were "Below Poverty Line", which came down to 11 in 2002. Today, not a single family in the village is "Below Poverty Line" (Phand, S. 2005).

Previously, most of land in the village was barren and it was difficult even to survive there, number of families had migrated to nearby villages and cities for their livelihood. These families returned to village and started farming. Thus today about 40 families have returned. Migration from the village in search of job has almost stopped.

WATER MANAGEMENT AND CONSERVATION

About five years of strenuous work of watershed development by the villagers resulted into prosperity in the village. Then the big challenge for Mr. Pawar was how this development will sustain in future? He found the way and took certain steps. He explained villagers about water management and conservation. If we use water carelessly then in future we may have to face problems again. Due to increased human activities and industrialization, nature is being destroyed day by day, which has resulted into the decrease and uncertainty of rainfall. Vagaries of monsoon will play its role in foreseeable future. Though, today we have enough water availability, but it should be used judiciously. Villagers realized and with the consensus they decided to follow certain norms, such as:

1. Water intensive crops like sugarcane and banana have been prohibited in the village by popular decree.

2. They also decided to use the modern irrigation methods of water conservation for other horticultural crops. As an effect, today 95 hectares of village land is under the drip and sprinkler irrigation. They have targeted that every farmer will have at least 1 acre of land under such irrigation system in near future.

3. Bore wells have also been banned for the purpose of irrigation as it has damaging effect to the underground aquifers and diminishes the water table level.

4. Due to availability of water some wealthy landlords from other villages turned to 'Hiware Bazaar' to purchase village land but they have passed strong rule that no one will sell his land resource to any non-citizen of the village.

As an impact of all such decisions water table level remained constant in between 60–120 feet throughout the year. In between 2000-2003 most of the part of Ahmednagar district suffered drought. Nearby villages of 'Hiware Bazaar' had to be provided drinking water by government tankers but this condition was not seen at 'Hiware Bazaar' (Phand, S. 2005).

INFRASTRUCTURAL DEVELOPMENT

Along with the watershed development and natural resource management they created several community assets in co-operation with the various government agencies and through labour donation (Fig. 10.6). Now the village has well-facilitated school up to tenth standard with trained teaching staff. Due to development of dairy farming, a veterinary clinic was set up in the year of 2000, which is providing animal health services promptly. A beautiful 'Memory Park' has been created in the memories of the persons, who had Lion's share in the development of village. Today thousands of people come to visit that economically, socially and culturally developed *Adarsh Gaon* from all over the Maharashtra and the neighbouring states. Therefore, a capacious and well-facilitated guest house of worth Rs 3.2 lakhs is constructed for the visitors in the village. Also the other structure includes: community hall, health club, library and a beautiful temple of village deity.

Entire village has been lightened by use of solar lamps. They have also established a "Market Information Centre" in September 2002, which helps the

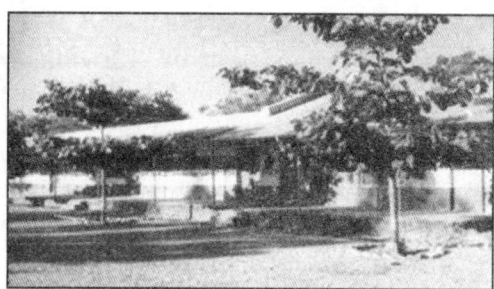
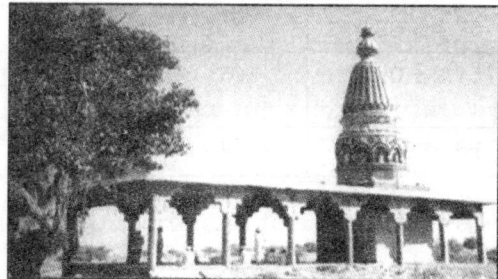
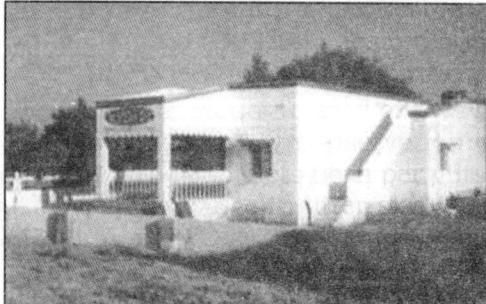
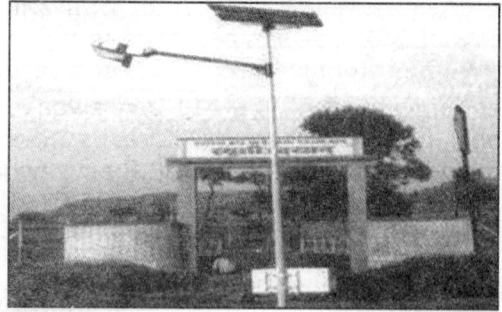

Fig. 10.6: Infrastructure development

farmers for getting correct and rapid information about market rates and other new agriculture technology. Recently, one of the training centre has been constructed to impart the training to the people about watershed management and natural resource management.

They planned to establish a small agro-processing and packaging unit in the village and also decided to establish devices of wind energy to produce electricity.

CONCLUSION

As village economy and development depend on natural resources of village and their successful management by the people. One of the biggest environmental challenges that, developing countries face in the coming decades is to balance their increasing demand with the natural resources. Drought and poverty will not subside by giving temporary help to the villagers, but the local community initiatives within the purview of *Panchayat Raj* system is the most important approach. Agriculture and livestock sector is the key component of rural economy. This particular sector has number of enterprises such as horticulture, floriculture, apiculture, pulses, nursery and also livestock enterprises like dairy farming, goat and sheep rearing, poultry, and piggery enterprises. There is vast scope for promotion of such enterprises in India but availability of water is most prerequisite factor for the development of these enterprises. Large irrigation projects and interlinking of the rivers will remains as 'dream' in foreseeable future. In fact there is no village in India which cannot meet its drinking water needs through rainwater harvesting. Even in an arid area with an annual rainfall of only 100 mm, one hectare of land can theoretically capture as much as one million liters of water. India has about 170 million hectares of waste and degraded land in which though 50 million hectares is very difficult to use like the Thar Desert, the Himalayan cold deserts, still 120 million hectares of land can be brought under productive use. India gets approximately 300 million hectare-meters of rainfall, but only 20% is captured. In fact rain captured from 1–2% of India's land can provide India's population as much as 100 liters of water per person per day.

It has been proved at village Hiware Bazaar that what could be done through mass cooperation and a devoted leadership within the purview of *Panchayat Raj* system. The single largest factor in the transformation of 'Hiware Bazaar' has been the reassertion of democratic responsive governance principles at the village level. By consistently calling upon every member of the society to consult with and participate in the process of their development, the *Grampanchayat* has succeeded in creating a sense of ownership and pride in 'Hiware Bazaar's remarkable achievements. What is today surprisingly noted that not a single family out of 211 families is below poverty line and not a single person in the village is unemployed? Therefore making good use of these waste land and water resources through community participation and along with the government assistance to enhance agricultural and livestock productivity, production and thereby the incomes and employment in villages is the answer to widespread poverty in India. Henceforth, there is a need to replicate 'Hiware Bazaar' pattern, which will not only results in promotion of entrepreneurships in these sectors, but also the way towards "Mahatma Gandhi's dreamed village"— 'self-sufficient, prosperous and peaceful'.

11

Sources and Utilization of Specialty Hair Fibres of Livestock

Sapna Gautam, Alka Goel

Sheep and various other animals have coats which produce natural fibres for providing warmth and protection to mankind and have been utilized since time immemorial. The principal component of hair, wool and fur is the protein keratin. Specialty hair fibres that have the qualities of wool are obtained from specific animals. These fibres are available in smaller quantities than sheep's wool. Hence, they are usually more expensive. Specialty hair fibres are of two kinds: the coarse long outer hair and the soft fine undercoat fibres. The former is used for interlinings, upholstery and the latter is used in luxury coatings, sweaters, shawls, suits and dress fabrics. These fibres can be blended into sheep wool of similar staple and fineness and this increases the durability and strength of yarn made from them and allows more economical use of these scarce and expensive materials. The other animals with coats are: commonly camel family alpaca and vicuna, rabbit family angora rabbit and others are Yak, musk oxen. Mostly specialty hair fibre animals are reared for their wool, meat, pelts by the small scale producers. All the fibres are not of same type, because they possess inherent qualitative differences and are specific to species.

The production and harvesting of luxury fibres is difficult and labour intensive as these come from remote areas having limited availability and requires special climate. So the prices are very high.

The seasonal weather changes cause corresponding changes in the texture and amount of fibre and its diameter is function of both genetic make up (genotype) and environment. For an animal to express its true genotype, the environment pressure must be minimized. These fibres are chemically protein fibres (keratin) similar to wool. The notable countries producing specialty animal fibres are China, South Africa, USA, Turkey, Australia, New Zeeland, France, Germany, Iran, Afghanistan, Mangolia, India, etc. The major users of specialty hair textile are USA, Germany, Italy, UK and other European countries. Fibres obtained from goat, camel and rabbit are also used by man either in pure form or blended with sheep's wool to produce special fabrics or articles of enhanced value. Nevertheless, these properties have secured firm places in the niche areas of luxury apparel and furnishing fabrics. The notable specialty fibres are Cashmere, Mohair, Yak, Angora rabbit hair, Camel hair, Alpaca, Vicuna, etc.

Vicuna is considered as endangered species because of over hunting in Andes area.

SOURCE AND UTILIZATION

The following animals are the rich sources of specialty hair fibres which are utilized for making value added products.

Cashmere Goat

Cashmere itself derives its name from the Kashmiri goats of Tibetan origin which are found in the mountainous regions and Himalayas. The hair obtained its fame through the beautiful cashmere shawls made from it in the mountain valleys of Kashmir. Cashmere goat (Fig. 11.1) is smaller than Angora goat. It is covered with straight coarse long guard hairs of outer coat with a fine soft under coat or down or under layer of hair.

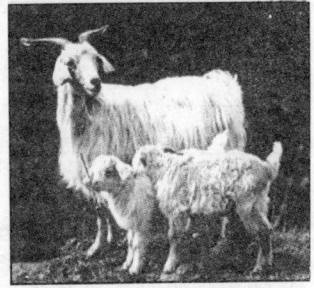

Fig. 11.1: Cashmere goat

The fibres vary in colour from white to gray to brownish gray. The specialty animal hair fibres are collected during molting seasons when the animals naturally shed their hair. Goats molt during second week period in spring.

The coarse hair and down hair of the Cashmere goat are separated by a mechanical process known as dehairing. Only a small part of the fleece is the very fine fibre, which comes up to 450 g of fibre per goat. Separation of the soft fibres from the long, coarse hair is tedious and difficult, contributing to the expense of the fabric.

Cashmere fibres have natural light weight and insulation without bulk. These hairs are extremely warm to protect goats from cold mountain temperatures. Fibres are highly adaptable and are easily woven into fine or thick yarns, with the end product as light to heavy weight fabrics. A high moisture content allows insulation properties to change with the relative humidity in the air.

The fibres are capable of dyeing to a broad range of colours and take dye equally as wool. The Knitwear Industry is the largest consumer of the Cashmere hair fibre. The soft hair is woven or knitted into fine garments and can also be blended with silk, cotton or wool. Shawls, dressing gowns, sweaters, dresses and long underwear have luxurious, silky, soft and triant texture, beautiful drape and rare wrinkles. The best quality Cashmere fibre comes from China.

Angora Goat: Mohair

Mohair is a hair covering of the Angora goat (Fig. 11.2). Angora goats originated in the Himalayas. Today the best raw material comes from South Africa. Australia currently contributes 4% and New Zealand only 2% of world Mohair production although the fibres produced in these areas is more lustrous than that obtained from more arid climate.

The brilliant, transparent texture of mohair has made it a valued material. The long, extraordinarily lustrous fibre is stronger and more resilient than sheep wool. Shearing time depends on the area of production. It dyes the best of all fibres and does not shrink. To improve fluffiness, it is blended with sheep wool or synthetics. One of the few natural fibres with multiple end-users, it can be blended into either upholstery, drapery or rugs, laces, wigs and hair piece, hosiery goods, shawls, suitings, etc. Mohair makes a better novelty loop yarn than wool or the other specialty hair fibres. It provides warmth during the winter months but also makes a cool suiting fabrics for the humidity of summers. One of the challenges facing the

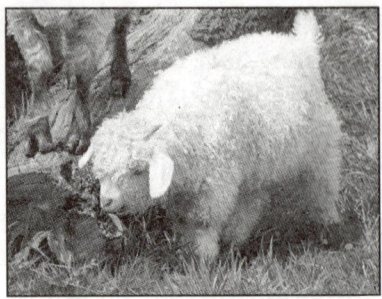

Fig. 11.2: Angora goat: Mohair

mohair industry particularly the knitting sector is that the fibre has been imitated by much cheaper acrylic yarns adulterating its high quality image.

Yak

Yak (Fig. 11.3) is widely used in mountainous region. Yak is found in China, India and Tibet. In India, Yak is an important animal of Ladakh region. It is also found in isolated pockets in Himachal Pradesh, Sikkim, Arunachal Pradesh and Garhwal hills of Uttaranchal. Yak also possesses two types of hairy coats, viz. outer coat long coarse hairs and under coat of fine wool fibres.

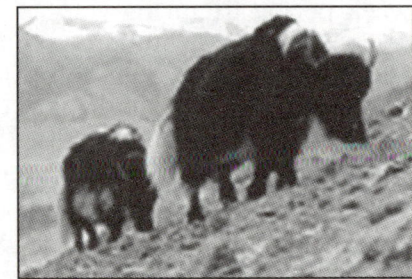

Yak hair is locally used for woven coverings for the huts, blankets, mats and sacks. Strong ropes are made from the tail hair. The fine down hair is also made into yarn comparable to cashmere hair fibres.

Fig. 11.3: Yak

Angora Rabbit

Angora rabbit hair fibre is finer and shorter in length as compared to woolen standards. Through blending, length of fibre can be increased. Angora rabbit have the characteristics of super whiteness, high bulk and warmth (Fig. 11.4). It is softer, finer and warmer than sheep's wool. China is by far the world's leading producer of Angora rabbit hair. Small amount is produced in East European countries. Individual yields are in average of 300 grams.

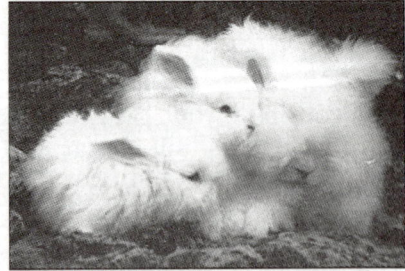

Fig. 11.4: Angora rabbit

The Angora fibre has a smooth silky texture which makes it difficult to spin. The fibre is preferred for its texture, warmth, light weight and pure white colour and it is primarily used for items such as sweaters, mittens and baby clothes. The international standard organization has given WA abbreviation for Angora wool where W stands for fine animal fibre and A for Angora rabbit. Therapeutic garments made from the blended yarn, are other sources of income to angora farmers.

Camel Hair

The camel hair is known for its natural colour and is comparatively coarser than other specialty hair fibres. The younger camels produce relatively finer and softer fibres. This fibre is mainly used for making *patties* for camel carts, rough floor coverings, etc. with appropriate technology and proper spinning techniques. Camel hair can be used for over coating, blankets and carpets through the combination of different fibre components which forms a blend.

FIBRE PROCESSING

Specialty hair fibres are finer, smoother and straighter than wool and lack cohesion which is due to absence of crimp that create problem in processing. This problem can be overcome by blending. Static charge development is also very high in these fibres. Flow chart 11.1 depicts their various stages of processing specialty hair fibres:

Flow chart 11.1: Stages of processing specialty hair fibre

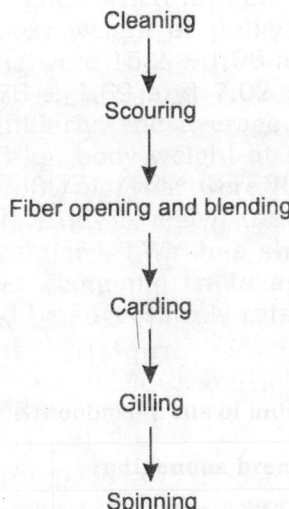

Cleaning
↓
Scouring
↓
Fiber opening and blending
↓
Carding
↓
Gilling
↓
Spinning

1. **Cleaning:** This is the first stage of process. Sand, dust and to some extent the vegetable matter are removed at this stage. This can be done manually.
2. **Scouring:** This process is done to remove the grease and suit present in the fibre. Less amount of detergent is used.
3. **Fibre opening and blending:** Fibres are opened and different fibers are blended at this stage in different ratios.
4. **Carding:** This is for making the fibres parallel or more parallel. The leftover material after scouring is removed as much as possible. After carding, wool opens up.

5. **Gilling:** Gilling straightens and aligns the fibres by drawing them through a bed of pins into the delivery rollers. Fibres are passed through gill box in order to prepare more homogenous tops for better spinning.
6. **Spinning:** In spinning operations of drawing/drafting, straightening of fibres, testing and winding of yarn into package of adequate shape and size are carried out.

Processing of fine wool is done on worsted system where fibre length is about 70 mm and diameter ranges 22–25 μ. If the length is shorter, there is a need to identify a system where such short and fine fibres can be processed. Ghandaria Charkha, Bageswari Charkha, Medlay and Electric spinner (Pant Charkha) are generally used in Indian Himalayas. With the advent of micro-processors and computer the control on yarn formation is possible. Some of them are siro spinning system, solo spun and self-twist spinning system, etc.

Weaving

Such prepared yarn can be woven into fabric on handloom or on a power loom. In either case, the fabric that is produced will be made by interlacing one yarn with another. Through weaving, aesthetic properties can be improved with reduction in cost which in turn will assure the availability of specialty hair fabric to more people at affordable rate.

These fibres are utilized in the cottage sector for manufacturing blankets, ropes, durries, etc. These fibres also have properties of warmth without weight. So sweaters, shawls, mufflers, tweeds, stoles are usually prepared from different specialty fibres and their blends.

USE OF SPECIALTY FIBRES FOR TECHNICAL TEXTILES

Technical textiles are the textile materials and products manufactured primarily for their technical and performance properties rather than their aesthetic or decorative characteristics. Specialty hair fibres provided for less versatile and economic for most industrial applications although it is still valued for its insulating and flame retardancy properties. It finds use in several high temperature and protective clothing applications. Wool and specialty hair fibres and their wastes in pure form or in blend with other fibres can be used in technical textiles.

It can be concluded that success of specialty fibres depends on the quality and productivity. Cost of production should be competitive with other countries with infrastructure for utilizing such fibres so that producer get remunerative price for their produce of specialty hair. Utilization of animal hair blends can be efficiently and profitably used in the decentralized sectors with the help of *Charkha* and other *Khadi* spinning units for enhancing small scale employment potential.

The market outlook for specialty hair fibre is good and can provide greater financial security. There are indications that fashion favours specialty animal hair fibres. Product and market development are priorities in various segments of the market, with developments in the furnishing textile sector holding exciting prospects for future demand. There is evidence of an increase in the use of specialty hair fibres in the production of hand knitting yarns. The introduction of new spinning technology could open new avenues for the use of specialty hair in weaving. The future prospects of these fibres, therefore, lies in exclusive, luxury *nitch* markets, quality conscious consumers at the very high income level. This market segment in term of specialty hair fibre is regarded as a growing market.

The specialty hair fibres have tremendous potential for encouraging the farmers revolutionizing the cottage industry and providing great scope for producing high value products by the industrial houses. It also helps in conserving the endangered species of various animals, which are proved to hunting sprees.

12

Entrepreneurship Development through Vermi-composting

KL Jeengar, Prakash Panwar, PM Khan

Entrepreneurship is a major component of economic development. Economic prosperity of any country depends on entrepreneurial competence. In India, about one-third of population lives under extreme poor condition and a large majority of them live under rural areas. Here, most of young people after basic education or matriculation search for employment in their areas but do not get the same. In order to improve their living condition and to increase their income, developing the capabilities of poor people for self-employment becomes paramount.

VERMI-COMPOSTING

Vermi-composting is a method of making compost with the use of earthworms, which generally lives in soil, eat biomass and excrete it in digested form. This compost is generally called vermi-compost or wormi-compost (Fig. 12.1). It is estimated that 1800 worms which is an ideal population for one square meter can feed on 80 tonnes of humas per year. Soil fauna play a prominent role in regulating soil processes and the termites and the earthworms play a vital role in maintaining soil quality and managing efficient nutrient cycling. In organic farming practices, the soil is considered to be a living component with physical,

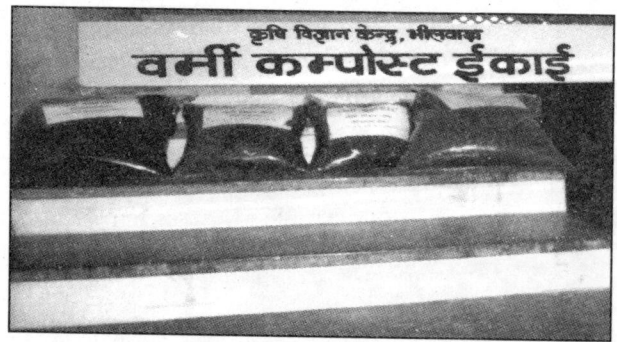

Fig. 12.1: Wormi-compost

chemical and biological characteristics. Vermi-composting and commercializing live material, indicate needs of developing mass earthworm culture. Vermiculture means scientific method of breeding and raising earthworms in controlled conditions (Figs 12.2 and 12.3). It aims at creating improved conditions artificially so that earthworms multiply in shortest possible time and space.

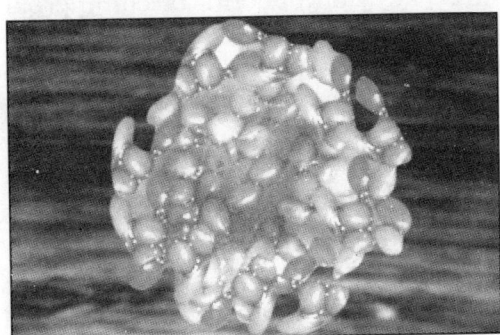 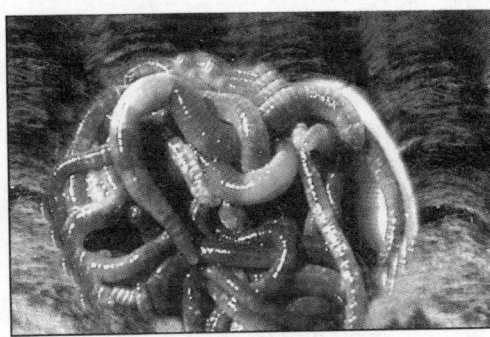

Figs 12.2 and 12.3: Vermiculture and earthworms

Some Facts about Vermiculture

- The art of composting has been part of our global culture since ancient time.
- Worms live where there is food moisture, oxygen and a favourable temperature.
- In one acre of land, there can be more than a million earthworms.
- Worms are cold blooded animals. They hatch from cocoons smaller than a grain of rice.
- Worms can sense light, especially at their anterior (front end). They move away from light and will become paralyzed if exposed to light for too long (approximately one hour). If worms skin dries out, it will die.
- Worms are hermaphrodites. Each worm has both male and female organs. Worm mate by joining their clitella (swollen area near the head of a mature worms) and exchanging sperm. Then each worm forms an egg capsule in its clitellum.
- Worms can eat their weight each day.
- Composting with worms avoids the needless disposal of vegetative food wastes and enjoy the benefits of a high quality compost. It is done with "redworms".

PROGRESS OF WORM INDUSTRY

Most people probably believe that worms are grown commercially for bait. While this has been the case for dozens of years, new applications for vermiculture - breeding earthworms - one now in use, and the demand for redworms is soaring. The tiny red worm, principally the species *Eisenia foetida*, is a powerful resource in waste reduction. Capable of conversing up to its own weight daily in organic waste, worms are now in use in the world at landfill diversion sites, converting yard trimming and other organic waste into worm casting—worm manure, which is highly prized soil amendment. Some sites are currently using 100,000 to 500,000 pounds of worms to convert tons of composted waste into vermi-compost—a highly valuable product, sold to nurseries, farmers, vegetable growers, orchard growers and gardens, etc.

Turning Garbage into Money

The money making potential of vermiculture is so attractive that it is rapidly becoming a growth industry. There are three key components of commercial vermiculture which explain its present and future potential.

1. Earthworms are capable of transforming huge amount of waste. For those who are raising worms for profit, the feed stock is generally plentiful and free. Typical feed stocks also consist of manure from a variety of animals: horses, cows, buffalloes, pigs, sheeps, etc.

2. The worms population can double in 2 to 4 months. Thus after acquiring an initial inventory as breeding stock, sales of worms can be realized in a relatively short time.

3. The production of vermi-compost is a highly prized soil amendment, sought by farmers, gardners and horticulturists. Studies about the nutrient-rich vermi-compost have proven its preferred value over ordinary compost and synthetic fertilizers. Vermi-compost dissolve slowly rather than allowing immediate nutrient leaching. The product has excellent soil structure, porosity, aeration and water retention capabilities. The product can insulate plant roots from extreme temperatures, reduce erosion and control weeds.

Earthworm farming can be done in a small, residential sized bin from recycling kitchen waste. An average of 5 to 10 minutes a day will do it. Nevertheless, one person can successfully manage quite a large number of worms, up to at least 3,000,000 to 5,000,000.

WHY VERMI-COMPOSTING?

Nowadays natural farming, such as organic farming, eco-agriculture, perma-culture, biodynamics agriculture, *Rizhi Kheti*, *Sadhu Kheti* is in vogue. They all agree in principle for least interference in nature system to raise healthy plants and animals. They all agree in limiting and in some cases eliminating use of artificial chemicals and heavy machinary in agriculture. They all aim at quality and nutritions nature of the farm produce.

The green revolution has resulted due to intensive agriculture with the extensive use of chemical fertilizer. The intensive agriculture practices boosted the production to feed the growing population in the underdeveloped countries. Farmers could harvest three crops in a year with good irrigation facilities. But there was no thought about its adverse effect in the long run on the soil condition in general and on the environment in particular for nearly four decades.

Fertilizers Use and Deterioration of Soil Environment

The fertilizers are the combinations of chemicals which are used to increase soil fertility. Nitrogen fertilizers that form the major components of the chemical fertilizers are usually the derivatives of petrochemicals. The run off from the fertilizer factories are carriers of atmospheric and water pollution. Precautionary measures have to be taken to avoid fire hazard and leakage of poisoning gases to atmospheric from these units.

The primary ingredient of the phosphorus fertilizer is the deposit in the earth crust. To minimize the cost of transport, the factories have to be setup near the mining sites. Only one-third of the raw material used in the production is recovered as the fertilizer and rest of the material is the waste, which causes disposal problem.

In general, the production of chemical fertilizers is leading to depletion of fossil fuel, causing environmental pollution and occupational hazards.

It is true that crops to nitrogen-based fertilizers show a spectacular response. But this is short lived and can result in subsequent crop failures unless it is followed by phosphorus and potassium fertilizers. In the years to come, the need for fertilizer quantity will increase to get the targeted yield. This clearly shows how the productivity of the soil is affected with indiscriminate use of fertilizers. These chemicals either leach or form complexes with metal ions to form undesirable complexes. Constant use of chemicals increases their leaching because of the depletion in pH of soils and they become less productive due to lack of good top soil. To restore the soil composition, farmers are now showing inclination to revert to organic farming. With this changing trend, it is necessary to produce the organic manure in large quantities from the available sources of organic matter to maintain the high level of produce in the available agricultural land. In this regard, because of the rapid organic fertilizer production locally at extremely low cost using all kinds of biodegradable waste materials, vermi-composting has great future.

NITROGEN AND HUMIFICATION IN VERMI-COMPOSTING

As regards total nitrogen, in all treatments and also at the different times, the net content decreased being more marked at the final stages when earthworm activity was higher. The different nitrogen fractions followed a similar tendency to the total nitrogen. In all treatments, at the final stages of the process, when the earth worm populations were bigger and active, important reductions of the organic nitrogen content and a high nitrification rate were observed.

VERMI-COMPOST—A QUALITY MANURE

Vermi-compost is the stable fine granular organic matter, when is added to clay soil it loosens the soil and provides the passage for the entry of air. The mucus associated with the cast being hygroscopic absorbs water and prevents water logging and improves water holding capacity. Sandy soil have less water retention capacity, the strong mucus coated aggregates of vermi-compost hold water for longer time. The organic carbon in vermi-compost releases the nutrients slowly and steadily into the system and enables the plant to absorb these nutrients. The soil enriched with vermi-compost provides additional substances that are not found in the chemicals. Vermi-compost improves physical, chemical and biological properties of soil in the long run on repeated application. The properties of vermi-compost which make it an ideal biofertilizer, enhance soil fertility in the long run on repeated application. The properties of vermi-compost which make it an ideal biofertilizer for the soil are:

- Vermi-composts have immobilized enzymes like protease, lipase, anylase, cellulose, lichenase and chitinase which keep on their function of bio-degradation of macro-molecules of the agricultural residues in the soil so that further microbial attack is speeded up.
- Vermi-compostings are rich in vitamins, antibiotics and growth hormones.
- Vermi-castings are free from pathogens.
- Vermi-castings have immobilized microflora which function in the soil to produce useful products.
- Vermi castings have earthworms cocoons and promote earth worm population in the soil thus ensuring continuous production of vermi-castings in the soil itself.
- Give structural stability to the soil.
- Absorb moisture from air.

Recycling of Wastes through Vermi-composting

Vermi technology is useful in recycling the agro-wastes. Nutrients present in vermi-compost are readily available and the increase in earthworm populations on application of vermi-compost and mulching lead to the easy transfer of nutrients to the plant providing synchrony in interfered ecosystems. The availability of biomass in the compost and the nutrients in soil tilled by earth worm are definitely more due to the formation of drilospheres.

Minimizing Pollution Hazard

Earth warm can minimize the pollution hazards caused by organic waste by enhancing waste degradation. The experiences of the farming community have shown that the exclusive use of chemicals to keep away the famine has turned out be a mirage.

Providing Growth Promotors

In the vermi-compost, some of the secretions of worms and the associated microbes act as growth promoters along with other nutrients. The multifarious effect of vermi-compost influences the growth and yield of crops.

Black Gold (Worm Casting) from Worms

Black gold (worm casting) is constantly in demand. Black gold is the most valuable type of fertilizer on the market, and because it is made of worm bi-product, it will continue to be an endless demand for consumers.

HOW VERMI-COMPOSTING

Vermi-composting Materials

The degradable and decomposable organic wastes commonly used as composting materials in vermi culture. Earthworm can be fed all forms of food waste, yard and garden waste leaves, grasses, straw and non-woody plant trimmings can be composted. Leaves are the dominent organic waste in most back yard compost piles. If grass clippings are used, it is advisable to mix them with other yard wastes, otherwise the clippings may compost and restrict airflow.

Animal Dung

Cattle dung, buffalo dung, sheep dung, horse dung and poultry dropping, etc. may be used for this purpose. The uses of horse dung should be done carefully because tetanus virus is common in horse dung and is lethal to humans.

Agricultural Waste

After harvesting and thrashing it may be used. It includes stems, leaves, husk (excepting paddy husk), peels, vegetable waste, orchard leaf litters, processed food waste, sugarcane brash and baggase and processing waste.

Forest Waste

These are wood clippings, peels, saw dusts and pulp. In addition of this, various types of forest leaf litter can also be used.

City Leaf Litter

The burnt leaf litter from residential areas may be used, however, reports are not available. If it is used, this would keep cities clean and would provide useful product. The leaf litter of mango, guava, grasses and certain weeds (free from seed) may be used, but we need more information on this aspect.

City Refuge

City refuge or garbage on daily production basis comprise important material which can be stored, recycled or composted. Most of household kitchen waste with little manipulation can be used for vermi-compost.

Biogas Slurry

After recovery of biogas, if not required for agricultural use, viz. in conventional composting can be used for vermi-composting.

Industrial Waste

The industrial waste from food processing, distillery, etc. can also be used in vermiculture with some manipulations.

More specifically following combinations can be used as feed for earthworms for vermiculture and vermi-composting. However, exact proportions may have to be adjusted with little pretesting.

- Biogas slurry with some leaf litters and some soil sprinkler over.
- Cow dung/buffalo dung + sheep dropping + horse dung mixed in equal quantities.
- Cow dung/buffalo dung + agricultural wastes in ration of 10:3.
- Mixed dung of cow dung + gram bran in ratio of 10:3.
- Cow dung or mixed dung + kitchen waste in ratio of 10:3.

- Cow dung or mixed dung + semi-flushed leaf litter in ratio of 10:3.
- Cow dung or mixed dung + sewage sludge in ratio of 10:3.
- Cow dung or mixed dung + vegetable waste in ratio of 10:3.
- Cow dung or mixed dung + wheat bran in ratio of 10:3.
- Old cow, buffalo dung of minimum 7 days.
- Weed leaves, grass clippings + cow dung or table waste + soil 70:15:15.
- Standard diet includes cow dung or mixed dung + gram bran + wheat bran + vegetable waste in ratio of 10:1:1:1 + some powdered egg shell.

Vermi-composting: General Procedures at Agricultural Farms

A 7–8 cm thick layer of hardy raw material, i.e. stovers, stubbles and locally available weeds (avoid seedling stage) is laid out in a bed of suitable size, i.e. not exceeding 3' in width and length according to materials availability. To this, a second layer of the same thickness comprising partially decomposed FYM or old cow or buffalo dung of 7 days, is added. A vermi-compost or vermiculture with dung carrier of 1.5 to 2 cm containing earthworm and cocoons (*E. foetida*) is spread on it. Now again 1' to 114' thick layer of cow or buffalo dung layer is added and provide light irrigation or sprinkle water to maintain a moisture of 60–80% and the last layer again 0.75' to 1' of partially decomposed bio-agri-waste material (3 to 4 days old cattle dung mixed with chopped waste of farm, vegetable, weed and plants, etc.) is spread at the top. This heap is then covered by jute cloth or gunny bags. Each layer is sprinkled with water and the frequency of water application be kept in such a way that 30 to 40% moisture can be maintained throughout the decomposition process. The temperature of heap must be monitored and it should not be exceeded from 35°C. The total height of the heap may be maintained about 2'–212' from the ground level (Figs 12.4 and 12.5).

Fig. 12.4: Vermi-compost heap

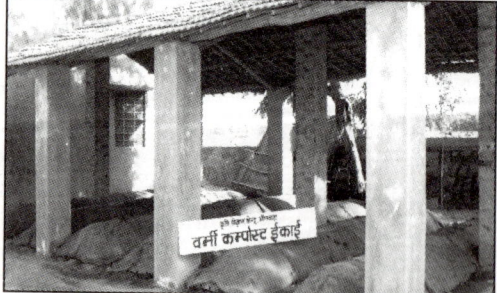

Fig. 12.5: Vermi-compost heaps covered with gunny bags

BUSINESS OF WORMS

The use of chemical fertilizers has increased the salinity of the soil, making it unpalatable to our worm, pesticides, in turn, kill indiscriminately, destroying the good with the bad.

Across the nation, farmers are developing their interest in vermi-composting because:

• Low start up costs—just worms and off the shelf supplies.
• No turning. Layout the manure, and the worms do the work.
• Completely natural biological process produces all organic material.
• Use existing equipment. It is simple, no special training required.
• Increase the value of manure to Rs 1500.00 per cubic yard or more.

Worms growing has been a commercial business for years. The industry started out for the fisherman but has since evolved for supplying worms to individuals who want to recycle their waste to fertilizer.

Comparing a large number of worm-related businesses, it is possible to categorize them according to three basic models the classic worm farm, the home vermi-composting business, and the resource recovery vermi-composting operations. Each one varies to the extent that it emphasizes production and sales of worm, supplies or castings.

First: The classic worm farm is primarily concerned with vermiculture, growing and raising earthworms for the huge fishing bait markets, as well as for home gardeners and farmers. Worm farms are often developed around a consistent source of animal manure. Today, the classic worm farm is still a thriving part of American economy. Worm farms are often maintained on small scale. Part time hobby farms are second sources of income for the farmers. The earthworm and castings farm are one of the largest vermiculture worm farms in North America.

Second: The increasing interest in home vermi-composting has given rise to another category of worm enterprise whose focus is on marketing worms, worm bins, kits, tools and educational materials for small scale vermi-composting.

Third: Vermi-composting for resource recovery, i.e. recycling of manure, yard and garden debris, food materials and biosolids, is one of the fastest growing sectors of the industry. Vermi-composting projects may be developed on site to manage organic wastes from a campus or other institution. As a commercial enterprise, vermi-composting operations depends on receiving revenue for managing the wastes and for the resulting vermi-compost.

A case study was carried out by two young farmers of village Nanudia, Panchayat Samiti (PS)-Banera of Bhilwara district. Before doing case study, training was imparted. For the purpose of imparting training, two young farmers from each PS were selected with the help of State Agriculture Deptt. who were interested to have training on vermi-composting at Krishi Vigyan Kendra. There were 11 PS. Thus total trainees were 22. One-week vocational training was given to the trainees in Oct. 2003.

During training programme, the trainees were motivated to take it as an enterprise so after 15 days two innovative young farmers of Banera Panchayat Samiti came back at KVK and asked for the establishment of units (Fig. 12.6). With the help of scientist, the units were established by use of 100 kg vermiculture.

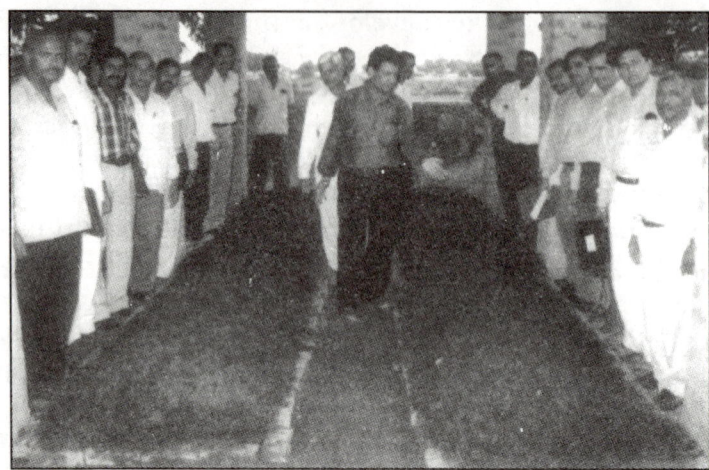

Fig. 12.6: Demonstration of Vermi-composting

The vermi-compost was ready after 45 days. After that they multiplied it and the detail record of income generation along with expenditure is given in Tables 12.1 and 12.2

Table 12.1: Income of units established during 2004-05

Name of the department	No. of units	Vermiculture kg/units	Rate/kg (Rs)	Amount (Rs)
1. Dept. of Agri., Rajsamand	50	4	250	50,000.00
2. Dept. of Agri., Bhilwara	100	2.5	250	62,500.00
3. Dept. of Agri., Chittorgarh	265	2.5	120	79,500.00
4. Dept. of Soil and Water Conservation, Bhilwara	45	2.5	250	28,125.00
			Total	2,20,125.00

Selling of vermi-compost: Sold 275 quintals of vermi-compost at the rate of Rs 4/00 per kg. and earned Rs 1,10,000.00. Thus total income = 2,20,125.00 (vermiculture) + Rs 1,10,000.00 (vermi-compost) = Rs 3,30,125.00.

Table 12.2: Expenditure during 2004-05

S. No.	Particulars	Quantity	Rate per unit (Rs)	Amount (Rs)
1.	Labour (assistant)	12 Months	1000.00	12000.00
2.	Cow dung with transport	24 Trolley	600.00	14400.00
3.	Water tanker	72 Tankers	150.00	10800.00
4.	Light and telephone	12 Months	1800.00	21600.00
5.	Extension activities (film show, pamphlets, folders, etc.)	12 Months	1000.00	12000.00

Table 12.2: Expenditure during 2004-05 *(Contd.)*

S. No.	Particulars	Quantity	Rate per unit (Rs.)	Amount (Rs.)
6.	Packaging materials	12 Months	–	19560.00
7.	Vermiculture and vermi-compost transportation expenditure	12 Months	–	10000.00
8.	Miscellaneous expenditure	12 Months	–	9500.00
			Total	**109860.00**

Net income = Income – Expenditure
330125.0 – 109860.00 = 220265.00

ECONOMIC VIABILITY

Vermi technology is popular because it is a simple methodology with low investment. This technology does not need sophisticated infrastructure. For composting yards all that is required is some pits or containers to initially decompose organic waste and tanks made out of stone slabs or wooden planks, trenches, plastic toughs to protect earth worms from pests and predators. Stone slab is subjected to availability, while plastic bins would be less durable and expensive. Thus, tanks built using cement and bricks could suit all situations. However, trenches without any cement are popular in low rainfall areas. Further, no or negligible cost is involved in developing vermiculture parks. The term park is used for the places which are different from composting yards. The park is an inventory of spaces over 1000 sq. meter with fencing and water supply facilities. They can be landscaped with tyres and the waste can be processed by earthworms under a cover of green manure (mulch). It does not smell any unpleasant odours. This method has been successfully tried at IIT, Mumbai, to convert the food waste from canteens into earthworm castings. The major benefit from vermiculture technology are:

- Effective utilization of non-toxic wastes as resource in meeting agricultural objectives.
- Has a potential to reduce dependencey on non-renewable input, i.e. chemical fertilizers, pesticides which also cost petro-dollars to the country.
- Potential for conversion of waste land into productive land.
- Optimum utilization of land, labour and water in agriculture.
- Effective environmental protection.
- Give quality produce which fetches better price in the market.

CONCLUSION

Entrepreneurship of worms is an eco-viable technology. It became popular because it is a simple methodology with low investment. This technology does not need sophisticated infrastructure. For composting yards all that is required is some area, bricks and roof. The method is also simple and can be easily understood by an uneducated person also.

13

Agriclinics and Agribusiness Centres for Promoting Agripreneurship

AK Thakur

Second half of 20th century witnessed the change of traditional and subsistence Indian agriculture into a commercial activity. Green revolution of sixties paved the way for entry of agribusiness companies selling seeds, fertilizers, pesticides and farm machineries. Today's farmer is different from yesterday. He is not depending upon agriculture for food alone, but to produce more marketable surplus to make more profit. He is depending on agriculture to meet his diversified growing needs born out of modernization, besides food. His expectations on extension are changing. There needs to be more extension focus on low cost technologies, high production technologies, value addition through processing, quality, price competitiveness and marketing. Revolution in information technology and role of mass media made the common men's access to the information easy and cost-effective. In light of this changed scenario, the expectation of the country from present extension system is also changing.

The pressure of changing role and additional responsibility on public extension has further added to its whole lots of existing problems like wide ratio between extension worker and farmer, inadequate infrastructure and finance. Hence, the existing gap is expected to enlarge. In the larger interest of the farmers, this gap has to be filled by private extension and already being filled to some extent. The extension services are mainly funded and delivered by government in Indian context. But, there are private players who also fund and deliver extension services. The process of funding and delivering the extension services by private individual or organization is called private extension. Today, considerable number of private extension service providers (PESPs) are there in the field who can influence the ultimate profit of the farmers. The genesis of private extension may be due to following reasons.

1. Inability of the public extension system to reach all the farmers, all the time, regarding all problems created the space which is gradually filled by private extension agencies.

2. The services which are not fully covered by public extension system are being covered by private extension system, e.g. input supply, market support and processing, etc.

3. The extension worker:farmer ratio is very wide, i.e. more than 1:1000.
4. Educational background and professional expertise of village level extension worker is very low.

Nowadays, the government is encouraging the participation of private sector in agriculture and animal husbandry research, extension, marketing, post-harvest management and human resource development (HRD). For public extension, it is very difficult to cater to the needs of all categories of farmers all the time. Thus, the gap created is field by public extension service providers (PESP) specially (1) in commercial crops like coffee, tea, grapes, and floriculture, (2) in areas like supply of inputs, processing and marketing, (3) in farmer's categories like commodity-based farmer's organization, big farmers and farmers in irrigated areas.

These sporadic activities are themselves product of either gap filling or substitution process. The space created by public extension is becoming as active ground for private extension. The gap filling/substitution process is expected to continue in the light of availability of huge space created by public extension services, World Trade Organization (WTO) and rapid commercialization in agriculture.

GENESIS OF AGRICLINICS AND AGRIBUSINESS CENTRES

In India through 32 agricultural universities and 4 deemed universities around 12,000 graduates in agriculture and veterinary sciences are passing out every year whereas only 2000 are getting employment in government and private sectors. Most of them go unemployed or search for jobs in private sectors or find avenues for self-employment. This is happening for many years in the recent past. With the announcement of the scheme on "agriclinics and agribusiness centres" by Govt. of India, it is now possible to utilize the potential of this large reservoir of unemployed agricultural graduates as private extension service providers (PESPs).

Agriculture is a key sector of Indian economy and plays crucial role in the livelihood of rural people. The development of trade, commerce and services in rural areas will depend on demand base arising from agriculture growth, faster industrialization and economy. The open as well as competitive agri-businesses take a pivotal place with its linkages to the world market. In this direction, a large pool of young agricultural graduates can provide a platform to establish a world market as well as the efficient services to farming community. The entrepreneurship development among the agricultural graduates is very essential to enable them to take up new ventures relating to agriculture. The entrepreneurial development programme (EDP) for agricultural graduates has three stages, viz.

1. Pre-training—identification and selection of potential entrepreneurs.
2. Training of potential entrepreneurs and
3. Post-training support and follow-up services (hand-holding facility).

Ideally speaking, separate training programmes have to be evolved to suit to the varying needs of different target groups. The justification for training is threefold. Firstly, to reinforce latent entrepreneurial spirit and to channelise it into new ventures; secondly, to build up confidence of 'first timers'; and thirdly to equip them to manage the units more successfully.

The Government of India recently announced the National Agricultural Policy which accords a very high priority in the areas, viz. application of frontier sciences, adequate and timely supply of quality inputs, strengthening of research and extension linkages and a broad base extension system to achieve a growth rate of more than 4% per annum in agricultural output. This gave an insight to launch a scheme for setting up of agriclinics and agribusiness. The scheme "Agriclinics and Agribusiness Centres by Agricultural Graduates" has been formulated by the Small Farmer Agribusiness Consortium (SFAC), New Delhi. The National Bank for Agriculture and Rural Development (NABARD) through its different branches is providing the financial assistance under the system. The National Institute of Agricultural Extension Management (MANAGE), Hyderabad is coordinating in organizing the training programme through selected institutes in the country.

The primary aim of launching the scheme is to supplement the extension network to accelerate the process of technology transfer to farmers; providing supplementary sources of inputs supply and services to needy farmers (for which farmers by and large presently depend upon state agencies) and providing gainful employment to agricultural graduates in new emerging areas in agricultural sectors.

The salient features of the programme are: (i) the participants should be graduate in agricultural science, (ii) should intend to start the agriclinic or agribusiness, (iii) should undergo two months residential training, (iv) providing free lodging and boarding facilities to participants (v) covering the contents relating to the financial and technical management and (vi) exposing the participants to the real agripreneur's situation. The project would provide the opportunity to take up the scheme to be stated as agriclinics and agribusiness by agricultural graduates either individually or on joint/groups basis. The outer ceiling for the cost of project by individual would be Rs 10 lakhs and for the project by group would be Rs 50 lakhs.

An ambitious yet pragmatic scheme of "Agriclinics and Agribusiness Centres" was launched on April 9, 2002. Being a centrally sponsored scheme, it has revolutionized the thinking in agricultural research, extension, marketing and in agriculture itself. Today's agriculture is witnessing commercialization and diversification at very rapid pace. Commercial agriculture needs more investment, high technology and various inputs which is opening up new opportunities for agri-business. Entrepreneurship development, innovation and value addition, processing and marketing outlets through agriclinics and agribusiness centres are going to make present extension system more responsive to farmer's needs, dynamic and rural employment oriented.

Aim of the Scheme

The programme aims at creating job producers rather than job seekers in agriculture sector. The scheme of agriclinics and agribusiness centres intends to provide financial assistance to unemployed agricultural graduates in terms of loan to launch agriclinics or agribusiness centres. Agriclinics are envisaged to provide expert services and advice to farmers on cropping practices, technology dissemination, crop protection from pests and diseases, market trends and prices of various crops in the markets and also clinical services for animal health as well as consultancy services for animal husbandry and dairying which would ultimately enhance the productivity of crops/animals. Thus, on the one hand, this scheme is bound to stimulate the agricultural growth and development, on the other hand it will tackle the growing problem of unemployment among graduates in agriculture/veterinary/animal sciences and other allied areas. With the diversification and modernization of agricultural practices, there is need to augment support and extension services for agriculture and its allied fields. For this purpose. a scheme for setting up agriclinics and agribusiness centres by graduates in agriculture/veterinary/dairying and allied fields has been launched with the support of NABARD. Agribusiness centres are envisaged to provide input supply, farm equipments on hire and other similar services. The Agriclinics centres would render consultancy services package of practices and clinical services for animal health, soil testing, protection of plants from pests and diseases, etc.

The scheme will strengthen transfer of technology and extension services and also provide self-employment opportunities to technically trained professionals in agriculture and its allied areas. Loans on attractive terms would be provided by banks, with reference from NABARD.

Demand Dimension

Finance Minister in his budget speech in 2001-02 announced "a scheme for financing and setting up of agriclinics and agribusiness centres by agricultural graduates has been formulated by NABARD. The scheme aims at supplementing the existing extension network to accelerate the process of technology transfer to agriculture and providing supplementary sources of input supply and services for which farmers by and large presently depend upon state agencies".

In order to accelerate the diffusion of agricultural technology there is a need for:
1. Supplementing the efforts of Govt. extension system to accelerate the process of technology transfer in agriculture.
2. Supplementary sources of input supply and services for which by and large farmers presently depend upon public sector agencies.

This scheme would lead to multi-sourced extension services and ensure input supply and support services on commodity basis. This scheme will supplement existing extension and technical support systems because of following reasons.
1. Government is not equipped for rendering location specific specialized crop-wise advice.
2. Field level staffs are neither exclusively available for extension work nor adequately qualified and trained.
3. Public sector input supply agencies are not able to cope with the needs of fast transforming and accelerated pace of agricultural production.
4. Specialized agri-services (e.g. soil and input testing, maintenance and repairs, seed/agro-processing, agricultural insurance, technology information, post-harvest management, etc.).

SUPPLY DIMENSION

These gaps can be filled by qualified private entrepreneurs.

1. The annual out-turn of graduates in agriculture and allied subjects is around 12,000.
2. The intake in post-graduate programmes is 5500, leaving about 6500 graduates of which about 2000 are able to find employment, both in government and in the private sector.
3. Thus, a huge qualified manpower of around 10,000 graduates every year is available for supporting agricultural production process, if viable business opportunities are made available.

FRAMEWORK OF THE SCHEME

Extension of equal opportunities to all eligible agricultural graduates to undertake economically viable ventures in identified areas through a network of agriclinics and agribusiness centres wherein the applicant graduate would be a stakeholder.

1. The scheme will provide opportunities for self-employment to agricultural graduates (in agriculture and allied activities).
2. The scheme will promote investment in agriculture and allied activities and create the support services required by the farmers and help in the application of productivity enhancing technologies in their areas of operation.
3. The NABARD through its system will facilitate bank credit for this purpose on priority sector lending terms.
4. Ministry of Agriculture, Government of India has envisaged extending credit linked back-ended subsidies for identified ventures. The subsidy is presently under consideration.
5. Funding of the scheme at present will be according to guidelines issued by NABARD.
6. SFAC will arrange training for 6/8 weeks duration free of cost to those who apply for loan under this scheme.
7. The training programme will comprise of entrepreneurship and business management training as well as skill improvement and propagation in the chosen area of activity.
8. The bank credit, as per the scheme, will be extended to the entrepreneurs on specific terms and conditions only on completion of training programme.
9. To begin with, a programme of supporting 5,000 ventures per year with investment up to Rs 10 lakhs per venture has been envisaged.
10. Group venture ceiling is Rs 50 Lakhs for a group of five, in which one could be a management graduate.

Activity Areas

In order to enhance viability of the ventures, agricultural graduates may also take up the projects in agriculture and allied areas along with agriclinics and agribusiness centres. Any graduate in agriculture or allied fields are eligible to avail the scheme. The project may be taken up by agricultural graduate individually or on joint/group basis involving maximum five entrepreneurs. The group could also involve a member who is a management graduate or persons with experience in business development and management.

Agriclinics and agribusiness ventures could provide specialized agri-services in the following areas.

- Soil and water quality cum inputs testing laboratories (with advanced analytical equipments, some including atomic absorption spectrophotometers, etc.).
- Crop protection services, including pest surveillance, diagnostic and control services (with culture rooms, autoclaves, microscopes, ELISA kits, etc. for detection of plant pathogens including viruses, fungi, bacteria, nematodes, and insect pests).
- Micro-propagation including through plant tissue culture labs and hardening units.
- Maintenance, repairs and custom hiring of agricultural implements and machinery including micro-irrigation systems (Sprinkler and drip).
- Seed processing units.
- Setting up of vermiculture units, production of bio-fertilizers, bio-pesticides, and other bio-control agents.
- Setting up of Apiaries (bee-keeping) and honey and bee product's processing units.
- Provision of extension consultancy services.
- Facilitation and agency of agricultural insurance services.
- Hatcheries and production of fish fingerlings for aquaculture.
- Provision of livestock health cover, setting up of veterinary dispensaries and services including frozen semen banks and liquid nitrogen supply.
- Setting up of information technology Kiosks in rural areas for access to various agriculture related portals.
- Feed processing and testing units.
- Value addition centres.
- Setting up of cool chain from the farm level onwards including small rural cold storage units.
- Post-harvest management centres for sorting, grading, standardization, storage and packaging.
- Setting up of metallic/non-metallic storage structures (group activity).
- Retail marketing outlets for processed agri-products.
- Rural marketing dealerships of farm inputs and outputs.
- Other activities like mushroom production, dairy farming, etc. too may be undertaken.
- Any combination of two or more of the above viable activities along with any other economically viable activity selected by the graduates, which is acceptable to the Bank.

AGRIPRENEURSHIP

With the success of an innovative approach for entrepreneurship promotion in agriculture, "Network of agriclinics and agribusiness centres by Agricultural

Graduates Scheme" of the Department of Agriculture and Cooperation, Ministry of Agriculture being implemented by SFAC, New Delhi and MANAGE, Hyderabad has covered different regions of the whole country.

The majority of the population in India is dependent on agriculture and allied occupations. In view of the increasing population and reducing opportunities in rural areas, the problem of unemployment has become severe among educated rural youths. In rural areas, since 25 years, majority of the educated young people came from agriculture community or background, but due to many reasons they have not been able to compete for available jobs, which demand specialized skills and knowledge. Even in their attempts to set up small entrepreneurial activities in non-farm sectors they face many problems generally not encountered by such youths in urban areas.

All these rural youths can now be supported for new opportunities of entrepreneurship in business activities related to agriculture. These rural youths have the basic understanding of agriculture, which can be utilized for promotion of business enterprises revolving around agricultural activities. Most of the unemployed youths are also willing to take up self-employment activities which is a definite positive sign. With support also coming from the Government, only small efforts with appropriate linkages can help them to be gainfully employed as agripreneurs.

It is now also realized that the agriculture during the last 10 years has been exploitative in nature. This has resulted in increased cost of cultivation. The solution to this problem can be provided by giving technologies which can improve on-farm-fertility management for the farmers. The recent development in biotechnology for agriculture is now offering many new innovative options to help the farmers in increasing their net income. The agribusiness enterprises would thus be able to provide linkages for processing for value addition.

CONCLUSION

The scheme of "agriclinics and agribusiness centres" has completed the first cycle of training programme successfully. It has already met the main objectives namely supplementing general public extension services while providing specialized extension services to farmers. In the process, it has created self-employment opportunities for unemployed agricultural graduates. The scheme has exploded many myths during its first cycle of training programme. More than 112 success stories have been recorded as a positive outcome of first phase of this scheme. It disproved the myth that agricultural graduates are waiting for government jobs forever and farmers are not in a position to pay for their services. Generally, the strategies suggested for entrepreneurship development amongst unemployed agricultural graduates consist of stimulatory, supportive and sustaining activities. The stimulatory activities refer to all such activities related to creating entrepreneurial awareness and entrepreneurial motivation. For creating entrepreneurial awareness amongst unemployed agriculture graduates and motivating them as agribusiness operators, vigorous efforts should be made by all concerned agencies in coordinated manner.

14

Gender Role in Animal Husbandry Enterprises

Prakash Singh, Anupam, B Mishra

In India livestock rearing is a subsidiary enterprise for many rural households for generating additional income along with crop production. Being a predominantly agriculture economy, India has the largest livestock population in the world. Presently, the livestock sector accounts for about 21% of the values of out put of the combined crops and livestock sectors. Women's role in livestock keeping is an old age tradition and play a major role for rearing animals as much of the work of livestock management is carried out by women. However, the development, extension and training programmes are generally much less for involvement of women and for extending the benefit to them (Singh and Vitanen, 1987).

In Indian economy, farm business including animal husbandry (AH) has been family enterprise in which male and female share both work and wages. Their roles are complementary, not only in physical participation at farm and home-related activities, but also in respect of decision making process concerning such activities. Role of males is dominant and authoritative while that of women is subtle and persuasive. Outwardly, decision making is the prerogative of male head of the farm family, but any such decision taken is strongly influenced by the attitude and opinion of the female partner. An example of block contribution of women in animal husbandry in Milkipur of Faizabad district of Uttar Pradesh has been presented under the following headings:

1. The socio-economic profile of the respondents.
2. The extent of involvement of gender in animal husbandry enterprise.
3. Problem of gender regarding their involvement in AH practices.

For this purpose, the scale suggested by Kanwar and Kharde (1994) was used with some modifications.

Socio-economic Profile of the Respondents

The mean age of the respondents was noted to be 43.35 years with literacy percentage of 26. About half of them belonged to scheduled caste category. Agriculture was the main occupation of maximum families of respondents having marginal land with an average of 1.28 acres. More than 50% were found residing in nuclear families having 6 to 10 members in their families with a mean of 7.72 members. Almost nil participation was observed in social organizations. The material possession was observed of medium level. Majority of respondents had herd size of 1.2 to 5. The mean score of socio-economic status (SES) was found to be 39.74. Social mobility was very low. The medium level economic motivation was observed with 24.99 mean of scores.

Overall Extent of Involvement in Animal Husbandry Practices

Table 14.1 indicates that more percentage of females was observed performing daily practices either actual doing or supervision while in occasional practices in which more involvement of males was observed. In decision making about animal husbandry practices, the involvement of males was more in comparison to females.

Table 14.1: Overall involvement of gender in animal husbandry practices

Gender	Involvement extent (%)					Average
	Actual doing		Supervision		Decision-making	
	DP	OP	DP	OP		
Male	44.00	70.00	44.00	63.00	61.00	56.40
Female	56.00	30.00	56.00	37.00	39.00	43.60
Total	100.00	100.00	100.00	100.00	10.00	100.00

DP—Daily practices, OP—Occasional practices

Practicewise Extent of Involvement in Animal Husbandry Practices

As far as practicewise role performance by the males and females was concerned (Table 14.2), the maximum percentage of involvement of males in actual doing (daily practices) was found in case of 'chaffing of fodder', 'tieing and untieing the

Table 14.2: Practicewise involvement of gender in animal husbandry practices

Practices	Extent of involvement (%)			
	Male		Female	
	Actual doing	Supervision	Actual doing	Supervision
(A) Daily practices				
Cleaning the shed	18.00	26.00	82.00	74.00
Bathing animals	47.00	49.00	53.00	51.00
Arrangement of green fodder	44.00	48.00	56.00	52.00
Bringing fodder from field for chaffing	50.00	51.00	50.00	49.00
Chaffing of fodder	55.00	54.00	45.00	46.00

Table 14.2: Practicewise involvement of gender in animal husbandry practices *(Contd.)*

Practices	Extent of involvement (%)			
	Male		Female	
	Actual doing	Supervision	Actual doing	Supervision
Feeding of animals	39.00	45.00	61.00	55.00
Offering water to animals	49.00	45.00	61.00	55.00
Tieing and untieing the animals	52.00	51.00	48.00	49.00
Milking	55.00	49.00	50.00	51.00
Selling of milk	56.00	46.00	44.00	54.00
Preparation of milk and milk products	-	1.00	100.00	99.00
Grazing the animals	79.00	60.0	21.00	40.00
Average	**44.25**	**43.75**	**54.75**	**56.25**
(B) Occasional practices				
Care of animal at calving	56.00	53.00	44.00	47.00
Care of animals after calving	56.00	54.00	44.00	46.00
Taking sick animals to vet. dispensary	97.00	76.00	3.00	24.00
Protection of animals from bad weather	58.00	56.00	42.00	44.00
Taking in-heat animals for breeding	99.00	69.00	1.00	31.00
Purchase of animals	99.00	81.00	1.00	19.00
Selling of animals	98.00	81.00	2.00	19.00
Feeding of calves	47.00	51.00	53.00	49.00
Care of neonatal calves	47.00	52.00	53.00	48.00
Littering	50.00	53.00	50.00	47.00
Average	**69.80**	**62.62**	**30.20**	**37.40**

animals', 'milking', 'selling of milk' and 'grazing the animals'. But, in other practices, females were found to be dominated for performing them. In case of occasional practices 'feeding of calves' and 'care of neonatal calves' were observed dominantly performed by the females' while other practices like 'care of animals at calving', 'after calving', 'taking sick animals to veterinary dispensary, etc. predominately performed by the males. The overall degree of role performance by males was found to be 44% in case of daily practices whereas, by females it was 55% and 50% for occasional practices. Almost similar pattern was observed in case of supervision of daily practices as well as occasional practices.

Involvement in Decision-making about Animal Husbandry Practices

Table 14.3 shows the involvement of males and females in decision-making regarding animal husbandry practices to be adopted by them. The males were found dominant in most of the management practices except 'care and feeding of livestock' and 'responsibility for cleaning of animal sheds'. The overall involvement of males and females in decision making was observed to be 58.30% and 41.70%, respectively.

Table 14.3: Involvement pattern of gender in decision-making about animal husbandry practices

Particulars	Male	Female
Livestock to be raised	71.00	29.00
Equipment needed	70.00	30.00
Size and location of housing	76.0	24.00
Fodder production	70.00	30.00
Marketing/consumption of animal products	50.00	50.00
Disposal of excess and non-productive animals	70.00	30.00
Care and feeding of livestock	45.00	55.00
Preventive measures to protect livestock	59.00	41.00
Type of disease treatment	60.00	40.00
Weaning and care of young ones	53.0	47.00
Responsibility for cleaning of animals shed	27.00	73.00
Milking of animals	52.00	48.00
Average	**58.30**	**41.69**

Problems of Gender regarding Involvement in Animal Husbandry Practices

The problems relating to involvement in animal husbandry (AH) practices as perceived by the respondents have been assessed and given in the Table 14.4 according to the ranks mentioned against each problem in descending orders.

Problems of Gender regarding Decision-making about Animal Husbandry Practices

In the same way, the problems relating to decision-making about AH practices have been mentioned in the Table 14.5 according to the ranks mentioned against each problem in descending orders.

Conclusion

On the basis of above data, it may be concluded that more percentage of females was observed performing daily practices either actual doing or supervision but in occasional practices males were dominant. In decision making, the overall involvement of males was more. Therefore, it can be said that there is scope for women to handle the animal husbandry as family enterprises to enhance the economic condition and well-being of their family.

Table 14.4: Problems of gender regarding their involvement in animal husbandry (AH) practices

S. No.	Problems	Percentage	Rank order
1.	There are gender specific tasks or degree of work specialization in outdoor activities of animal husbandry like taking 'in heat' animals to breeding, purchase and selling of animals, taking sick animals to veterinary dispensary, etc.	100.00	I
2.	Lack of technical know how.	93.00	II
3.	Since, the male spent more time with the animals at the animal shelter therefore, there is more involvement of male, in comparison to female	70.00	III
4.	Men think that women is meant for only indoor house work	63.00	IV
5.	Drudgery in many practices of animal husbandry like chaffing of fodder, bringing fodder from field for chaffing, etc.	45.00	V
6.	Higher educated male and female do not want to participate in animal husbandry practices.	44.00	VI
7.	Presence of old women for doing work relating to animals.	36.00	VII
8.	The women are too busy in raising their children and household activities and therefore, cannot participate as much as they would like to do work relating to animal husbandry.	30.00	VIII
9.	Less exposure of women to outside world.	16.00	IX
10.	Women are not allowed to work because of family prestige.	13.00	X
11.	Presence of more member of males in the family hence, they do not give opportunity for doing work and supervise various activities.	5.00	XI

Table 14.5: Problems of gender regarding their involvement in decision-making about animal husbandary (AH) practices

S. No.	Problems	Percentage	Rank order
1.	Due to some gender specific tasks, the decision are taken accordingly which restricts the involvement of female.	98.00	I
2.	Women's thinking is that 'men know better than us' or it's men's job.	74.00	II

Table 14.5: Problems of gender regarding their involvement in decision making about A.H. practices. *(Contd.)*

S. No.	Problems	Percentage	Rank order
3.	Since, the male spent more time with the animals in the animal shelter therefore, there is more involvement of male, compared to female in animal husbandry practices.	70.00	III
4.	Men think that women's work is cooking, caring of children and other household activities. They can take decisions about these matters but not in animal rearing.	63.00	IV
5.	Women are not self-dependent. They are dependent on men for their livelihood	43.00	V
6.	Presence of old/senior women in the family, works as barriers to women's involvements in decision making.	36.00	VI
7.	Males usually go outside for their daily works hence, they could not take part in decision making.	35.00	VII
8.	Less exposure of women to outside world, hence, they lag behind the men.	16.00	VIII
9.	In the male dominating society, it hurts man's ego when they take advice from women.	15.00	IX
10.	The husbands mostly have works outside the village. Therefore, most of the decisions are taken by the women after consulting her children.	13.00	X
11.	Presence of more number of male in the family hence, they do not give opportunity for giving decisions on various aspects.	5.00	XI

Some Suggestion based on Findings

On the basis of results, following suggestions may be made to accelerate the involvement of gender in actual doing, supervision and decision making about animal husbandry practices so that animal husbandry can be established as family enterprise in rural areas:

1. There is a need to devise an educational/vocational training programme especially for women in the society to enhance the technical know-how about animal husbandry enterprise.

2. Importance of self-employment through animal husbandry should be realized and acknowledged by the development personnels and the farmers should be motivated accordingly.

3. The appropriate animal husbandry technologies should be developed for farm women to increase their involvement, if innovated to emancipate women from the drudgery in undertaking animal husbandry operations.

4. The value of money for family survival should be propagated among rural women so that they may be motivated towards animal husbandry enterprise to have more money.

5. There is a need of women oriented development programmes for improving the status of women in rural areas and make them more meaningful member of the society.

6. There is a need to make the menfolk in particular aware with the work load being carried out by women so that they may be more conscious of it and to strike out a balance.

7. The participation of females in the social organization seems very low in comparison to males. Thus, organisational and institutional infrastructure facilities should be created for active participation of females.

8. The females should be provided more opportunities by the males for more involvement in outside activities. The women should get freedom in decision making and supervisory role in their families especially in animal husbandry enterprise. For creating such environment, some of the old conservative cultural values, social customs and systems must give way to modern values and working milieu.

15

Women Empowerment: Systems and their Effect on Development of Women Entrepreneurship

Nirmal Kaur, Deepa Vinay, Shalini Agarwal

It is believed that economic strength is the basis of social, political and psychological power in the society. Thus, the lower status of women mostly stems from their low economic status and subsequent dependence and lack of opportunity for decision-making power. Therefore, if women gain economic strength, they gain visibility and voice.

Among the various approaches, the empowerment approach in development programmes is considered best. This approach is modeled to 'power' itself and gain control over the self, the resources and freedom to decide. This process of gaining control over the self, the resources and the decision-making power may be termed as empowerment. Ideally, the empowerment process should aim at "women finding time and space of their own" and should provide mechanisms for their active participation in the development process.

Entrepreneurship can help women's economic independence and improve their social status. Automatically, the women get empowered once they attain economic independence. The development of women entrepreneurship enables society to understand and appreciate their abilities. It enhances their status and leads to integration of women in nation building and economic development. It provides the needed psychological satisfaction and imbibes a deep sense of achievement to create their enhanced identity in society.

A woman entrepreneur is a recent phenomenon of late 1960's. Earlier women were involved in self-employment, mostly making home products like pickles, papad or handicrafts items which could be produced on a very small scale at home to earn money to support the scanty family income.

But self-employment is different from the entrepreneurship. Self-employment does not provide employment to others. An enterprise provides employment for self (entrepreneurs) as well as to others thus helping to reduce the unemployment problems of the nation.

A woman entrepreneur can be defined as a confident innovative person capable of organizing production, undertake risk and handle economic uncertainty to achieve self-economic independent individual or in collaboration generate employment opportunities for others through initiating and running of an enterprise by keeping pace with her personal family and social life.

Some called an entrepreneur an agent of change—a catalyst who transformed physical, natural and human resources into production possibilities. In recent years, managerial aspects of entrepreneurship are being emphasized.

A person involved in a business activity where the person sells a product/service and makes profit is an entrepreneur. This may include manufacturing, trading or service oriented business (i.e. laundry, restaurant, petrol pump, etc.). Whatever may be the activity, entrepreneurship has two distinct aspects – one is the entrepreneur herself and the other is the enterprise.

It has to be stressed that people are the most valuable resources within any country. There appears to be a strong linkage between the training, attitude and goals of people and the level of economic growth of a country. An essential ingredient in the economic growth of any country is thus the key individuals who promote change and development. These persons may be called entrepreneurs.

An entrepreneur may be defined as a person who is able to scan the environment, marshall resources and implement action to bring into existence a commercial venture. A commercial venture is profit oriented and which adds value to inputs in an economic sense. In its broadest turn, entrepreneurs (men and women) are persons who initiates and establish larger/medium/small enterprises. They may set up co-operatives for production of goods or even run their own cottage industries. They are all engaged in the business activity of selling products and services and making profit.

Whereas entrepreneurship can be described as a creative and innovative response to the environment. Such responses can take place in any field- business, industry, agriculture and the like. Doing new things or doing things that are already being done in new ways.

ENTREPRENEURSHIP

When taking up the task of establishment of a venture—whatever may be the activity, whether manufacturing, trading or service, there are two distinct aspects: one is an entrepreneur and the other is the enterprise. The process of creating an enterprise by creating an entrepreneur is entrepreneurship.

Entrepreneur + Enterprise = Entrepreneurship

On the basis of so many definitions given by different authors it may be stated that the entrepreneur is perceived as an individual with certain characteristics helpful in conceiving, initiating, establishing, running and finally managing an enterprise. An enterprise can vary from starting a small shop to establishing an advanced technology based industry. An entrepreneur therefore, may be differentiated not only in terms of the kind of activities he/she pursues but in the context of his lifestyle, attitudes, values and behaviours, which together go to make the entrepreneurial personality.

For developing women entrepreneurs in the last decade, the analysis of the development process that helps women to opt for entrepreneurial carrier and finally succeed in setting up and running of the enterprise, reveals that it follows a sequence of development in individual ability and capability.

The first generation women entrepreneur requires (Fig. 15.1):
a. Knowledge for enterprise building
b. Managerial skills
c. Entrepreneurial attitude and behavioural skills/competencies
d. Motives and motivation.

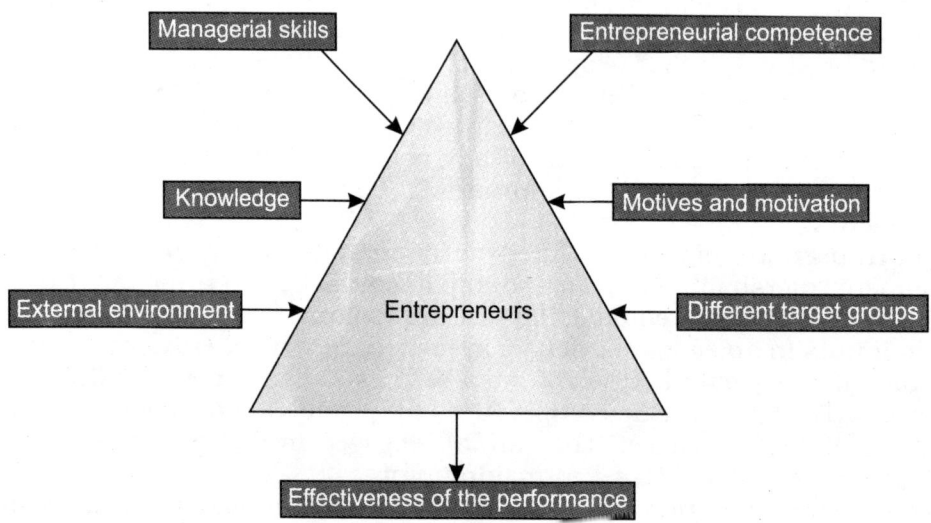

Fig. 15.1: Rational for selecting women entrepreneur

Characteristics of an Entrepreneur

Entrepreneurship development is an accepted, well-known tool for small industries/business development. The traditional approaches to entrepreneurship adopted by scholars and practitioners, regard it as being a personality type, and as a spontaneous reaction to the presence of economic opportunity. By implication, these approaches view the quantity and quality of entrepreneurial activity at any given place and time to be relatively fixed. As such, these approaches have little to contribute to the strategy for stimulating and promoting entrepreneurship other than to suggest broad reforms intended over time to alter the nature of the entrepreneurial environment.

The new approach regards entrepreneurship as a set of behaviours and practices which can be observed and acquired. The proclivity and facility, with which an individual evidences these behaviours and practices, might indeed be strongly conditioned by his or her genes, family background, culture or economic environment, but the behavioural approach to entrepreneurship suggests that such proctivities and facility can, however, be strengthened in individuals by approtiate exposure and training.

Critical to any effort to detect and strengthen entrepreneurial potential is a clear accurate identification of the specific and observable behaviours associated with successful entrepreneurship.

Drive and Energy

Entrepreneurs have a tremendous amount of personal energy and drive. They possess a capacity to work for long hours and in spurts of several days, with less than a normal amount of sleep.

Self-confidence

There is also agreement that successful entrepreneurs have a high level of self-confidence. They tend to believe strongly in themselves and their abilities to achieve the goals they set. They also believe that events in their lives are mainly self-determined, and they have a major influence on their personal destinies, and have little belief in fate.

Long-term Involvement

This is one of the characteristics, which distinguish the entrepreneur – the creator and builder of a business – from the promoter or fast – buck artist. Entrepreneurs who create high potential ventures are driven to build a business, rather than simply get in and out in a hurry with someone else's money. They make a commitment to a long-term project and to working towards goals that may be quite distant in the future.

Money as a Measure

Money has a very special meaning to the successful entrepreneur; it is a tool and a way of keeping score. Profits, capital gains and net worth are seen as measures of how well the entrepreneur is doing in pursuit of self-established goals.

Persistent Problem-solving

Entrepreneurs who successfully build new enterprises possess an intense level of determination and desire to overcome hurdles, solve a problem and complete the job.

Goal-setting

Entrepreneurs are very goal-oriented. They have an ability and commitment to set clear goals for themselves. These goals tend be high and challenging, but they are realistic and attainable. Entrepreneurs are doers; they are goal and action oriented.

Moderate Risk-taking

The successful entrepreneur prefers to take moderate, calculated risks where the chances of winning are neither so small as to be a gamble nor so large as to be a sure thing.

Dealing with Failure

Entrepreneurs are not afraid of failing. Being more intent on succeeding, they are not averse to the possibility of failing. The persons who fear failure will neutralize whatever achievement motivation they may possess. They will tend to engage in a very easy task, where there is little chance of failure; or in a very difficult situation, where they cannot be held personally responsible if they did not succeed.

Use of Feedback

Entrepreneurs, as high achievers, are very concerned about doing well. This concern is responsible in part for this entrepreneurial characteristic. Use of feed-back without information or feedback about performance, the entrepreneur cannot know how well or poorly he or she is doing. Successful entrepreneurs demonstrate a capacity to seek and use feedback on their performance in order to take corrective action and to improve.

Taking Initiative and Seeking Personal Responsibility

The entrepreneur has historically been viewed as an independent and highly self-reliant innovator, the champion of the free enterprise economy.

Use of Resources

Several studies have emerged in recent years, which show that successful entrepreneurs know when, and how to seek outside, as well as inside, help in building their companies. Successful entrepreneurs seek expertise and assistance needed in the accomplishment of their goals.

Competing against Self-imposed Standards

Competition with self-imposed standards is an internalized kind of competition. High performing entrepreneurs also possess this internalized competitive spirit in which he/she continuously engages in competition with himself/herself to beat their last best performance.

Internal Locus of Control

The entrepreneur does not believe the success or failure of a new business venture depends mostly upon luck or fate, or other external personally uncontrollable factors.

Tolerance of Ambiguity and Uncertainty

Entrepreneurs have long been viewed as having a special tolerance for ambiguous, situations and for making decisions under conditions of uncertainty.

Initiative

Does things before being asked or forced to by events. Takes action that go beyond job requirements or the demands of the situation. Acts to extend the business into new areas, products or services.

Sees and Acts on Opportunities

Sees and acts on new or unusual business opportunities. Seizes unusual opportunities to obtain financing, equipment, land, work space or assistance.

Persistence

Takes repeated actions to meet a challenge or overcome an obstacle. Switches to an alternative strategy to reach a goal.

Information-seeking

Takes action on her own to get information to help achieve objectives or clarify problems. Personally seeks information on clients, suppliers, competitors. Uses personal and business contacts or information networks to obtain useful information.

Concern for High Quality, Innovation and Efficiency

Looks for or find ways to do things better, faster, or cheaper. Acts to do things that meet or exceed standards of excellence or improve on past performance.

Commitment to Work Contract

Places the highest priority on getting a job completed. Accepts full responsibility for problems in completing a job. Makes a personal sacrifice or expands extraordinary effort to complete a job. Pitches in with workers or work in their place to get a job done.

Systematic Planning

Develops and uses logical, step by step plans to reach goals. Plans by breaking a large task down into sub-tasks. Keeps financial records and uses them to make business decisions.

Persuasion

Uses deliberate strategies to influence or persuade others. Uses business and personal contacts as agents to accomplish own objectives. Asserts strong confidence in one's own products or services.

Use of Influencing Strategies

It uses a variety of strategies to influence or persuade others to accomplish their own objectives and acts to develop business contracts.

Women entrepreneurs, because of the peculiar socio-cultural background, especially in the developing countries, need all the more attitudinal and behavioural changes in order to succeed in entrepreneurial activity. The WEDP designed by ICECD has, therefore, being upgraded from the one existing for a long time, without considering the women specific issues and approach needed.

Different Kinds of Systems and their Effect on Entrepreneurship Development

Self-sphere System

Self-sphere system is composed of personal characteristics, qualities and capabilities of self-employed women, such as age, education experience, etc. which can never be identical with other self-employed women. Usually, the middle age group persons enter in this system.

Socio-psycho Sphere System

Socio-psycho sphere is conceptualized as a specific set and social conditions and particular psychological characteristics and will include motivation, social participation, SES and caste, etc. Socio-psycho sphere system consists of socio-economic scale, family occupation, land holding, cost, possession, etc. Does not have much effect or does not guaranty even although it facilitates and help a person to participate in entrepreneurial activities. The study reveals that involvement of medium income and low income level are more in entrepreneurial activities, they might have been motivated by the need to overcome deprivation of basic needs or they might be seeking self-employment to fulfill there desire to be independent. The studies also revealed that majority of the respondents were forced self-employed rather than as a trained person. Since they started the business at a very small scale, the business premise was their own huts or houses.

Usually, it is found that although an entrepreneur want to start some enterprise of its own at large scale but very few of them were aware about the support system which is available in the form of governmental help or schemes for loan, finance, etc.

A strong need was felt to organize trainings which can enhance the knowledge regarding the benefits of the support systems. If support system can be strengthened, the entrepreneurship can be developed among the women in any situation.

Resource System

This system will include all the means and ways, which are used for achieving the desired goals in self-employment, viz. time, finance, raw materials, machinery equipment, etc. The institutional support in the form of training and financial assistance affects the entrepreneurial characteristics to a great extent.

Support System

It is operationalised as the extent of assistance or aid provided by the institution and persons. It includes institutional support, training support and manpower support. Support system profile has edge over self-sphere system. By strengthening the support system and by giving the emphasis to the resource system, a successful entrepreneur can be developed (Fig. 15.2).

ENTREPRENEURSHIP DEVELOPMENT

Entrepreneurship development is a human resource development task, for it deals with aspirations, motives, frustrations, creativity and therefore behaviour and psychology of the target groups with all their strengths and weaknesses to make an entrepreneurial movement. The first step in assessing the feasibility of an entrepreneurship development programme is to recognize the critical components in an entrepreneurship development process.

Long and comprehensive experiences in locating and building entrepreneurship through training-cum-development programmes, in India, point towards seven critical variables in entrepreneurship development function as shown in

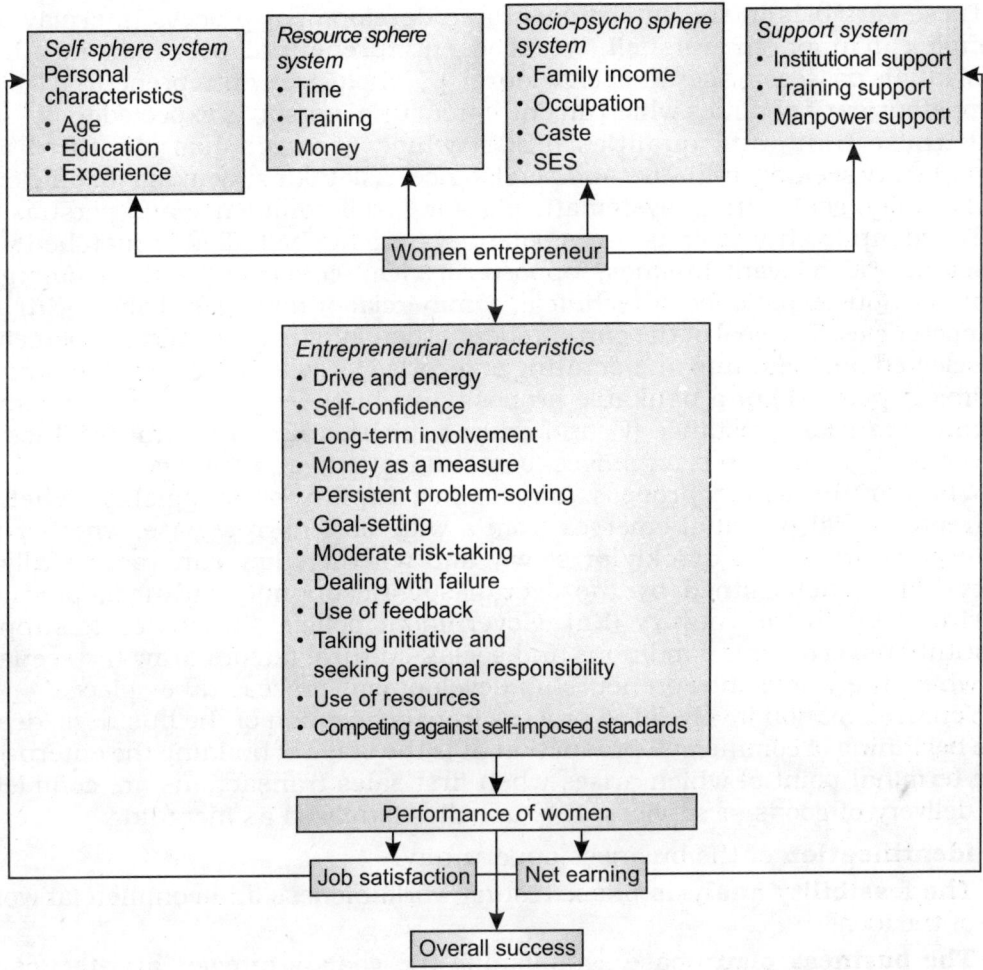

Fig. 15.2: Effect of systems on women entrepreneur

Chart 15.1 in which human resources potential interacts with the business/ economic environment in the region with the ultimate objective of converting a sound business opportunity into a successful profit making enterprise.

Chart 15.1: Entrepreneurship development function

ED	=	f (Et, Op, SK, PP, F, If, En)
ED	=	Entrepreneurship development
Et	=	Entrepreneurial traits/qualities
Op	=	Buisness opportunities
SK	=	Skills/competencies
PP	=	Project plan
F	=	Finance
If	=	Infrastructure
En	=	Environment

These variables in the entrepreneurship development process interplay in a complex manner. In nutshell, we need entrepreneurial potential, i.e. those individuals possessing certain behavioural, psychological, entrepreneurial traits/ competencies or qualities which an entrepreneurial person is expected to possess (Et): these traits and qualities (PECs) which research has identified are: opportunity seeking, initiative and persistence, risk taking, demand for efficiency and quality, goal setting, systematic planning, self-confidence and persuasion.

The identified human resources potential needs to be linked or matched with a sound and relevant business opportunity (Op) consistent with or emerging from previous experience or technical, commercial or managerial skills (SK) and competencies. The goal of the entrepreneurs thereafter is to convert the perceived or selected business into an operating enterprise for which they need to prepare a project plan (PP) or a bankable proposition which becomes an instrument to secure financial assistance (F) and other support. Infrastructural facilities (If) particularly land, factory premises, communications and transport.

Whether the whole process takes place rapidly or sluggishly, whether entrepreneurial potential emerges from a wide or a narrow base, whether the enterprise are set up quickly or slowly and whether they run successfully or they fall, is determined by the overall socio-economic, cultural, political, environment in the country (En). Government policies, existence of support institutions, economic conditions and social, cultural factors draw the scenario in which the whole entrepreneurship development process takes place.

Venture creation involves the process from conception of the business idea to the beginning of commercial production. It is the stage of building the enterprise, the terminal point of which arises when first sales transactions are completed by delivery of goods or services. It is usually visualized as including:

1. **Identification** of the business opportunity.
2. **The feasibility analysis** phase testing workableness and commercial worth of the idea.
3. **The business plan** phase establishing the goals strategies and tactics for initiating and operating the business.
4. **The resource acquisition** phase involving assembly of inputs (including finance).
5. **The activity initiation** phase implementation of operations.

Entrepreneurship is thus a chain of functions and decisions at different stages of venture/enterprise building. These functions are:

1. Searching for and discovering new information.
2. Translating new marks, techniques and goods.
3. Seeking and discovering economic opportunity
4. Marshalling financial resources necessary for enterprise
5. Making time-bound action schedule
6. Taking ultimate responsibility for management
7. Providing leadership for the work group
8. Taking risks for ultimate uncertainly

9. Status for enterprise building
10. We can very distinctly classify these functions into four phases (chart 15.2).

Chart 15.2: Stages of enterprise building

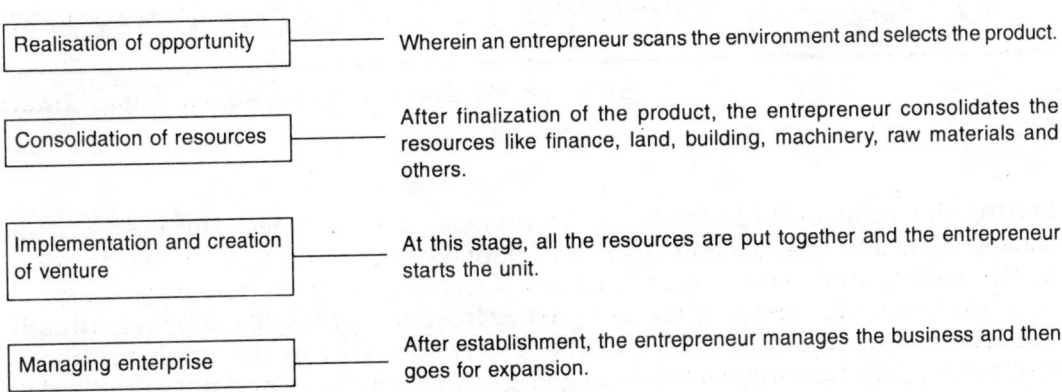

Realisation of opportunity —— Wherein an entrepreneur scans the environment and selects the product.

Consolidation of resources —— After finalization of the product, the entrepreneur consolidates the resources like finance, land, building, machinery, raw materials and others.

Implementation and creation of venture —— At this stage, all the resources are put together and the entrepreneur starts the unit.

Managing enterprise —— After establishment, the entrepreneur manages the business and then goes for expansion.

CONCLUSION

"When women move forward, the family moves, the village moves and the nation moves". These words of Pandit Jawaharlal Nehru are an accepted fact. Employment gives economic status to women. Economic status gives way to social status and there by empowerment to women.

In present scenario due to modernization, urbanization, globalization and development of education, with increasing awareness, women are now seeking gainful employment in several fields.

Women are entering into entrepreneurship even while facing socio-cultural, economic, technical, financial and managerial difficulties. Women entrepreneurship movement can gain momentum by providing an encouragement, appropriate awareness, training and support. This would definitely enhance their socio-economic status, a prerequisite of women's empowerment.

16

Entrepreneurship through Self-help Groups of Women in Livestock Sector

SK Singh, MC Sharma, Pankaj Kumar, Rupasi Tiwari

During the Vedic and Mughal periods, women were exploited. However, during the medieval and post-second World War periods, women enjoyed greater freedom in the society and family. All important decisions of the family were taken in consultation with women. They had greater freedom of mobility, which gradually suppressed and finally neglected by the society as well as by the family members. Gradually, they were restricted from going out of the house and not permitted to attend any social functions, religious ceremonies, political meetings, etc. They have been facing intolerable physiological, psychological, social, economic, political and cultural problems. These problems still exist in the form of female foetus termination, infanticide, wife beating, oppression of SC/ST women by the upper caste people, dowry deaths, rapes, suicides, etc.

After independence, eminent women and other reformers in the society started massive campaigns for women's emancipation and liberation. These movements helped women to attain constitutional backing for assuring equality, dignity, justice, stability and prosperity. The contribution of women has to be viewed in a wider perspective. Religious values and male chauvinism are the end products of patriarchal society. So, unless patriarchal values and structures undergo change, the male attitude towards women would continue to be one of domination.

The Constitution of India has guaranteed the right of equality to all its citizens irrespective of their sex, caste, creed and religion. Indian democracy, right from the days of independence, has been thriving on these basic principles for the last more than five decades. The national movement under the leadership of Mahatma Gandhi was one of the first attempts to draw Indian women out of the restricted circles of domestic life into equal role with men. Writings in "Young Indian" in 1918, Gandhiji said, *Woman is the companion of man gifted with equal mental capacities. She has the right to participate in the minutest details of the activities of man. She has the same right of freedom and liberty as he.*

Hence, in order to make women economically and politically empowered, it is essential to make them realize their role in building up a new set of values through education and employment, which would ultimately make them attain a better status in the society. Present level of employment does not yield adequate income for the survival of their family. So it is necessary to create new employment avenues for higher income generation. Thus, developing different types of entrepreneurial activities among women in order to generate high income has enormous potential.

In India, the majority of people lives in rural areas and involves almost half of the women folk. Today, rural women have acquired a secondary status in social life, economic activities and decision-making among their families. Their role in productive work, employment generation and income-oriented activities is hindered by many socio-economic constraints. The statistical data shows that of the world's 1.3 billion poor, nearly 70% are women. Out of the world's one billion illiterate, two-thirds are women and nearly two-thirds of 130 million children worldwide, who are not in school are girls. In most countries, women work approximately twice the unpaid time men do and on an average rural woman produce more than 55% of all total food grown in developing countries. The value of women's unpaid housework and community is estimated at 35% of GDP worldwide. Not only this, women hold only 10.5% of the seats in the world's parliament and only 24 women have been elected as heads of governments in the last century.

Hence, it has become strikingly clear that political and social forces that resist women's rights in the name of religious, cultural or ethnic traditions, have contributed to the process of marginalization and oppression of women. The basic issue that prevents women from playing full participatory role in nation building is lack of economic dependence.

Hence, there is a need to formulate policies, which aims for the empowerment of women. The planners and policy makers are eagerly searching for certain alternatives leading to the enactment of National Policy for Empowerment of Women in the Tenth Plan (2002-07). Empowerment is a multi-dimensional process, which should enable the individuals or a group of individuals to realize their full identity and powers in all spheres of life. It consists of greater access to knowledge and resources, greater autonomy in decision-making to enable them to have greater ability to plan their lives and free them from the shackles imposed on them by custom, belief and practice.

Empowerment of women also means equal status to women. Empowering women socio-economically through increased awareness of their rights and duties as well as access to resources is a decisive step towards greater security for them. Empowerment includes higher literacy level and education for women, better health care for women and children, equal ownership of productive resources, increased participation in economic and commercial sectors, awareness of their rights and responsibilities, improved standards of living and acquiring self-reliance, self-esteem and self-confidence.

WOMEN ENTREPRENEURSHIP THROUGH SELF-HELP GROUPS

Alleviation of poverty is the core of all developmental programmes, but early experiences of such poverty alleviation programmes have not achieved the required success. It has been found that rural poor women requires small but regular urgent loans whereas their options are restricted to programmes designed and approved by government, which do not cater their need. Hence, to bridge the gap between the demand and supply of funds in the lower runs of rural economy, the micro-finance schemes of NABARD have made a smoother foray into the role played by micro-finance in eradicating poverty and empowering women to manage the enterprises.

Micro-finance

Micro-financing is an enabling, empowering, bottom-up tool to poverty alleviation that has provided considerable economic and non-economic externalities to low-income households in developing countries. Micro-financing is being hailed as a sustainable tool to combat poverty, combining a profit approach that is self-sustaining and a poverty alleviation focus that empowers low income households. Micro-financing is increasingly becoming a tool to exercise developmental priorities for government in developing countries.

According to World Bank, 1997, it is a programmes that provides credit for self-employment and other financial and business services (including saving and technical assistance) to very poor persons.

As per UN, 1998, the world micro-credit programmes have succeeded in generating self-employment by providing access to small capital and people living in poverty and has proved to be an effective tool in freeing people from poverty.

According to NABARD, micro-financing is provision of thrift, credit and other financial services to the unserved poor enabling them to raise their income levels and improving living standards.

Thus, we find that micro-financing or micro-credit is a very effective tool for combating poverty and exploitation, create confidence for the economic, self-reliance of rural poor, particularly among women who are mostly invisible in the social structure. This group concept enables all the members to come together for a common objective and gain strength from each other to deal with exploitation which they (or an individual) are facing in several forms. A group thus becomes the basis for action and change.

The micro-finance initiative of NABARD has evolved as a sustainable social movement over a decade by now. The design and content of these innovations have remained dynamic in tandem with the changing needs of the micro-finance sector in the country. These initiatives have attracted the attention of a wide range of stakeholders, large number of formal and informal agencies have partnered with the NABARD in this unique process of socio-economic engineering. The relevance of the micro-finance programme was greatly enhanced for all the partners through the core strategy of SHG bank linkage, which was built around a simple but basic concept of human nature –the feeling of self-worth.

ENTREPRENEURSHIP DEVELOPMENT THROUGH SHGs

SHG is a small voluntary association of poor people, preferably from the same socio-economic background which becomes a platform for exchange of experiences and ideas, and better mechanism to reduce poverty as well as effective medium to tackle social and gender issues of the society. It can also be defined as a small voluntary association of poor people, preferably from the same socio-economic background which come together for the purpose of solving their common problems through self-help and mutual help. The SHG promotes small savings among its members which are kept in bank in the name of SHG.

The SHGs are formed around the theme of savings and credit. A small group of individuals become members and pool their savings on a regular basis to form a collective fund. This fund is then rotated as credit amongst the members through some system and self-generated norms. Hence, the basis of SHG is the mutuality and trust in depositing individual savings in a groups fund.

Concept of SHG

The concept of SHG is based on the following principles:

1. Self-help supplemented with mutual help can be a powerful vehicle for the poor in their socio-economic development;
2. Participative financial services management is more responsive and efficient;
3. Poor need not only credit support, but also savings and other services;
4. Poor can save and are bankable and SHGs as clients, result in wider outreach, lower transaction cost and much lower risk costs for the banks;
5. Creation of a common fund by contributing small savings on a regular basis;
6. Flexible democratic system of working;
7. Loaning is done mainly on trust with a bare documentation and without any security;
8. Amounts loaned are small, frequent and for short duration;
9. Defaults are rare mainly due to group pressure.

MICRO-ENTERPRISES

Micro-enterprise may be defined as any legitimate economic activity taken up with a view to increasing income. Micro-enterprise development is seen as a holistic approach, embracing poverty alleviation, human development and economic development strategies. For this reason, a wide range of institutions— including stand-alone micro-enterprise development organizations, community development corporations, loan funds, community action agencies, women's organizations, community development banks and credit unions, housing and social service programmes, and government agencies at the local, state, and national levels—are involved in micro-enterprise development.

After a decade of operation, micro-enterprises programmes in India are creating jobs, generating income, building assets and enhancing skills. These results are particularly impressive considering the fact that a significant proportion of assisted micro-entrepreneurs are individuals facing barriers presented by race, gender, ethnicity, income, job market fluctuations, or location. Whether the business is the sole source of family income or a crucial supplement to family earnings, micro-enterprise development has put many low-income families on the road to self-sufficiency. Four key elements, viz. training and technical assistance, credit and access to credit, access to markets and economic literacy and asset development must be kept in mind for micro-enterprise development.

GOVERNMENT EFFORTS TO PROMOTE WOMEN'S ENTREPRENEURSHIP

Women welfare is an integral part of the planning process in our country but for the first time in India's planning history, a chapter on *Women and Development* was included as late as the Sixth Five Year Plan. It is clear from the recent experiences of women's development that a woman like a man can represent an economic unit or do business or service thereby giving more opportunities for women's development. The government has introduced many development and welfare programmes for women. These programmes are aimed at providing financial and technical assistance to poor women to start self-employment units. Integrated Rural Development Programme (IRDP), Training of Rural Youth for Self-employment (TRYSEM) now renamed as Swarna Jayanti Gram Swarojgar Yojana (SGSY), Socio-economic Programme (SEP), Support to Training and Employment Programme (STEP), Development of Women and Children in Rural Areas (DWCRA), etc. are some of the important programmes implemented by the Government with reference to women's development. Likewise Women Development Corporation, Central Social Welfare Board and State Social Welfare Boards and state are also entrusted with women development schemes through financial assistance and generate employment for women.

The major drawback of these self-employment programmes was that group entrepreneurship approach was not followed in them. DWACRA was the only self-employment programme that was based on the group approach, covering 10-15 poor rural women in a group. The programme aimed at developing income generating skills and promoting activities among them. However, due to lack of literacy and entrepreneurial skills among the rural poor women, the programme could not succeed in achieving the objectives for which it was made.

Women development corporations were established in 11 states and union territories to improve the economic conditions of women by organizing training and generate employment. The Central Social Welfare Board through its programmes established agro-based productive self-employment units and ancillary units. Apart from these programmes, some other incentive schemes were also started like the TEP centres, Mahila Samriddhi Yojana, Rashtriya Mahila Kosh, etc. However, the expected results have not been achieved till date, because majority of these programmes had aimed at creating employment by starting production centres or big factories. It is very difficult for small and cottage industries in marketing their products, because consumers are attracted towards wide publicity and colourful advertisements, which need huge investments.

Another drawback was seen with TRYSEM, where the trainees were only interested in the stipends; they did not apply the training inputs for their self-employment prospects. But, the SGSY aims at establishing a large number of rural micro-enterprise by organizing rural poor into self-help groups (SHGs), capacity building, planning of activity clusters, infrastructure build up, technology, credit and marketing, etc.

ACTIVITIES SUITABLE FOR WOMEN ENTREPRENEURS

A number of sectors are having enormous service and business opportunities for self-employment of poor women, both in rural and urban areas. A number of service-oriented activities identified suitable for women at household level include agri-related services like implements repairing station, sprayer (pesticides) hiring, tractor hiring, seeds sales centre, animal health care, rice and flour mill and cereals processing, chairs and vessel hiring, oil extracting, cashew nut processing, grading of agricultural and livestock products, fish processing and selling, nursery schools, cycle repairing and vegetable sales.

Other services include petty shops, hotel running, beauty parlor, selling of consumable items, firewood shop, tailoring, spinning and weaving, dying and bleaching, embroidery works, washing and ironing, balwadi and crèche running, pulse dehusking, electronics and electronic goods, public telephone services, telephone cleaning, typewriting institute and computer training centres.

Agri-related services outside the household sector include commission mandi, horticulture nursery, services like soil testing, transportation of agricultural goods, organizing daily and weekly markets and milk vending.

Other services outside the household sector include lodging services, travel agency, pandal decoration works, marriage brokering, yam supply, masonry services, real estate, medicinal plants, collection counter services, law services, health clinic, voluntary service and motion picture distribution and projection.

INSTITUTIONS HELPING THE WOMEN ENTREPRENEURS

The efficient and entrepreneurial women waste their energy and talents by being simply engaged in the household work. Lack of finance hinders them from entering the field of self-employment. Majority of educated women are not aware of the schemes available from government meant to help entrepreneurs or to become entrepreneurs. The following institutions are available for benefit of entrepreneurs in the areas of finance, training consultancy and technical guidance along with schemes for concessions and subsidies for self-employment.

Financial Institutions

1. Industrial Development Bank of India (IDBI)
2. Industrial Financial Corporation of India (IFCI)
3. Small Industries Development Bank of India (SIDBI)
4. National Small Industries Corporation (SSIC)
5. Commercial Banks
6. Cooperative Banks
7. Regional Rural Banks
8. Gramin Banks
9. State Financial Corporation (SFC)
10. State Industrial Development Corporation SIDC)

Institutions for Technical Guidance

1. State Industrial Development Organization (SIDO)
2. District Industrial Centres (DIC)
3. Technical Consultation Organization (TCO)
4. Small Industries Service Institute (SISI)
5. Small Industries Development Corporation (SIDCO)

6. National Research and Development Corporation (NRDC)
7. Khadi and Village Industries Commission (KVIC)
8. Department of Science and Technology (DST)
9. Technology Development Cell (TDC)
10. LIC, GIC, and Unit Trust of India

Training Institutions

1. District Industries Centre (DIC)
2. National Bank for Agriculture and Rural Development (NABARD)
3. Council for Advancement of Peoples Action and Rural Technology (CAPART)
4. Small Industries Service Institute (SISI)
5. Indian Institute of Packaging (IIP)

Schemes Available

1. Refinance scheme for industrial loans for small and village industries
2. Composite Loan Scheme
3. Scheme for SC/ST and physically handicapped entrepreneurs
4. National Equity Fund Scheme
5. Special Scheme of assistance to ex-serviceman
6. Seed Capital Scheme
7. Single Window Scheme
8. Scheme for Women Entrepreneurs
9. Mahila Udhayan Nidhi Scheme
10. Scheme for Incentives for Exports
11. Equipment Refinance Scheme
12. Assistance to Small Road Transport Operators
13. Foreign Currency Refinance Scheme
14. Refinance Scheme under ADB Line of Credit
15. Refinance Scheme for Industrial Estates
16. Sampoorna Gram Swarojgar Yojana (SGSY)

Subsidies and Concessions to Entrepreneurs

1. Technical subsidy
2. Know-how subsidy
3. Power subsidy
4. Generator subsidy
5. Relief
6. Sales tax exemption
7. Octroi duty exemption
8. Electric duty exemption
9. Stamp duty exemption

FACTORS AFFECTING WOMEN ENTREPRENEURS

The following socio-economic, cultural and political factors affect women entrepreneurship.

Immobility of Women

Women are prohibited to move to long distances. Even short distance movements are allowed only for highly educated middle class family women. But, as far as entrepreneurship section is concerned, the owner may need to move to various places often to gain knowledge and to get things done. The commanding men tend not to bear it. Therefore, this hurdle of immobility to the development of women finally leads to idleness of women.

Lack of Training and Technical Assistance

Usually trainees face the difficult task of teaching complex business skills to women entrepreneurs who have little formal training, limited time to engage in learning and have various levels of literacy level.

Immoral Behaviour of Men towards Women

In the entrepreneurship field, women are facing a number of problems. The administration and management of industries or services requires close and continuous watch over work in progress and demands mutual relationship with workers irrespective of sex. Sometimes, the proprietor has to stay with management to solve the problems or to take some important decisions; even she may have to stay during night. The traditional society having orthodox men doubting the moral behaviour of women, ultimately leading to lot of problems in the family such as separation, divorce, etc.

Traditional Value System

In the patriarchal society, men still dominate over women in all walks of life. Even educated women are simply sitting in the house after complition of housework. They are wasting their energy in reading storybooks, playing with housemaids and gossiping with neighbours. Skilled and professional women also need to obey the decisions taken by their husbands. The effective traditional value system and writings like Manu Smriti, Vedas and other literatures are still focused on suppression of women. Indian culture bothers more about safeguarding virginity of women. So women are not allowed to go out of the family to take any job or to attend higher studies or to get professional training.

Low Level of Literacy

Illiteracy or low level of education is another important barrier to the entry of women in the entrepreneurship sector. Only after independence, because of various measures taken by the government as well as by the individual reformers, the importance to impart education to female children has been realized. Parents face problems in searching bridegrooms, inspite of being ready to pay the demanded dowry. Therefore, parents are not interested to send the girl child for higher studies. Even in schools, the ratio of dropout is higher for females. The low literacy leads to lack of awareness and courage to get into employment field.

More Household Responsibilities with Women

Women do not find time to think of their individual economic freedom. The wealthy women and women of higher status think that entering the risky field of entrepreneurship is waste of energy and money with the limited available time.

Lack of Awareness

It is true that lack of awareness hinders women entrepreneurship. There are number of factors responsible for the lack of awareness among women. Illiteracy, ignorance, lack of proper propaganda by agencies, corruption among government functionaries, etc. are some of the important factors responsible for this problem.

Access to Markets

In order to provide better services in the global competitive market, the women entrepreneurs must have access to latest market views which may include: regular sophisticated training on marketing and sale concepts, development and distribution of joint catalogs, internet access and e-commerce, participation in trade shows and innovative concepts, etc.

Non-availability of Proper Guidance

A number of schemes and programmes have been introduced and implemented for the socio-economic emancipation of women at various levels irrespective of caste, class, race, place, affluence and indigence. But, these provisions and facilities are not known to majority of women who are to be the beneficiaries. The government has initiated measures to propagate the same through media, but it has not reached the majority of women living in rural areas, especially uneducated women. The better-informed people also do not come forward to guide and help them to start self-employment and to climb up the economic ladder.

Difficulties in Availing of Loan Schemes

It is well known that women do not derive any assets from their parents. In the husband's family also, they have no property in their names. Often women are not willing to ask for the property rights because of the binding family relation and social custom prevail in the society. This condition does not permit women to avail any benefit from the financial institutions and this hinders their economic prosperity.

MEASURES TO STRENGTHEN WOMEN'S ENTREPRENEURSHIP

Empowerment of women is the prime objective of all development programmes and policies. These programmes could be planned properly and implemented effectively in order to attain self-sufficiency and self-reliance. The following measures can strengthen self-employment in the service sector, which will generate additional income leading to economic independence of women:

1. Effective producer-industry-consumer linkage is the need of the hour to develop strong linkages between micro-enterprise production system and marketing.

2. Identification and organization of innovative and high income generating activities suitable for women.
3. Development of entrepreneurial abilities of women by organizing special types of training on product planning, market information, preparation of produce for marketing via group action, improved marketing practices, rules and regulations, processing, etc.
4. Encouraging women to take up part-time jobs while being in the house itself, to earn additional income to support the family.
5. Effective planning at the micro-level in consultation with all the members of the SHGs.
6. Adequate representation of women experts in the case of women related development planning.
7. Central and state government to place more emphasis on untouched areas in the entrepreneurial sector to involve women.
8. Government can establish a separate mechanism at the centre, state and district levels to look after women's employment and their problems.
9. Development of infrastructure facilities and supportive services like land, building, transport and also to look after the children.
10. Encouraging women through formal and non-formal education to involve themselves in the service sector.
11. Organizing women labourers in the service sector through women's associations, cooperative societies or Mahila Mandals, etc.
12. Establishment of supervisory bodies to monitor the implementation of constitutional provisions related to women.
13. Steps to make women aware of technical and financial assistance available to women entrepreneurs, and to encourage them through concessions and incentives to enter into the service sector.
14. Government should encourage research and development in the service sector to find out high-income generating activities suitable for women.
15. Wide publicity about the training programmes in the service sector.
16. Creating awareness among educated and uneducated youth about the availability of facilities and concessions for entrepreneurs.
17. Special attention to grading and packaging of the commodities.
18. Government must have at least one channel on Doordarshan specially meant for services of women entrepreneurs, in order to have easy access to relevant information as well as better communication and also reduces transaction costs.
19. Strong infrastructure support must be developed in terms of roads, electric supplies, telecommunication, etc.
20. Efforts should be made to involve grassroot based NGOs, private or rural institutions for better credit worthiness.

17

Women Empowerment and Entrepreneurship Development through Self-help Groups

Prakash Panwar, PM Khan, KL Jeengar

Women constitute half of the world's population. According to the United Nation's report, they account for 60% of the working hours, contribute up to 30% of the official labour force, receive 10% of the total income and own less than 1% of the world's property. Out of 1.3 billion people living in absolute poverty over 70% are women.

Women are vital and productive workers in the Indian economy. Nearly 84% of all economically active women in India are engaged in agriculture and allied activities. Agriculture employees 4/5th of all economically active women, they constitute one-third of all agriculture labour force and 48% of self-employed farmers. There are 75 milllion women against 15 million men in dairying and those engaged in animal husbandry, accounts for 20 million as against 1.5 million men.

There is no denying the fact that women do not have equal access to beneficial change and their status in society is not identical to that of men. This is specially true in villages. Several studies have shown that the women employee, whatever job she holds, is equal in efficiency and performance to the male employee in identical employment situations. Some of the studies even indicate that in certain aspects the woman employee is even more efficient. In the matter of reliability, promptness and punctuality, she had been found to have an edge over her male counterpart.

Although our constitution has recognised the right of equality for women yet the findings on women towards equality are disappointing and discouraging. They have dual responsibility of shouldering the household chores and contributing to the family income but have limited access to resources and simultaneously lack of control over income, credit, land, education, training and information.

Role of home science for development of this important half of the society is crucial. Being an important segment of Krishi Vigyan Kendra, the home scientist has positive contribution in development of rural women. Empowerment of women can be done by empowering them both technologically and economically. For this purpose, self-help groups play an important role. Under this, the group enterprise provides an organizational framework for pooling up capital, technology, market and labour, thus facilitates participation of women in self-employment and income generating activities.

WOMEN EMPOWERMENT

Gandhiji once said "Women must not look to men for protection. They must rely on their own strength." It is definite that if appropriate skills and opportunities of decision-making are given to women, they can prove that they are, if not superior, at least equal to men. Recent trends in India and other parts of the world also indicate that women are far more superior to men in various aspects of development. Even at the global level, various developmental agencies have come to the conclusion that women are far more reliable in almost all types of development projects. Only problem is that so far the society has given little chance to women to enter into the fields of various economic activities where many have proved themselves as leaders. Hence, it is necessary today to empower women by providing the facilities to enter into various economic activities to make themselves economically independent and socially confident in their endeavour.

Women's ability to find innovative solution could be used to benefit cooperatives and influence their development. Empowering women to take a greater part in decision making is necessary both to cooperative efficiency and its sustainable development. Women are considered to be good leaders in matters requiring collaboration, group integration and ability to listen and motivation.

The economic activities may be various enterprises, viz. processing and preservation of fruits and vegetables, mushroom culture, papad making, processing of spices, cereals and pulses, handicraft making and various other enterprises where rural women can make their presence felt in earning extra money and doing the things for themselves and their family. This will not only help them to establish themselves in their families and societies as equal to their male counterparts but also help them to decide their own future as an equal partners in the family and in the society.

Many women in business have made success in many areas by running a variety of industries and enterprises. The success ratio of women is 47% (Kapur, 1993). A great number of women in India have taken up and are successfully running their own industries.

KRISHI VIGYAN KENDRA AND FARM WOMEN

Women play an active role in rural development schemes. Training of farm women is thus important to increase their involvement in the development process and to enhance their skills and make them equal partners in national development. The major objectives of training for rural women should be to equip them with better skill and enhance their knowledge so as to prepare them to face new challenges due to technological development.

Recent experiences have shown a strong link between education and development, particularly in case of developing countries as education is vital to human resource development. Education and training will help in raising their status, enable development of their potential as independent and equal partners.

The education to women should enable them to think critically identify their strength and take conscious decision, empower them to play a positive role on their own in the development of the nation. By and large they have remained as "invisible worker". Therefore, there is a need to allow them to breakout of stereotyped roles.

As both men and women constitute farming community, it is important and necessary to consider both of them as potential farmers. The institutional training for farm women is a prerequisite to make them aware about their role and contribution in the home economics and farm production process and to prepare them to utilize the inputs and information available through extension and other developmental agencies.

Fortunately KVKs have shifted their focus towards farm women by organising need-based training programmes like various farm management activities, home improvement and income generating projects. The main thrust in all these programmes is to enhance the socio-economic status, expose them to improved agriculture and related technologies and further their innovative proneness.

There is no doubt that rural development is a complex and challenging process in which women generally play a predominant role in most of the countries in Asia, Africa and Latin America. However, while questions of giving credit, rewards and recognition come they are generally ignored and their male counterparts hob the limelight.

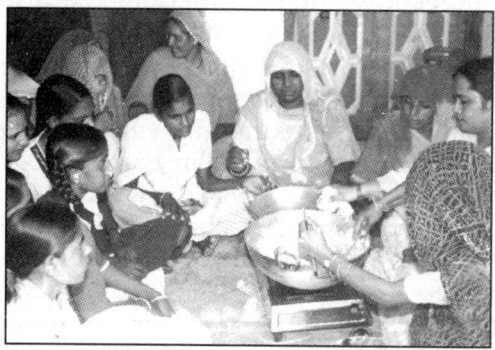

Fig. 17.1: KVKs and women

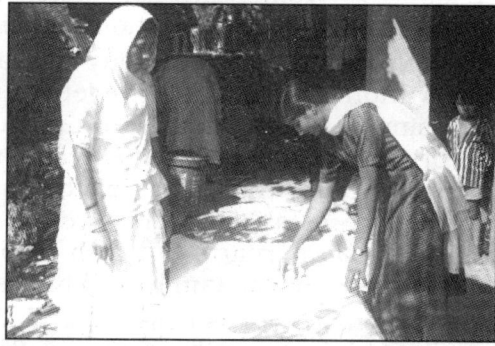

Fig. 17.2: Training of women

The practices all over the third world generally have that the women are designated as wives, mothers, sisters and home makers. However, in the recent time, this trend is changing with the changing socio-political and economic scenario throughout the world. Now the society has started recognising the women's ability in decision-making in developmental activities relating to agriculture, forestry and its allied areas and economic aspects of house and family management and also community development. It is widely recognised that apart from managing household, bearing children, women bring income with productive activities ranging from traditional work in the field to working in the factories or running small business. They have proved that they can be better entrepreneur and development managers in any kind of activities. Therefore, it is important and necessary to make women empowered in taking decision to enable them to be in

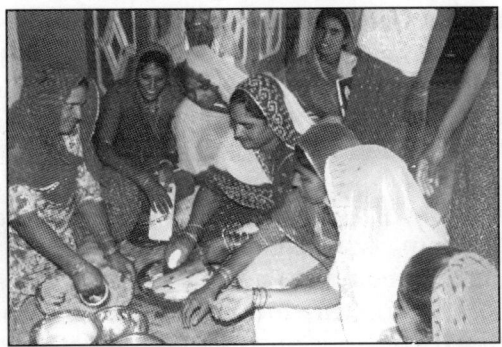 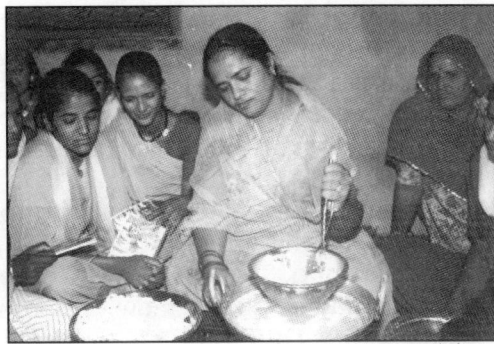

Figs 17.3 and 17.4: Women being given training in entrepreneurship

the central part of developmental process. There is no two opinion that women should be put in country's development agenda to achieve its desired goal.

ENTREPRENEURSHIP DEVELOPMENT

Prosperity of any developing country depends upon the prosperity of its rural areas and that is possible only when the villages become self-sufficient. There is frustration and feeling of insecurity among the villagers especially youth due to unemployment, under-employment, idleness, etc. Villagers tend to migrate to urban areas because of rural push due to hard boring work, long working hours, little money due to low wages, few services, no prospects and dwindling land holdings due to division of lands among family members and on urban pull due to better chances of jobs, higher income, better health care and education facilities, etc. Avenues of gainful employment have to be found out and they have to be found right in the villages themselves. To create more employment opportunities, there should be even expansion and diversification of agricultural production. Rural industrialization with development of suitable agro-processing models/complexes is therefore a patent tool to prevent the migration of these surplus manpower to the urban areas and boosting developmental activities at the village level for socio-economic up lift of rural masses. The processing of agro-food material into value added products will not only increase the income of the farmers, but will also provide significant employment opportunities to the rural youth. In addition, a huge amount of post-harvest losses, especially in cereal, fruits and vegetables can be reduced by establishing such agro-processing complexes at the village level/at the focal points in districts. The problems of post-harvest handling are generally location specific and thus require development of technology suited to such situations. India has all the makings of an agricultural super-power. The Indian agriculture is the largest producer of pulse crops, cashewnut, coconut, sugarcane, milk and tea in the world. From the stage of struggling to take care of basic food requirements of its increasing populations since independence, the country has come a long way towards visualizing the tremendous potential for commercial and export oriented agri-business. Exploitation of this potential can bring about an era of prosperity with the right mix of employment generation and profits.

On-farm primary processing of agricultural produce has now become a very important tool of boosting our economy through scientific conservation of food, feed and fibre materials, efficient and appropriate use of wastes and by products of agriculture and generation of appropriate technologies, which leads to the development of rural agro-processing industries enabling the farmers to settle their value added products.

Almost all the items of agricultural produce which are used by human being are consumed only after some kind of processing which is the important post-harvest operation. Traditionally, processing was being carried out in the village itself on a small scale but slowly, a trend of shifting this industry from its rural base has set in. This trend started only with the advent of commercial methods of crop processing because these new methods saved the human beings from the drudgery and tardy nature of traditional methods. In order that Indian agriculture becomes competitive nationally and globally, it should be highly productive, intellectually stimulating to youth and profitable. Another feature of our agriculture is that except in irrigated areas, it is largely mono-culture and thus very seasonal, leaving the farmers and farm labourers without any job for most of the year as a result of which the capable youths move towards towns/cities for a better job prospect and in that process creates many municipal problems like high pressure on public utilities and facilities.

SELF-HELP GROUPS (SHG)

SHG is a voluntary association of 10–20 members with common interest, formed democratically without any political or religious affiliation to mobilize savings, to manage credit, encouraging group members to take loan for appropriate productive income generating activities and to solve family financial problems with low rate of interest. The basic objective is to develop saving capability among the poorest sections of the society, which in turn reduce dependence on financial institutions and develop self-reliance.

Several surveys and researches have reported that the farm and rural poor women from small and marginal farm families and agricultural labourers need less amount of credit loan, but on regular and urgent basis for their day to day consumption for which the bankers do not take much interest. Apart from this formal rules and regulations also kept the poor away from formal credit institutions.

As a result, they often approach village or nearby town's private money lenders and are exploited by paying heavy interests, even they have to sell or mortgage their lands and gold/silver ornaments to repay their debts. Under these circumstances, it is widely accepted by many that formation of SHG is essential and perhaps the only alternative to reduce drudgeries and to solve socio-economic problems of rural women of farming community.

ADVANTAGES OF SELF-HELP GROUPS
- Through the SHGs, it is possible to reach large number of small borrowers.
- Reduction in transaction cost.
- Ensure better quality lending and need based credit.
- Cuts time lag between application and actual sanction/disbursement of loan.

Flow chart 17.1: Self-help group formation process

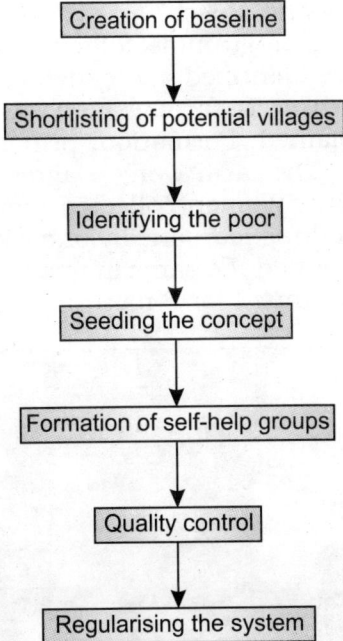

- Helps to bring the disadvantaged people within the folds of some organisational format which they can understand and operate.
- It enables simultaneous undertaking of social development also.
- Develops the habit of saving among the rural poor..
- Helps the poorer to escape from the crunches of local money lenders.
- Improves the employment opportunities through easy availability of finance.
- Financial empowerment among the women category.
- Improvement in social and educational status in the society.

It is expected that within the group there is true democratic culture in which all the members must participate actively in the decision-making process by taking part in the discussion. Collective work, leadership with fixed tenure, mutual trust and cooperative philosopy would be the driving force for SHGs. These groups are called "Solidarity groups" as they provide monetary as well as moral support to individual members in times of difficulties.

Case Study of a Self-help Group

Vocational training is one of the important mandate of Krishi Vigyan Kendra. The main purpose behind conducting vocational training is to provide new knowledge and new skills so that the participants may be able to generate additional income by performing a particular vocation successfully.

With the financial assistance from Indian Council of Agricultural Research under National Agricultural Technology Programme, Krishi Vigyan Kendra, Bhilwara (Maharana Pratap University of Agriculture and Technology, Udaipur) organised four vocational training programmes of 10 days each. Each training was given to the group of 30 farm women in their own village on processing and packaging of cereals, pulses and spices.

After 15 days of the training programme, follow-up was done and 10 innovative and active farm women were identified and convinced to form a self-help group in one village. A meeting of these 10 farm women was organised and importance of self-help group was explained. Formation, principles and rules of self-help group were also explained. The farm women agreed and started collection of money @ Rs 20/- per month. Women collected money every month and after three months they started taking loan one by one who was in urgent need from the money collected and refunded the same in monthly installment with interest @ 10% per annum. This continued for 6 months.

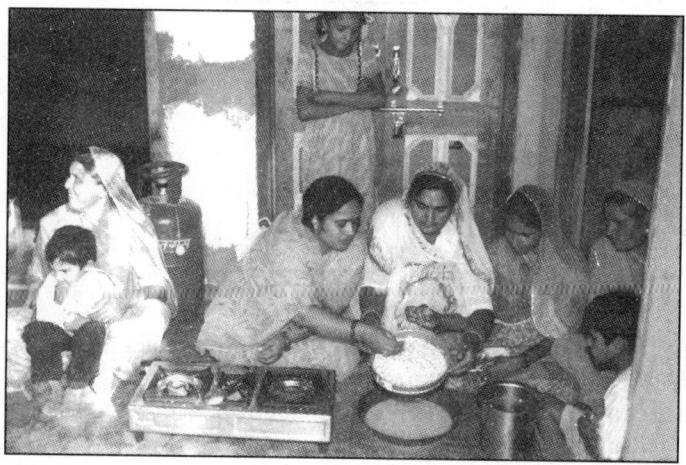

Fig. 17.5

In monthly meeting, women were more technically backed up in other areas of home science also. After 6 months, they opened accounts in bank and as a result of regular follow-up and persuation they were convinced to start enterprise or processing of cereal, pulses and spices.

Masala chakki, weighing balance and packing machine were provided to the SHG free of cost under NATP.

The group started processing and packaging in January 2005 with the help of machinery provided by KVK, the capital collected by the group and additional contribution to purchase raw material time to time and the profit was also distributed according to the amount/percent of capital investment by the individual.

They sold their products on their own in nearby places and in Bhilwara city through KVK. They also sold the products by putting stall in Gramin Hat Bazar, Bhilwara and Kisan Mela held at Udaipur.

The economics of this activity from January 2005 to September 2005 is presented in Table 17.1.

Processing of cereals, pulses and spices is a simple technology which does not need much expertise and therefore, it was adopted easily by farm women.

Table 17.1: Economics of processing and packaging of cereals, pulses and spices—Income Expenditure Statement (January to September, 2005)

S. No.	Particulars	Expenditure (whole)	Income (proceed)	Expected profit	Net profit
1.	Red chilli	600 × 40 = 24000.00	600 × 60 = 36000.00	12,000.00	10,800.00
2.	Turmeric	100 × 30 = 3000.00	100 × 54 = 5400.00	2,400.00	2,160.00
3.	Coriander	200 × 20 = 4000.00	200 × 40 = 8000.00	4,000.00	3,600.00
4.	Cumin	20 × 52 = 1040.00	20 × 80 = 1600.00	560.00	504.00
5.	Maize + wheat	200 × 7 = 1400.00	200 × 12 = 2400.00	1,000.00	900.00
6.	Pulses (urd.+ moong)	300 × 18 = 5400.00	300 × 30 = 9000.00	3,600.00	3,240.00
7.	Miscellaneous (electricity, polythene + oil, salt)	1960.00	–1960.00	–1960.00	–1960.00
	Total	**41,400.00**	**62,400.00**	**21,000.00**	**18,900.00**

It is clearly evident from Table 17.1 that within a period of 9 months, without putting much extra efforts, labour, investment and time, the group earned a sum of Rs 18,900. It is because of this fact that they are now thinking of going to the enterprise of papad making also which is a more technical enterprise.

Impact of Self-help Group

The participation of women in SHGs made a significant impact on their empowerment both in social and economic aspects.

- Most of the women were able to increase their income level and contributed to the development of the family. In the process, many of the women reported that they were participating in the final decisions of the family, which earlier they were not allowed to do. All the members were getting support from their husbands, which was not available before they joined the group.
- Women members expressed full satisfaction over their performance and wanted to continue their association with the groups.
- The group dynamism helped the women to pressurise the authorities in laying of roads, getting electric connection and providing drainage. Women are coming out in the open to discuss their common problems, which would not have been possible in the absence of such group activities. This type of social impact would definitely go a long way in improving the quality of life of the members.

Social impact: Regular interaction of the group members through periodical meeting and sharing of common problems with them, with requisite training from KVK ensured effective participation of all the members in the programme.

Economic impact: Additional employment generated through the groups collective functioning has provided scope for increasing the household income.

CONCLUSION

Empowerment of rural women is an important aspect today and self-help group is an important tool for it in which specialists have to provide technology and also motivation. Self-help groups have successfully developed a system of revolving credit for the benefit of group members on their own savings. The linking of these self-help groups with formal financial institutions has further enhanced availability of micro-credit financing to the groups. The SHGs have successfully maintained a high rate of loan repayment and successfully generated income, jobs and small enterprises for their members.

18

Business Acumen and Business Communication for Establishing Livestock Enterprise

Debashish Sengupta, Manish Sharma

According to a recent census, India has perhaps the largest number of youths in the world, also representing the biggest percentage of Indian population. However, the fact remains that large section of these youth force remains unemployed and unused. No wonder India ranks 127th in the UN Human Development Index. Rural youths are perhaps the worst affected caught not only in the dilemma of urban and rural opportunities but also facing a huge shrinking of job opportunities in the rural areas. Under such circumstances, generation of self-employment opportunities, especially for the rural youths, is a must for ensuring true development of the rural masses. Livestock sector offers a very attractive opportunity for such entrepreneurial ventures. Some of the lucrative options in the livestock business include:

1. Dairy sector
2. Poultry sector
3. Piggery sector
4. Meat industry
5. Sheep rearing (only in certain areas), etc.

There is plenty of financial assistance available from the government and its agencies for the development of livestock entrepreneurship. However, most of the funds remain unutilized, largely because of the lack of initiative among the rural youths. ***Where low motivation is one of the factors, the main reason is the lack of business acumen and business communication skills among the rural youths.***

BUSINESS ACUMEN FOR LIVESTOCK BUSINESS

Business acumen, defined in simple terms, is the ability to understand and judge things quickly and clearly the activity of making, buying, selling or supplying goods or services in return for money. In the discussion to follow, we shall attempt to identify and analyze the various business acumen needed to set-up and run livestock business by budding entrepreneurs:

However, before that we shall attempt to expose and break certain myths associated with livestock entrepreneurship.

Myth 1: Successful entrepreneurs inherit their father's business.

Myth 2: Family status plays a significant role in ensuring success of an entrepreneur.

Myth 3: Age makes a difference in the business acumen of an entrepreneur.

Myth 4: Technical education and training is must to ensure success of an entrepreneur.

Myth 5: Work experience in related field is must to ensure success of an entrepreneur.

The findings of the empirical analysis conducted by KRG Nair and Anu Pandey in the Trissur District of Kerala on entrepreneurs will be very helpful in proving these myths to be just wrong notions (Table 18.1).

Table 18.1: Findings of the empirical analysis on entrepreneurs

Entrepreneurial background	Business running	Business closed	Total
Father's occupation			
In business	11	8	19
Not in business	19	8	27
Family status			
Better-off	13	2	15
Worse-off	17	14	31
Age			
Less than 35	11	11	22
35 or more	19	5	24
Entrepreneurs technical education			
Some	18	4	22
Nil	12	12	24
Related work experience			
Some	17	4	21
Nil	13	12	25

(*Source:* Nair KRG, Pandey Anu, Characteristics of Entrepreneurs: An Empirical Analysis, Journal of Entrepreneurship, Sage Publications (2006))

Reality Check about Entrepreneurial Acumen

Based on the above findings we can replace the following myths with the prevalent realities (Table 18.2).

Table 18.2: Myths and realities about entrepreneurial acumen

	Myths about entrepreneurial acumen	**Realities about entrepreneurial acumen**
1.	Successful entrepreneurs inherit their father's business	Inheritance creates no difference to entrepreneur's chances of success
2.	Family status plays a significant role in ensuring success of an entrepreneur	Entrepreneurs coming from poor backgrounds have been as successful
3.	Age makes a difference in the business acumen of an entrepreneur	Young as well as not-so-young people, both make equally good entrepreneurs
4.	Technical education and training is must to ensure success of an entrepreneur	People with no formal technical knowledge have done well too. Skills are more important than knowledge
5.	Work experience in related filed is must to ensure success of an entrepreneur	Experience come from work and not the vice-versa (i.e. work does not come from experience)

BUSINESS ACUMEN INVENTORY FOR A LIVESTOCK ENTREPRENEUR

Acumen for management of various business issues is essential for an entrepreneur. The following inventory will help one to assess the relative strengths and abilities that will be expected out of him/her for taking-up the entrepreneurial role.

Organizational Acumen

Ability to plan, organize, direct and control the various resources is the basic requirement for setting-up any enterprise. The entrepreneur must be able to:

- Choose a right location for his business.
- Choose the right breed of animals.
- Choose the right kind of people for his enterprise.
- Manage the various resources to facilitate optimum utilization.
- Handle legal issues.
- Understand partnership agreements and other contracts.
- Comply with government regulations.
- Obtain appropriate business licenses and permits.
- Comply with tax laws.
- Comply with labour code.
- Insure the business

Financial Acumen

Financial acumen refers to the ability of borrowing money, managing money, analyzing the financial statements and handling credit and collection primarily. The entrepreneur must be able to:

- Determine how much money is needed to start his business.
- Forecast the need for additional capital or cash.
- Identify appropriate sources for short-term-long-term financing.
- Negotiate loans.
- Do book keeping
- Establish and use financial records.
- Set-up a cost control system.
- Analyze overhead cost.
- Prepare basic profit and loss statement.
- Prepare an annual or quarterly budget.
- Understand profit-loss statement and balance sheet.
- Understand current credit policies of the government and private agencies.
- Use various collection techniques.
- Know how to go to small claim court.

Marketing Acumen

Marketing acumen refers to the ability to identify and target customers and being able to successfully push one's product into the market. It includes the ability to:

- Determine the territory in which he wants to operate.
- Determine the market and sales potential.
- Determine the type of customers he will serve.
- Assess the size of the market.
- Determine the needs and expectations of the customers.
- Distinguish his product from other products.
- Create awareness regarding his product.
- Motivate the customers to buy his product.

Competing Acumen

In this fast track world, competition is inevitable and hence the acumen to compete with others is must, no matter operating at whatever small level. It includes the ability to:

- Find out how the competitors are doing.
- Analyze how the competitors attract and retain their customers.
- Determine how one's firm will be different from the competition.
- Set a competitive hourly labour rate.
- Prepare an estimate of the costs for providing the services.

- Negotiate contracts or deal with other parties.
- Develop an adequate promotional strategy.
- Design promotional materials.
- Prepare and decide a budget for advertising.
- Use of quality of workmanship and customer service as a promotional tool.

Operational Acumen

Operational acumen refers to the smooth conduction of business operations especially with the management of the channel partners and the supply chain. It includes the ability to:

- Buy supplies from the best source, at the best price possible.
- Buy reliable equipment with adequate warranties.
- Negotiate contracts with suppliers.
- Use techniques for controlling material inventories.
- Set-up quality control techniques.
- Coordinate own work schedule with the convenience of other parties.
- Set-up a system for recording orders.

Knowing the Basics—Foundation Acumen

One of the foundation acumen or abilities that should be present in any person interested to establish a poultry or dairy unit is the various components of such business and the estimated cost of creating that infrastructure. This is the very foundation for starting any enterprise and hence before all other abilities, acumen to judge the structural and financial framework is an absolute prerequisite. Tables 18.3 and 18.4 describe these points.

Table 18.3: Ability to judge poultry enterprise requirements

S. No.	Component	Maximum total project cost* (Rs in lakhs)
1.	Establishing poultry breeding farm with low input technology birds and also for ducks/turkey/guinea fowl/quail/emu/ostrich, etc.	30.00
2.	Establishment of feed godown, feed mill, feed analytical laboratory	16.00
3.	Marketing of poultry products (Specialized transport vehicles, cool room storage facilities and retention sheds for birds, etc.)	25.00
4.	Egg grading, packing and storage for export capacity	80.00
5	Retail poultry dressing unit (300 birds per day)	5.00
6.	Egg/broiler carts for sale of poultry products	0.10
7.	Central grower unit (12,500 birds per batch and 4 batches per year)	20.00

Table 18.4: Ability to judge dairy enterprise requirements

S. No.	Component	Maximum total project cost* (Rs in lakhs)
1.	Establishment of small dairy farms—Ten animal unit (buffaloes/cross-bred cows) for milk production	Rs 3.00 lakhs per unit (up to ten animals) - Any non-operation flood areas. - The total cost depends on the infrastructural facilities required.
2.	Purchase of milking machines/milk tester/bulk milk cooling unit, etc.	Rs 15.00 lakhs Milking machine, milk-o-tester, bulk milk cooling units (up to 2000 lts capacity).
3.	Purchase of dairy processing equipment for manufacturing indigenous milk products.	Rs 10 lakhs per unit - Unit cost depends upon the quantum of milk to be handled and the type of products to be manufactured. - The total cost depends upon the investment on civil structures, type and ource of machinery.
4.	Establishment of dairy product transportation facilities including cold chain.	Rs 20 lakhs per unit - Unit cost depends upon the quantum of milk/milk products to be transported/handled and the type of products to be transported. - The total cost depends upon the investment on type and source of transport vehicle and machinery.
5.	Cold storage facilities for milk and milk products.	Rs 25 lakhs per unit - Unit cost depends upon the quantum of milk/milk products to be stored and the type of products to be stored. - While the cost depends upon the investment on type and source of machinery used.
6.	Establishment of private veterinary clinics.	Rs 2.00 lakhs per unit for mobile clinics and Rs 1.5 lakhs for stationary clinic - Area of operation from 8 to 10 villages having 5000 to 6000 cattle units.

(* *Source:* Website of Deptt. of Agriculture and Animal Husbandry, Government of India)

An entrepreneur who has high level of administrative capability, flair and ability for decision-making, computational skill, delegation skill, organizational skill, good at communication and has a basic level of technical knowledge stands a much better chance of success than his counterpart who possesses none or low level of these basic abilities. It is the possession of these scarce abilities, which confers an advantage on some people in becoming an entrepreneur. Besides these abilities, however, the entrepreneur also needs to be himself a generalist so that he can discharge his function without delegation, or to possess delegation and organizational skills. The characteristics of an entrepreneur that contribute to success are the result of achievement motivation. A successful entrepreneur must be a person with technical competence, initiative, good judgement, intelligence, leadership qualities, self-confidence, energy, attitude, creative thinking, fairness, honesty, tactfulness and emotional stability.

Mental Acumen

Mental acumen includes intelligence and creative thinking. An entrepreneur must be reasonably intelligent and should have creative thinking and must be able to engage in the analysis of various problems and situations in order to deal with them.

Visionary Acumen

A small entrepreneur like livestock entrepreneur cannot be expected to be very highly visionary but he must be able to set clear objectives as to the exact nature of the business, the nature of the goods to be purchased and subsidiary activities to be undertaken. A successful entrepreneur may have the objective to establish the product or to make profit or to render social service.

Confidentiality Acumen

An entrepreneur must be able to guard the business secrets; leakage of business secrets to trade competitions is a serious matter, which should be carefully guarded against by an entrepreneur.

Relationship Acumen

The most important personality factors contributing to the success of an entrepreneur are emotional stability, personal relations, consideration and tactfulness. An entrepreneur must maintain good relations with his customers. He must also maintain good relations with his employees if he is to motivate them to perform their jobs at a high level of efficiency and commitment. An entrepreneur who maintains good relations with his employees, customers, channel partners (suppliers and distributors), creditors and the society at large has much higher chances of success.

Technical Acumen

An entrepreneur must have a reasonable level of technical knowledge. This is necessary to have proficiency over the business operations and to tide over the change.

Business Communication Acumen

Communication is said to be the process by which a sender sends a message across a media to the intended receiver. Communication ability is the ability to communicate effectively. Good communication also means that both the sender and the receiver understand each other and are being understood. An entrepreneur who can effectively communicate with customers, employees, suppliers, creditors will be more likely to succeed than the entrepreneur who does not. In order to understand the essentials of effective business communication, one has to have a fair idea of the world of business itself. Business communication is distinct from personal communication as it has a different set of objectives. In the discussion to follow, we shall be focusing on the various characteristics and features of business so that the needs of business communication become clear. Any business has certain distinct characteristics. This set it apart from other activities such as personal affairs, religion and charity.

Any business has certain distinct characteristics. These set it apart from other activities such as personal affairs, religion and charity.

Profit Motive

Any business is known by its commercial character, i.e. the profit motive. At the end of the day, every business looks at its net earning. It looks to a healthy bottom line that is responsible profits, and generally not to exorbitant profits. There may be times when it incurs losses and will have to live with such losses. While seeking profits is a necessary trait for any business, profiteering or seeking exorbitant profits from the customer is inimical to any business. Customers are the essence of any business and when they are no customers, there is no business. Customers are the source of income and profits for any business. Business communication should, therefore, aim at keeping the customer base intact and ever expanding.

Competitive Nature

Today's business world is in intensely competitive world. Competition means that there are many players in the market offering identical products and services. As a result, have substantial choice of products, services, markets and sellers. In a competitive scenario, the producer or the service provider has to emphasize on the quality, price, durability and such features, which has product, or service provides in order to attract and retain customers. This competitive situation is in contrast to the monopolistic situation where there is only one seller and hardly any choice. Business communication has to necessarily take cognizance of the nature of the market and evolve strategies appropriate to the competitive situation.

Sustainable Results

Businesses operate generally with a long-term objective. Barring some types of players and services that are short-term in nature, most other in business on a sustainable basis. Those players who are in business to make fast money and disappear are referred to as fly-by-night operators. They are distinct from the majority of players who wish to be in business today, tomorrow and the day-after. Large business organizations tend to acquire a perennial character. Business communication, to be effective, should recognize the long-term sustainability of results.

Business Relationship

Like any individual who has personal relationship, a business has its business relationship. These relationships are with customers, buyers, suppliers and others with whom one has to interact on an ongoing basis. It is these relationships, which sustain the business in the long run. Every business strives to make much relationship not only profitable, but also mutually beneficial. An important objective of any business communication would be to established, nurture and sustain such mutually beneficial long-term relationship.

Business Ethics

Every business has its set of principles of a code of conduct. This code often outlines the dos and don'ts of its approach to business and customers. The code also articulates its duties and responsibilities as well as expectations. Every profession similarly has ethical values governing its business conduct. There are also wail laid down and understood fair practices for any business. Again effective communication aims at articulating business either and related qualitative aspects.

Every connected with communication should take note of such characteristics of the business and use appropriate methods and approaches.

MASTERING THE SKILLS OF BUSINESS COMMUNICATION

Business the world over, have come to recognize the need for fast, accurate and effective communication in a common language. Skill relevant for ensuring effective communication in the new business world includes the following.

- Communication skills
- Listening skills
- Grammatical structures, vocabulary, idioms and pronunciation
- Presentation skills
- Interpersonal communication
- Negotiating skills
- Social language for business
- Business writing skills
- The art of good speaking
- Business simulation
- Telephone techniques
- Cross culture awareness
- Electronic communication

A good communicator has to master numerous skills.

COMMUNICATION NEEDS

Any business organization will have to communicate with the several of people on an ongoing basis for a variety of reasons. They include the following:

Stakeholder

The process of communication should, as we have already discussed, effectively cover all the stakeholder, viz. owners, employers, customers and the community. Employers and customers are particularly related in any organization and a wide variety of methods, types, channels and strategies will have to be adopted to effectively address their communication needs.

Government Agencies

Every business, in some way or the other comes within the ambit of Government and agencies may be national or central, provincial or state or local in nature. Quite often every business will have to comply with various government rules and regulations. Inadequate reporting could result in penalties. Every business has to necessary respect the law of the land. Communication between any business organization and the government has to be recognized.

Trade Organization

Every business generally has certain affiliation or membership with a trade organization or an association. It may be functional or geographical in nature. Such organizations generally work with the large interest of its member in mind. Communication with this segment becomes necessary.

Competitor

There may be various players who operate within the market and the marketplace. There are often occasions for them to communicate with each other. Notwithstanding the competitive nature, different players may arrive at some understanding to respond to the customers. They may even be occasions where there is a clash of interest that needs sorting out. For different reasons, a business organization may have to communicate with its competitors and other operators in the market.

Media

Businesses also often the need for communicating or interacting with the press, television and other media. It may be for the purpose of advertisement or announcement or clarification or image building.

Not all communication that takes place between individual and groups is effective. Barriers apart, there are several factors affecting communication. These are conceptual clarity of the communicator, language used in communication, moods, and receptivity of the sender and the receiver and the timing of the communication.

Good communication is not a matter of an accident or a happening especially in any business situation; it calls for planed, organized and coordinate efforts.

There are several essential ingredients contributing to the success of the communication. These are:

- Clarity of purpose
- Understanding of the process
- Addressing the right target audience
- Requisite communication skills
- Adequate information
- Proper planning
- Positive approach
- Sincerity

Effectiveness of communication also calls for avoiding extreme feelings, consistency, timeliness, use of appropriate modes and channels, cost consciousness and finally for feedback.

Communication takes place among human being. Therefore, the behaviour dimension assumes much signification. Human behaviour gets reflected through perceptions, attitudes, beliefs, values, norms and experiences. That is why it is said, "Meaning is in people, not is words." Perception is described as the process of making sense out of events. It is essentially a matter of personal judgment. A good communicator has to realize that perception tend to vary from person to person and accordingly factor this realization into his or her communication.

Attitudes exert a strong influence on human relationships and consequently on the process of communication. They can be both positive and negative. A good communicator should recognize the importance of positive attitudes.

Values and value systems also influence communication. Values are seen as standards of behaviour communication becomes effective only when values shows congruence.

Norms and experiences too impact communication. People tend to interpret messages it terms of this facets. A good communicator develops a clear insight into human behaviour and uses it to his or her advantage.

Language is the vehicle of communication. According to an estimate, there are more than 3500 languages in the world. Each language has its own idioms, expressions, phrases and nuances. A good communicator masters and uses the language, which the addressee understands.

Business communication is distinct from personal communication and has certain specific characteristics. It has to be in tune with the business objectives. It should support the profit motive. It should recognize the competitive nature of business. It should work towards sustainable results. It should strengthen relationships. Finally, business communication should articulate business ethics.

Each business has its four major stakeholder—owners, employees, customers and community. Business communication should encompass all these sections. Additionally, it should also address government agencies, trade organizations, consumer forums and the press and media as well.

Business communication has many non-verbal dimensions as well. The several dimensions of non-verbal communication discussed in this chapter include the following:

- Body language
- Personal space
- Gesture and posture
- Facial expressions
- Timings, examples and behaviour

FEW MORE BUSINESS ACUMENS

Innovation

Innovation, by its very nature, disrupts the equilibrium of a competitive market and causes uncertainty. To confront it, the enterprise must innovate further. The competition driven innovation (Canter, Guth, Nicklisch and Weiland, 2004), central to technical progress and responsible for keeping large corporation vibrant, however, creates peculiar difficulties for the new farm. As research and design budgets and technical change accelerates, innovation becomes even more focused and competitive. Markets take unanticipated paths hammered by the onslaught of innovators. New products spring up and disappear before people have a change to look at them and the inventors have time to exploit the gain of their creation. The scale of creative destruction wrought by entrepreneurs trying to break into rival markets using the innovative edge of their products and processes has been, of late, growing increasingly discomforting. No wonder, the closure rates are mounting and the steady advancements in knowledge continue to leave behind entrepreneurial mass graves.

It seems, new enterprise in the next century is going to awaken to a competitive reality that is both overwhelming and scary. Entrepreneurs everywhere are now facing the classic.

As efficiency standards rise, survival becomes increasingly difficult for new enterprises. Effective management and exploitation of change of this magnitude and complexity is extremely difficult. Under such intense uncertainty, there seems to be no guarantee of payoffs from any programme to improve technology.

To innovate or not is the question which haunts the new business.

Due to the random and accidental nature of inventions and innovations, even in a non-competitive research milieu, there can be no formula for success from innovation, which depends on information for which the requirement cannot be anticipated on definitive terms and therefore, cannot be programmed. Calculating profitability of a new process is more difficult than is usually acknowledged. The failure to manage innovation is the most discouraging part of its history. The issue central to successful innovation is most merely to run fast, but also to run in the right direction. You cannot come back if you follow a wrong lead because before that one of your rivals must have already reached the goal. Failure, thus, could be costly many times over. For a start-up, following multiple leads is difficult due to both resource crunch and inability to develop and market an unintended discovery. The small business thus must be both competent to have inventive genius and fortunate to be groping in the right darkness. In competition with a large corporation which has the advantage of some illumination due to its past groping experience and has resources to fumble simultaneously in several alleys, the new enterprise is handicapped. It is one thing to operationalize a principle, but totally different to refine, make it cost effective, and put it successfully in a market of increasingly discerning customers. The new realities of competitive innovation have enhanced the uncertainty facing small business and have raised the chances of its failure. In such a state, to stake your fortunes on innovation is a difficult and discouraging option. Not to innovate is equally daunting, since the productivity, profit, and growth of enterprise are all closely linked to an organization's ability to innovate successfully. The survival is an aim more urgent than all above, however, is too obvious to be stressed. Though it would be churlish to claim that all start-ups must survive and grow, high fatality of nascent business is both undesirable. Every failed enterprise leaves in its wake a large number of entrepreneurial hopes and despairs are contagious. Budding entrepreneurs are affected by the fate of previous entrepreneurial attempts. It is true that entrepreneurial plunges are not always discouraged by prospects of failure and if only the mathematical probability of success were to be the basis of enterprise formation, no new enterprise would ever be formed.

The essence of that strategy is outline here. Imitate the technology that has proved itself, sell the product that is a winner and accumulate the experience of administrating a success. Learn to understand and handle the economy, financial and legal complexities of business when you do not have to bother about technical change and marketability. Then slowly change gear, invest in R and D and bring under scrutiny both your buyer and technology to see how and where to they are changing. Concentrate on one fundamental issue. In which way the technology at your command can be marginally molded to create a slightly different variant of the products to cater to an emerging or hitherto unfulfilled need. Once you have done that, you have broken away from your umpteen peers who spend a lifetime imitation. This incremental change should be the mainstay of your strategy unit you have the resources, skill and experience to break new grounds.

Attitude

It was the legendary George Bernard Shaw who once wrote, *The reasonable man adapts himself to the world; the unreasonable one persists in trying to adapt the world to himself.* All progress thus depends on this unreasonable person.

Entrepreneurship is generally understood as a pursuit of opportunity without limiting oneself to the accepted within the existing norms and confines of an organization.

A viable alternative to the personality and demographic approaches is the use of attitudes in predicting behaviourial tendencies. Social-psychological theories view attitude as the predisposition to respond in a generally favourable or unfavourable manner with respect to the object of the attitude.

The set of attitudes measured by this scale therefore covered a total of five dimensions: innovation business, perceived personal control in business, achievement in business, perceived self-esteem in business and taking advantage of opportunities in business.

The importance of risk-taking in business has been emphasized by many. Attempts to distinguish entrepreneurs on their risk-taking propensity have produced conflicting. These results highlight the significance of loss an important aspect in risk-taking, which is often ignored in entrepreneurial and managerial studies. The riskiness in business ventures, which has been the main stumbling block for many, is not the low probability of success but the high stakes involved in entrepreneurship.

Research on the risk-taking propensity of entrepreneurs has also produced conflicting results. Hull, Bosley and Udell (1980), in their study of university alumni, found risk-taking to be an important factor influencing an individual's likelihood of starting a business. Risk-taking is inherent in entrepreneurship (Dickonand Gigillierano, 1986, Knight, 1979; Palmer, 1971). However, studies on the risk-taking propensity of entrepreneurs have indicated that entrepreneurs and managers do not differ significantly in this regard from managers (Brockhaus, 1980, Sunderr, andKamalanabhan, 1996). Atkinson and Raynor (1974) and McCelland (1961) have advanced the explanation that people high on achievement motivation, prefer moderately risk ventures.

Social Capital

Social capital is an attribute that is created in interactions among people, which increases the strength and value of personal qualities like intelligence and work experience and is manifested in norms and networks that enable people to act collectively. Social capital is commonly defined as "information, trust and norms of reciprocity inherent in one's social networks." This social capital may have positive effects on entrepreneurial activities. A scholar makes a distinction between two specific dimensions of social capital, namely, bridging (or inclusive) and bonding (or exclusive). The bridging networks are open for access to external assets and facilitate information diffusion, whereas bonding social capital is good for mobilizing solidarity but may 'create strong out-group antagonism', which could limit entrepreneurial potentials. Social capital related to sub-cultures and ethnic enclaves often seems to combine the bonding qualities and non-acculturation with bridging networks to related ethnic group in other geographical settings. This can be observed among trade diaspora in various parts of the world.

Social capital is spread and exchanged through social networks. Social capital of various groups or sub-cultures may reflect different levels of trust in social relationship and have an impact on information search and transaction costs. Social capital is also responsible for creating norms of behaviour and forms the basis for accumulation of human capital. A social capital that is conducive to entrepreneurship is closely related to social skills. Authors have argued that a high degree of social perception and adaptability, ability to induce liking and a favourable first impression and to persuade and influence others are of social importance for entrepreneurial endeavour. Social skills provide an entrepreneur with a competitive advantage in the networking process, and like the social network, they are an integral part of the social capital. Social skills are seen to develop due to factors like in-group solidarity, pride, mobility, and education.

Another important aspect of any business culture is the extent to which it promotes intra- and inter-community trust. Social networks are ways which entrepreneurs to reduce transaction costs and risks. They also aid in the process of learning and information dissemination.

Managerial Resourcefulness

Managerial resourcefulness, as defined, is a set of generic competencies that enable adaptive reponses to the demands of the managerial role. Conceptualized in the manner, competencies are basic, critical components of a successful manager's repertoire. They can be considered as inner resources that managers possess which help them to deal with non-routine and often stressful or challenging situations. Such situations require a variety of adaptive response ranging from emotional control in the face of strong emotions, to cognitive in information processing (planning, problem solving, decision-making, etc.), perseverance in the face of hurdles and distractions. Managers who possess these competencies are considered more resourceful than managers who do not possess them. The resourcefulness framework outlines three types of generic competencies that constitute managerial resourcefulness. The first, affective competence, deals primarily with emotional control in situations that can provoke strong emotions. Specific examples include control of aggressive tendencies against goal-blocking agencies, control of fear of failure or consequences of goal directed actions, control of hopelessness or depressions, of excitement that many interfere with goal attainment, developing equanimity, and coping with the delayed gratification. The second, intellectual competence, in problem solving and the capacity for self-reflection. Specifically, it refers to capabilities dealing with information gathering, analytical and synthetic thinking, analogical reasoning goal analysis in terms of components and linkages or dependencies among components, planning and evaluation of alternative courses of action, etc. The third, action oriented competence, refers to task related capabilities like attention to deal, persistence, concern for the time-frame, and people-oriented capabilities sensitivity and empathy.

Thus, a resourceful manager is one who shows competence in regulating his/her emotions or feelings, thoughts and actions. Although resourcefulness involves self-control procedures to regulate one's emotions, thoughts and action orientation, at the deepest level, self-control producers represent a set of cognitions regarding one's own that ultimately determine the emotion, thoughts and behavioural processes.

Acumen to Manage Human Resource

Owner-managers and senior managers of small enterprises have often expressed that the main problems related to human resource management (HRM) in their enterprises are attracting talent, motivating employees and retaining key employees. They reason that small enterprises lack resources to advertise for positions, pay salaries in the range of large organizations and train employees. They face the addition problem of not having enough hierarchical layers to regularly promote employees. It has also been said that employees complain that they cannot learn much and find the job content monotonous. Hence, owner-managers of such enterprises are hesitant to provide external and costly training to their employees because they fear that after such training, will either demand very high salaries or leave the organization for better prospects. Human resource management in small enterprises has not got the attention it deserves from both researchers and entrepreneurs. In small enterprises, owner-managers are responsible for decisions related to human resources (Matlay, 1999). Their managerial style has a direct influence on the HRM practices (Koch Andde Kok, 1999). Owing to the small size of the organization, the motivation and morale of each employee has a direct and visible influence on the productivity of the organization. It has also been found that at a certain point, entrepreneurs are reluctant to give up control because of the belief that formalization might take management of the enterprise beyond their capacity (Mac Mahon and Murphy, 1999) and out of their hands. However, lack of attention by owner-manager in developing and formalizing HRM systems create barriers to organization growth.

CONCLUSION

Livestock business like all other small enterprises requires an optimal degree of business acumen among the entrepreneurs. Not all the abilities may be present in a budding entrepreneur, however, with persistence and guidance these acumen can be developed. Conclusively one thing can be said for certain that the success of any enterprise depends largely on the development and exhibition of business acumen.

19

Economics of Disease Management for Entrepreneurs

Umesh Dimri, MC Sharma, D Swarup

The persistence of widespread poverty and hunger are the principal disappointments with the post-independent India. More than five decades later, when the government claims that a change would place India on a new growth trajectory, the importance of public action to deal with poverty and vulnerability has only increased. Even official estimates, estimate the number of poor in India at 260 million.

The country being predominantly rural and agriculture still being the principal source of livelihood of a majority of the population; alleviating poverty requires special attention to rural livelihoods. The agriculture's share in gross domestic product (GDP) has fallen from 38.1% in 1980 to 31% in 1990 and 24.7% in 2001. Of the total population residing in rural India, agriculture accounted for 57% of total employment in 1999-2000. A trend analysis of GDP growth prior to and after the reforms points to a deceleration in the GDP growth in agriculture from 3.1% (1981-82 to 1990-91) to 2.5% (1992-93 to 2002-03). Even to the extent that growth did occur during the 1990s, the available evidence suggests that the impact of this growth on employment was limited. National Sample Survey (NSS) estimates indicate that the average annual rate of growth of aggregate rural employment growth stood at just 0.58% over the period 1993-94 and 1999-2000. This is the lowest rate of increase observed since the NSS first began reporting employment data in the 1950s.

The decline in the overall rate of growth of employment was largely due to the stagnation of employment in agriculture, that earlier had been a major source of incremental employment. With a substantial part of employment in the unorganized sector being reflective either of a process of agricultural "involution" or of a distress-driven spill-over into low-paid, casual and insecure employment, it appears that the ability of the current process of growth to adequately impact on poverty and deprivation is indeed limited.

An entrepreneur is an individual who accepts financial risks and undertakes new financial ventures. The word derives from the French "entre" (to enter) and "prendre" (to take), and in a general sense applies to any person starting a new project or trying a new opportunity. Many societies place great value on the entrepreneur. To encourage their activity, they may be offered access to inexpensive capital, tax exemptions and management advice. An entrepreneur has the greatest chance of success by focusing on a market niche either too small or too new to have been noticed by established businesses. To help new technologies come to market, many universities establish business incubators for entrepreneurs hoping to turn leading edge research into marketable products.

Characteristics of an entrepreneur include spontaneous creativity, the ability and willingness to make decisions in the absence of solid data, and a generally risk-taking personality. An entrepreneur may be driven by a need to create something new or build something tangible. In the Austrian school of Economics, entrepreneurs are described as being engaged in the *creative destruction* of existing products and services. As new enterprises have low success rates, an entrepreneur must also have considerable persistence.

Entrepreneurs are generally highly independent, which can cause problems when their ventures succeed. In a small company, the entrepreneur is able to personally manage most aspects of the business, but this is not possible once the company has grown beyond a certain size. Management conflicts often arise when the entrepreneur does not recognize that running a large stable company is different from running a small growing company. The problem is often resolved by the entrepreneur either leaving to start a new venture, or being forced out by shareholders. At Apple Computer, for example, one founder, Steve Wozniak, left to pursue other interests, while the other, Steve Jobs was ultimately fired and replaced with a CEO from a much larger company. Note that many years later, jobs returned to the helm.

An *intrapreneur* is an individual who acts like an entrepreneur but from inside the confines of a large organization or corporation.

In the present era, most of the activities are diverted in a way such that maximum income is generated from them. One of the basic aims of animal rearing is to improve the economic status of the human. Health status of the animal significantly affects the animal productivity and income generated from them. In animal rearing, a significant part of the input expenditure is spent on disease prevention or cure.

THE ECONOMICS OF ANIMAL DISEASE CONTROL

Economics is a social science dealing with the production and distribution of goods and hence of wealth. It analyses how meager resources are allocated between different uses and groups within the economic framework. Initially, economic thought was developed under the name "political economy" and examined the production and distribution of money in a society comprising people from varied economic groups. Industrialization made people to view the economic relationship between industrialists, workers and landowners. This was the attitude of Marx and indicates the Marxist economics. Capitalist economies view the economic interactions as the inter-relationship between producers and consumers, who meet in the market place and try to satisfy each others need. It targets at critically analyzing the "positive", i.e. the real or observable aspects of this relationships in the market and to derive generally applicable theories. It does not associate itself with the "normative" aspects which relate to value judgments about how the economic process ought to function.

The study of economics is conventionally divided into two areas. *Micro-economics* analyses the individual producer and consumer behaviour, emphasizing the factors affecting the production and consumption. *Macro-economics* analyses the overall economy. It considers national income, balance of payments, overall savings and investment.

Development economics deals with the specific problems of the under developed economies. It evaluates their economic policies (price control, subsidies, taxes, channellising funds into specific areas, aimed at overcoming their economic problems and improving the living standard of their people. The topics covered include an analysis of the reasons, implications and remedies of poverty and division of economy between the agricultural and the industrial sectors in Third World countries. It economically examines the type of technology, employment scenario, and movement of people, trade and market.

Project appraisal is economically analyzing the project prior to undertaking it. Project evaluation involves economically evaluating the projects after its start and at specified intervals till its completion. The project is evaluated for its practical implications considering economic principles for decision-making based on a social benefit-cost analysis. It ultimately finds whether the project would be profitable. Budgeting and accounting may also be utilized for this economic analysis.

SCIENTIFIC AND TECHNICAL REVIEW

There is sometimes a degree of hesitation before economics are taken into account in decisions concerning investment in animal health programmes. Preference is often given to the use of biological criteria of efficacy and expected outcomes. However, the challenge for the future is to develop an appropriate balance between the biophysical and economic criteria in rational decision-making. This is particularly important for countries contemplating major disease control or eradication programmes, to relieve the burden of a given disease on livestock production, or to open avenues to increased trade in a particular livestock product.

To reduce the costs on disease prevention/cure, methods to reduce the expenditure on antiparasitic drugs (both against endo- and ectoparasites), antibiotics and vitamin/mineral preparations and to minimize the diseases/conditions against which such therapies are required need to be looked into.

APPLICATION OF ECONOMIC ANIMAL DISEASE CONTROL POLICY

For better animal health projects and programmes, principles of economics contribute at the following levels towards the improvement of policy and decision-making:

i. In the livestock sector, it explains how economic factors influence producers (their decisions on what, how and when to produce; the acceptable prices; whether to expanded or contract the business and production and investment, etc.); factors determining demand for livestock products, how these affect the quantity and quality of products bought, and how prices are fixed in different circumstances (micro-economics). The economic aspects of the different livestock production systems can be described by collecting relevant information on producer-consumer behaviour—its overall effect on price structure and economic outputs and how producers and consumers interact. A particular livestock production system can be described in economic terms by looking at the value of output, the cost of the inputs, calculating the income received by the producers, butchers, traders and other middlemen, and examining the final price paid by the consumers.

ii. Once the production system as well as the interaction between the consumer and producer is identified, it becomes feasible to evaluate and predict the likely economic effects of any changes introduced into the sector. Such changes would include both changes affecting prices of inputs or outputs, income of consumers, demand and qualitative and quantitative fluctuations in the output due to introduction of improved inputs, changing the management and animal health scenario.

iii. Ultimately, economic analysis makes it possible to arrange this information for evaluating, categorizing hence comparing different programmes or projects and assessing their overall economic feasibility.

Thus, for an animal health project, economic theory can help explain and describe producer-consumer behaviour, the production systems involved, predict and quantify the effect of the project on output, prices, demand and incomes. This information may be arranged in the form of a benefit-cost analysis. Then, having sequenced and compared the alternatives, a decision can be made whether to implement the project or not.

The technical feasibility of any proposed measure must be examined by the relevant specialists (veterinarians, animal husbandry experts, sociologists, economists, management professionals, etc.). Then, its overall compatibility with the stated policies and goals of the livestock sector must be ensured, and, ultimately, its feasibility from an organizational and social point of view needs to be verified.

Here, economic (cost-benefit) analysis is made about long-term decisions on animal health programmes. Some of the basic economic principles are:

Demand and Supply

Money is the "unit" in terms of which prices of goods are given in a cash economy, although barter can fix their relative values. Price is an item used in economic decision-making. An understanding of how they are derived and what they represent is crucial. For example, if a kid costs rupees 700, an adult sheep costs rupees 1400, 2 kids could be exchanged for 1 adult sheep in the absence of money, or both could be paid for in dollars, pounds or any other acceptable currency.

Concept of price theory emerged with the concept of goods with a limited supply and a constant demand or which needed labour for its production and consequently, the labour charges. Presently, prices are determined by the status of demand, depending upon the prices acceptable to producers as well as the consumers. For most goods, the quantity offered increases with increasing price, but the quantity demanded decreases. If demand equals supply, the market is said to be "in equilibrium" at a particular price. This price is also called the *market-clearing* price, and it represents the point at which all that is produced is sold. At a higher price, supply exceeds demand, since production is more than demand. The reverse is true if the price is lower than the market-clearing price, in which case consumers are eager to buy but producers are reluctant to sell or produce, and, ultimately, the quantity demanded exceeds the quantity supplied. If the individuals bargain in a real market place, they would continue to offer each other prices until they arrived at a mutually agreeable price, or else the consumer would decide not to buy or the producer not to sell.

If the government fixes a maximum price for an effective and much needed antibiotic with the objective of ensuring that low-income consumers can afford it. If this price is below the market-clearing price, producers would like to charge more, demand outstrips supply, and a black market develops where the drug is sold at prices nearer to, or even exceeding, the market-clearing price to those consumers who can afford it. Contrarily, if a government fixes a minimum price which is above the market-clearing price, supply will tend to outstrip demand at that price and suppliers will be forced to sell off their medicine cheaply, avoiding the government regulations.

The discussion of price theory has raised several points which need to be considered when deciding which prices to use in various economic studies.

i. Since for most goods the quantity demand falls as the price rises, government can stimulate demand for an item by setting a low price. Conversely, they can lower demand by setting a high price. A low price can be supported by a subsidy; a high price may be enforced by a purchase tax. For example, the consumption of milk may be encouraged by setting a low price for consumers, backed up by a subsidy to producers. Similarly, new inputs into production systems, such as fertilizers, improved breeds of livestock, ploughs, etc. may be encouraged by subsidizing their cost to whoever is prepared to use them. In the absence of a support for artificially high or low prices, black markets tend to emerge. With medicine production, sometimes a very commonly needed medicine may involve a low cost of production, but because of its high utility, consumers may purchase it even at high costs.

ii. Different consumers may pay different prices for the same medicine. For example, because of the costs of transport, medicines may cost more in isolated rural areas or if they are imported from another region or country. Products may be more expensive when bought in retail outlets with high overheads, while items sold in large quantities are usually cheaper.

iii. A variety of prices, affected by a government subsidy or tax, exist for each item. These may be the price paid by the consumer, which may include a purchase tax or is the portion of the cost after the subsidy has been removed; the price received by the producer, which is the price before purchase tax is added or, in the case of a subsidy, the equivalent to the price paid by the consumer plus the government subsidy; the cost to the government of the subsidy or the revenue brought in by the tax; the cost to the nation, which is roughly equivalent to the price paid to the producer.

Elasticity

In order to be able to measure precisely how supply and demand respond to changes in prices, the concept of *elasticity* was developed, which is expressed by the formula given below.

$$\text{Price elasticity of supply (or demand)} = (-) \frac{\text{The percentage change in quantity}}{\text{The percentage change in price}}$$

Elasticity should be expressed as a positive number. A minus sign is placed before the equation in the case of the price elasticity of demand, since demand falls as price increases, making the overall result positive. Thus, if the demand or supply changes by the same percentage as price, the elasticity is I. If a price increases by 10% and elasticity is 2, supply will increase by 20%. Goods are said to be *inelastic* if the demand for them changes very little with price, in which case the calculated elasticity is less than 1. Such goods are generally necessities, for which demand is very stable. For luxuries, demand is generally more elastic. Similarly, for essential and commonly used medicines which have no substitutes, the demand is very stable.

Sometimes, producers have a target income rather than trying to maximize their profits, and once this income is reached, they cease to supply more goods. Thus, beyond a certain point, price increases may lead to a reduction in supply. This has been alleged to be the case with some nomadic cattle keepers, who only sell their animals to meet their fixed cash needs for such items as school fees, taxes, clothing, veterinary expenses, etc.

$$\text{Income elasticity of demand} = \frac{\text{The percentage change in quantity}}{\text{The percentage change in price}}$$

Changes in income must be taken into account when trying to project how the demand for livestock products will evolve over the years. Generally, the demand for good increases with increasing incomes. However, as people get wealthier they reduce the consumption of goods that are considered inferior, such as very cheap cuts of meat and/or clothing.

The concept of elasticity thus has the following practical applications in the formulation and assessment of animal disease control policy:

i. It helps in determining what the future supply and demand are likely to be in response to changes in prices and incomes.

ii. It is crucial in determining what prices to charge producers for various veterinary treatments. We may consider a hypothetical relationship between the demand for deworming and its price. The elasticity of demand varies, being very elastic as the price of an individual deworming falls from rupees 0.60 to about rupees 0.12 and relatively inelastic at rupees 0.85 per deworming. Therefore, to ensure a deworming coverage of about 90%, it will be necessary to provide the deworming free of charge. To increase the coverage further, livestock owners might actually have to be persuaded. If dewormers cost more than rupees 1.00 each, less than 5 to 10% of the livestock would be dewormed. Suppose that a coverage of 685 is thought necessary for a voluntary deworming campaign to be effective, then the maximum amount that can be charged by the veterinary service is rupees 0.10. If the dewormer costs rupees 0.12 per dose and the average cost of distributing and administering the distribution is rupees 0.30, it will be necessary to subsidize the campaign to the extent of rupees 0.32 per dose. The dewormer might be cheaper if purchased in bulk, and the cost per dose for distribution and administration might go down as more animals are presented at each deworming session.

However, experience has shown that this analysis of livestock producers' response to opportunities for deworming may not always correspond to reality. In some cases, producers avoid having their animals dewormed when the deworming is free but present them when a fee is imposed. This does not reflect a failure of economic theory to cope with reality; rather the belief of producers that free deworming may be inferior to those that are charged for.

ORGANIZED FARM STUDY

The expenditure incurred on the disease prevention/cure at the Sheep and Goat unit of the Indian Veterinary Research Institute, Izatnagar, Bareilly, Uttar Pradesh, India, was analyzed (average rain fall = 50–70 cm/yr; average temperature = 6.9–37.3°C; average humidity = 29.5–87.3%). The maximum expenditure was incurred on antiparasitic drugs (both against endo and ecto parasites) followed by antibiotics and vitamin-mineral preparations in the descending order.

Antibiotic Resistance

Significant increases in prevalence of resistance to antibiotics have been observed in common pathogens of humans in the United States and worldwide. The consequences of the appearance and spread of antibiotic resistance have included increasing morbidity, mortality, and cost of health care. The fundamental cause for the appearance and spread of antimicrobial resistance has been increasing antimicrobial use. However, other factors contribute in both inpatient and outpatient settings. Recognizing the important causes of increasing antibiotic resistance in these settings has led to practical recommendations, which health care facilities and outpatient practitioners will need to review, adapt, and apply for maximum local effectiveness for progress to be made in addressing one of the most challenging problems facing modern medicine.

As hard as it is to believe, antibiotics are also used in agriculture on plants rather than mammals. They are applied sprays to fruit tree farms, for preventing bacterial infections of the fruit. The concentrations may kill all the bacteria on the trees at the time of spraying, but the residual antibiotics can encourage the growth of resistant bacteria that later colonize the fruit during processing and shipping. The sprays randomly are carried by the wind and air for considerable distances to other trees and food plants, where the concentration is too low to eliminate infections but are still capable of killing off sensitive bacteria and thus giving the edge to resistant versions. These resistant bacteria work through the food chain, ending up in the intestinal tract of the host after the produce is eaten.

Another use of antimicrobial agents is the use of disinfectants and antiseptics. These agents are now used in everything including household cleaners, soaps, detergents, baby toys, cutting boards and even bedding! They are often bacteriostatic agents although some are bactericidal, and include quaternary ammonium compounds and triclosan (the most common) which mostly select for resistant strains, rather than permanently reducing the bacterial load in household items. Since these products are often used in food preparation, they increase our intake of resistant bacteria.

There are currently some major pathogens like *E. faecalis, M. tuberculosis* and *P. aeruginosa* of which certain strains exhibit total resistance to all currently used antibiotics. For instance, *E. faecalis,* which is normally resistant to cephalosporins, heavy use of these agents in immuno-compromised patients allows overgrowth of the organism, in the past one would have administered antibiotics, but some are now resistant to all antibiotics, and so become lethal agents. One major fear is that since *E. faecalis* is resistant for vancomycin, that this will get passed via plasmid to other organisms, especially *S. aureus.*

Dealing with Antibiotic Resistance

After determining that resistance is a major crisis, we need to come up with strategies to fight it. The 1st strategy is to return to the bacterial control methods used before the widespread use of antibiotics; in other words, patient isolation with multi-drug resistant infections, gowning and gloving, hand washing and other antiseptic techniques.

The 2nd strategy is to culture hospitals for resistance to antiseptics and antibiotics, and rotate antiseptics and antibiotics on a regional basis, to assure maximum effect of antimicrobials. Reductions on the use of non-essential antimicrobials, such as the antiseptic soaps, detergents and toys should be implemented as well.

The 3rd strategy is to perform rational design of new antimicrobial agents that share no similarity with the current naturally derived antibiotics. Some interesting agents are under development, including a pump inhibitor for tetracycline resistance.

The 4th strategy is the reduction in the prescription of antibiotics in cases where they are not necessary. When veterinarians prescribe, they should culture and perform a minimum inhibitory concentration whenever practical, so that targeted drugs, rather than broad-spectrum drugs that encourage resistance and alteration of normal floral composition.

The 5th strategy is the cessation of sub-therapeutic administration in animal feeds and agriculture. Limit the use of major antibiotics for non-therapeutic uses.

The 6th strategy, perhaps the hardest one, is to educate owners to follow the prescribed regimen of the chosen antibiotic. Owners often stop giving antibiotics as soon there is improvement, thinking that the disease has been cured; this behaviour often selects for resistant bacteria. This behaviour may also lead to veterinarians giving more potent antibiotics, assuming that the owners may not give the full course. Since owners often demand antibiotics for what are truly diseases of viral aetiology, the incomplete course will often select for resistance. It is imperative that veterinarians educate owners on the appropriate use of antibiotics. The appearance and spread of resistance in aerobic gram-negative pathogens, such as Enterobacter, against broad-spectrum, third-generation cephalosporins was reported in the 1980s, shortly after the introduction of those medications. Resistance in these pathogens is often mediated by broad-spectrum beta-lactamases, which can inactivate most penicillin and cephalosporin antibiotics. The genes for these enzymes can be carried on plasmids, which may contain genes for products that inactivate other classes of antibiotics, such as aminoglycosides; these plasmids can sometimes be spread between different species and genera of aerobic gram-negative bacilli.

The appearance and spread of antimicrobial resistance has not been limited to bacteria. Since the introduction of fluconazole, strains of Candida causing hospital-acquired fungal infection have changed from ones with predictable fluconazole susceptibility to those with significant resistance. Most important in this regard is *Mycobacterium tuberculosis*. The appearance and spread of resistance in aerobic gram-negative bacilli to multiple beta-lactam antibiotics has been observed worldwide as has quinolone resistance in both *Staphylococcus* and gram-negative bacteria.

Increase in Anthelmintic Resistance

The prevention of parasitic relies on regular anthelmintic dosing to suppress faecal worm egg production and to reduce the build up of infective larvae on the pasture. A common cause of failure in worm control programmes is the development of anthelmintic resistance. Fenbendazole resistance was found to be widespread.

Benzimidazole resistance seems to develop in stages.

- Individual worms are still susceptible to higher doses of the drug. In this case giving a 5-day course of fenbendazole may overcome the resistance.
- Increased level of resistance—the worms are no longer susceptible even to repeated doses, as in the animals in this study.

For parasitic control, rotational grazing must be adhered to. For optimization of parasitic load there is need for regularly changing the anthelmintic and using them in a cyclic manner so that each time we do deworming, it should be different from the drug used for the immediate earlier deworming.

For using vitamin and minerals, it is essential that scientific calculations be made for their prevailing levels in the animal body and accordingly the deficient micronutrients may be supplemented in the diet or administered through the other routes. To reduce expenditures, it would be advisable to use appropriate, feeds rich in those micronutrients, which are deficient in the animals of a particular area.

Prices of Factors of Production and of Durable Goods

Prices for durable goods and the various inputs of production are slightly more complex unlike prices as though they were for consumer goods that were purchased outright. There are three factors of production to be considered for durable goods:

i. Labour, which can be divided into various grades;
ii. Land, which includes natural resources; and
iii. Capital, which covers both money itself and production goods such as livestock and machinery.

A fourth factor, entrepreneurship or management, is sometimes added to cover management and risk taking.

The factors of production are subject to the laws of supply and demand in the same way as other goods, but the demand for them is described as *derived demand*, since it depends on the demand for the products the factors are used to make. Given sufficient information about the production conditions, prices and the demand for final products, input-output models can be constructed for the whole economy to determine the demand for the different factors of production.

The many inputs of production and most durable goods can usually be bought in two ways:

i. Outright purchase, which confers on the owner all the incomes that can be earned from using a particular input or all the benefits from a particular durable good.
ii. Renting or hiring, this enables the purchaser to use the item for a stated period of time.

Underlying all investments or project appraisals is the concept that the various inputs or factors of production at the disposal of an individual or a nation should be used so as to earn that individual or nation the highest possible income. Thus, just as an individual should not borrow money at an interest of 10% per annum to finance an investment from which he expects a profit of 8% per annum, a nation should not invest resources in projects with a return of 8% when alternatives yielding 10% exist.

OPPORTUNITY COST AND THE CHOICE OF PRICES IN ECONOMIC ANALYSIS

In a project appraisal or budget, the main economic input lies in the choice of prices, since it is assumed that the technical inputs which give the main physical components of costs and benefits have been derived by the professionals responsible for ensuring the technical feasibility of the project. In the same way as all the assumptions necessary for deriving the physical parameters must be clearly stated, so the origin or derivation of every price or group of prices chosen must be given as well as the justification for using them. A simple rule determining which prices can be used in a particular analysis is that the prices chosen should approximate, as far as possible, to the opportunity cost of the relevant items to the individual, firm, institution or country from whose point of view the analysis is being made.

The opportunity cost of making a particular economic choice is given by the cost of whatever alternative production or consumption had to be foregone as a result of that choice. The allocation of labour in a village production system means that new projects introducing new work patterns need to take into account opportunity costs. The opportunity cost of capital, i.e. of using money or investment funds, is the rate of return or interest rate that can be earned in alternative uses.

From the concept of opportunity cost, the idea of shadow prices can be derived. Shadow prices are used with the broad objective of bringing prices to values nearer their true opportunity cost and thus, in project analysis, they lead to the selection of projects which use up the different resources at rates reflecting the real cost to society. Shadow prices can be defined as artificial prices calculated for certain items in order to ensure that their real opportunity cost is taken into consideration when making decisions. These shadow prices may be different from the money actually received or paid for the items at the time they are used.

Shadow prices are generally used in the following circumstances:

i. Where market prices do not reflect real opportunity costs. This is often the case when prices are fixed by the government or are affected by speculators indulging in monopolistic trading.

ii. To accomplish particular policy objectives by encouraging the use of some items by setting artificially low prices for them and discouraging that of others by setting artificially high prices.

Thus, in project appraisal, shadow prices will present the costs and benefits of the projects at prices that: (a) reflect, as far as possible, the real opportunity costs of the choices being made and the policies being proposed; and (b) follow government policy by making those projects that use a higher proportion of the inputs whose use or production the government wishes to encourage, seem relatively more profitable. This is because shadow prices give such inputs an artificially low cost and such outputs an artificially high value.

Shadow prices are most commonly used in the case of labour and foreign exchange. Shadow prices can be used for any commodity if the need arises. For instance, if the objective of government policy is to raise the living standard of a particular group of people in a country, shadow prices can be used to give a higher value to incomes gained by that group as compared to those of another group.

Generally, it is not recommended that individuals working within a government framework attempt to use a variety of shadow prices that they have calculated themselves. Ideally, the ministry in charge of planning and appraisal should give clear guidelines as to which shadow prices are acceptable. In the absence of this, individuals should make their initial calculations at market prices, and only if they feel that there is a strong case, should they apply their own shadow prices, stating clearly what these are and how they have been derived. Because the issue of shadow pricing is a complex one, the advice of a professional economist should be sought before attempting to assign shadow prices to goods and resources.

Choice of Prices for Financial and Economic Analyses

In economic studies, a differentiation is made between financial and *economic* analyses. Financial analyses evaluate the monetary implications of any particular activity by an individual person, enterprise or institution, looking at the actual expenses and receipts from the point of view of the individual or firm concerned. The prices used in these analyses are usually market prices.

Economic analyses works upon the effect of a particular activity on the whole economy. The prices used should approximate to their opportunity cost, so they may be shadow prices. Since the analysis is undertaken from the point of view of the whole economy, all prices are net of purchase taxes and subsidies.

As a study undertaken from the point of view of an individual person (firm or institution) examines the implications of a particular activity to that individual, the prices used must be those that the individual faces. Thus to a farmer who ends up buying all the supplementary feed for his cattle on the black market, the application of the government's subsidized price makes no sense. Supplying supplementary feed at subsidized prices costs the government the handling and distribution expenses plus the value of the subsidy. Whereas if a trader is involved, the feed brings him a profit if he sells it at a higher price, less his own costs of transport, handling, storage, etc. These are all *financial* viewpoints.

From the nation's *(economic)* point of view, the cost of the supplementary feed is probably best estimated using the price paid by the livestock producer, if the feed is sold on the open market. In economic evaluations involving most agricultural and livestock products, the so called "farm-gate price", which is the price paid to the producer, should be used. The retail price paid by consumers includes the profits of middlemen, transport and handling charges, etc. which do not form part of the real value of the product. Where the farm-gate price is artificially fixed, a shadow price reflecting the black market price may be used. World market prices for particular items should only be applied if these prices are being used throughout and if the government or agency for whom the evaluation is being undertaken desires this.

Adjusting for Inflation-price Conversions and Price Indexes

The principle of compounding, which will be of use in estimating the effect of an annual rate of inflation on prices over a number of years. For the purposes of project appraisal, making budgets or other economic or financial activities, it is often necessary to convert prices at current levels (i.e. for the year in which they occur) to constant values, i.e. to those in a chosen base year.

Any project manager, planner or individual planning his finances must make it a priority to collect not only information on costs but also on prices. Ideally all quantities, prices and expenses should be recorded. In fact, since the objective is to compare expenditure or receipts at constant prices, a record of total costs and unit prices would be sufficient. Expenditure and receipts could then be converted to the base year by making price indices out of the price series. This is the most practical approach. An alternative approach is to note all quantities purchased or sold. When the moment for comparing expenditure and receipts comes, these can converted to current costs for all items since the quantities and current prices are known.

Simple vs. Compound Growth (or Interest) Rates

If a given number (a livestock population, a sum of money, a price) is said to increase at a percentage rate per annum (population growth, interest or inflation rates), this increase could be interpreted as simple or compound growth. *Simple growth* is calculated by applying the percentage rate only to the initial sum, so that the numerical value of annual growth is always the same.

Compound growth is calculated by applying the percentage rate each year to the initial *sum plus* the previous year's growth, so that the annual growth rate also increases each year. Thus *compound interest* is paid not only on the principal but also on the interest that has accumulated.

In practice, almost all forms of annual increase are calculated on a compound basis. Interest is always paid on the full amount of money in the account, so simple interest would generally only apply if the individual removed the previous year's interest leaving the original sum in the bank. Human and livestock population growth rates apply each year to the whole of the population existing in the previous year, so the growth rate is again compound. The same is true of the annual inflation rate. If the present value (PV) and the annual rate of increase (i) are known, the future value (FV) can be calculated from the formula: $FV = PV (1 + i)^n$.

Discounting and Compounding

Discounting is the process of converting future values to present values. It is used in project appraisal, when considering a stream of future costs and benefits in order to determine what their total present value would be. Items for different years are "discounted" separately by calculating their present value and then the total present value of all items is calculated by adding these together. Compounding is the process of converting present values to future values.

It might be argued that the greatest impact of economic approaches to disease control and management has been in the more intensive production systems of the developed world, particularly the intensive poultry, pig and dairy industries, where widespread use of computerised economic-based decision support aids are in use daily and have contributed considerably to improving efficiency. However, there has also been increasing use of economics in decision-making in most other spheres of livestock production, although not necessarily through the use of sophisticated computerised techniques. In the developing world, the requirement for improved quality of decisions on resource allocation is driven not only by the need to enhance efficiency in the livestock industries, but also by the need to prioritise public expenditures in response to the diverse and sometimes competing needs of rapidly growing human populations, compounded by declining financial resources and declining public sector involvement in animal health service delivery.

To secure funding for new programmes of disease control or eradication, the benefits to the different beneficiaries, and to society as a whole, often need to be quantified and compared to the benefits to society that might accrue from other investments. This is particularly important in the developing world, as donors and international organisations place greater emphasis on activities that contribute to poverty alleviation and sustained food security.

There is need to realize the relevance of economic impact assessments in animal disease control, and identify methods that can be used under different circumstances and present selected examples.

In recent years, the livestock sector has been hit by a number of high-profile diseases, such as BSE, foot and mouth disease and avian influenza. These have had a devastating economic impact on livestock producers and the broader livestock industry. One key response has been a growing interest in livestock disease insurance. However, there is a need for greater understanding of private incentives, market impacts, and public policy perspectives on regional, national and international levels, if livestock insurance products and complementary risk management programmes are to be developed.

MAIN AREAS FOR ANIMAL HEALTH ECONOMICS

- Effects of globalization and consumer demand on risk and risk management in agriculture and the food chain with particular reference to the changing nature and perception of risks associated with farm animal disease.
- Optimal strategies to promote farm animal health within the context of whole farm management.
- Implementation of these strategies through education, training and decision support, etc.
- Development of economic weights for selection indices to be used in dairy cattle breeding programmes with particular emphasis on health and fertility traits.
- Impact of bovine infertility on resource management in agriculture.

The disease surveillance and control section of any animal rearing system must give information about the *notifiable diseases, zoonoses* (diseases which can spread between human and animals), *other diseases* (diseases which are not notifiable or zoonoses), *animal pathogens* (organisms and associated derivatives which cause disease), *disease control* (gives the background information on disease control and includes advice on *biosecurity, veterinary surveillance* (covers proposed strategy for enhancing veterinary surveillance), *endemic disease surveillance* (provides quarterly surveillance reports of endemic diseases), *international disease monitoring* (qualitative hazard assessments and reports on major animal exotic disease outbreaks), *dog and cat travel and risk information* (a scheme to find out about the occurrence of exotic diseases in dogs and cats in Great Britain).

THE ANIMAL HEALTH AND WELFARE STRATEGY

The animal health and welfare strategy should work to improve the health and welfare of kept animals. It should be a strategy for all who have a role to play— government, the food and farming industry, vets, consumer groups and many others. It covers animals kept for pleasure or profit—pets, livestock, game and wildlife where it impacts on kept animals.

The strategy aim should be to develop a new partnership in which we can make a lasting and continuous improvement in the health and welfare of kept animals while protecting society, the economy, and the environment from the effect of animal disease. It must set out a *vision for animal health and welfare* showing where we want to be at a specified time in the future.

Literature on costs and benefits of preventing animal diseases aims to use evidence from the literature to assess the best ways to measure the real benefits of improvements in farm animal health. With such evidence, it will be possible to estimate the full relative investment potential of animal health and use such information to encourage farmers to adopt good practice in support of achieving desirable strategy for animal health and welfare.

Livestock systems are important in India, vulnerable to policy reform and concentrated in fragile regions. There is also evidence that they offer most scope for benefit from increased investment in disease prevention. Furthermore, the responsibility for controlling endemic diseases rests with farmers rather than the state.

In order to assess the true potential benefits from improvement in disease prevention it is necessary to assess the avoidable losses (as opposed to total costs) from disease. Simulation modelling can provide a solution to this problem. The approach has the added potential advantage of allowing results to be adapted to the individual circumstances of decision-makers. Several mechanistic models of the epidemiology of important endemic diseases of various animal have been published that exploit scientific advance to provide the necessary adaptability. There is therefore a need for interdisciplinary systems research in this area.

Static deterministic evaluations of avoidable losses are useful at regional or sectoral level but do not reflect the main impact of disease as experienced at the farm level. Here it is important to capture the risk that disease represents to farm business viability as it varies over the course of an epidemic. The interactions between diseases and between disease control and other farm management activities are also important. As well as establishing the opportunity cost of investing in animal health and welfare, more holistic long-term studies will reveal the impact of disease on the sustainability of an agricultural business. This aspect of animal health economics requires focus on the impact of animal disease on the land and hence the environment. The use of decision analysis techniques in animal health economics has helped to progress this aspect of research and should therefore be encouraged. Knowledge transfer to farmers should emphasize the role of animal health in risk management.

Voluntary health schemes, particularly those that offer certified health status provide a ready-made system to enhance the health and welfare of farm animals. Such costs could be considerably reduced if farmers in a region co-operated with each other. However, the problem of 'free-riders' makes it difficult to achieve the consensus necessary. This situation indicates a need to re-assess the role of state in such schemes.

An important aspect of this strategy is the promotion of farm animal health and welfare through disease prevention rather than cure. It encourages animal keepers to adopt good practice in this regard, there is a need to identify and assess the real benefits of improvements in animal health and welfare. How best to measure the economic impact of farm animal disease, gaps in evidence, areas for future research and implications for future farm management practice.

Basically why epidemic and zoonotic disease control should remain the responsibility of government while endemic disease prevention and control may be a private matter. The latter are considered private goods because vets and farmers who chose to control them can easily exclude others from any benefits gained. Also there is strong competition (rivalry) for the services concerned. Neither of these attributes applies to the control of epidemic or zoonotic diseases. However, overlap exists where endemic disease gives rise to significant externalities or control efforts for specific diseases interact. Farmers are generally slow to adopt disease prevention (biosecurity) strategies.

Direct Costs of Farm Animal Diseases

Large Animal Disease

Estimates of disease costs based on the output of epidemiological models can draw on scientific knowledge of the mechanisms that govern disease spread. They may thereby escape any bias inherent in studies based on empirical observation. More likely, they will be used in the absence of data necessary for economic analysis.

The problem of infertility in dairy cows (and even some disease problems) is in part due to negative genetic correlations with milk yield and therefore progressive deterioration in response to selection for milk yield. It must therefore be tackled at national level by widening breeding goals. It will be important to include the benefits of improved fertility in any economic evaluation of such diseases. These are often seen in the short-term as greater output of milk per unit time and reduced replacement costs. However, fertility has a long-term benefit at whole-herd level as it allows the productive animals to be supported by a smaller replacement rearing herd. Production targets can therefore be met from fewer animals, putting less pressure on the land and resulting in a more sustainable agricultural system. It also facilitates the maintenance of a closed-herd which in turn reduces the risk of introducing disease. By incorporating the long-term effects of fertility on land value, the apparent benefits of fertility will be much enhanced.

It is important to put the cattle disease costs into the context of returns from the associated farm enterprises. By doing so, the relative economic importance of animal disease to farmers can be gauged. The power of such figures to persuade farmers to invest in disease prevention strategies can then be assessed.

Small Animal Disease

Footrot is one of the most important contagious diseases affecting sheep and should be a high priority for farm-level economic analysis and associated knowledge transfer to farmers.

The main risk factors for lamb mortality are low birth-weight and low serum immunoglobulin concentration. Both factors will be influenced by disease in the pregnant ewe and in the newborn lamb. Rather like fertility in cattle, lamb mortality may be a useful key performance indicator on which to base a knowledge transfer programme to farmers aimed at disease prevention.

Economics of Animal Disease; Total Cost or Avoidable Losses

The main reason for discrepancy between published disease costs and farmer experience is that most published estimates give the total cost and not the avoidable losses. For many endemic diseases, most of the output loss and some of the control costs will be unavoidable even under best practice. For exotic diseases, it may be prudent to incur some recurrent expenditure in order to reduce the risk of an outbreak. Such costs are already part of farmers' income calculations. Total disease costs are therefore inappropriate for direct knowledge transfer to farmers because they give a false impression of the investment potential of disease prevention. However, it may at least provide a first crude, though imperfect, indication of which diseases might give the greatest potential economic benefit from control. Total costs are justified because they can be estimated within inherent livestock disease information constraints.

In general, the greater the expenditure on disease control, the lower the output loss from the disease. However, at any given level of disease control expenditure, there is a wide range of output losses. Strategies that give the lowest output loss at each level of control expenditure form the loss-expenditure frontier. The point on this frontier that gives the lowest total cost is found on the iso-cost line tangential to the loss-expenditure frontier.

Health Schemes

Private health and productivity schemes need to be developed in response to the realisation that most diseases are multifactorial in nature and therefore required a more holistic approach based on herd health rather than 'fire brigade' attention to individual animals by the veterinary surgeon. Early initiatives in the dairy sector involved regular planned health visits from the veterinary surgeon to individual farmer clients. More recent initiatives have extended into the sheep and beef sectors and may involve more formal planning, perhaps as part of a multi-farmer group. The importance of these schemes is likely to grow given the emphasis on disease prevention and the shortage of large animal veterinary practices to carry out 'fire brigade' work. The goals of these schemes are to identify disease problems, priorities them and then plan, implement, monitor and control a programme of remedial actions that are technically and economically efficient. The activities associated with this type of health scheme are referred to as 'farm health planning' in the outline health and welfare strategy. In the dairy cow at least, early signs of disease may be very subtle, involving disruption of the normal association between weight change and production rather than a sudden drop in productivity. By using developments in information technology to spot such changes, health scheme members may be able to react more quickly and hence more effectively to impeding health/welfare problems.

As well as or instead of 'farm health planning', some health schemes aim to detect, eradicate and then demonstrate continued freedom from specific diseases in the members' herd/flock. If such schemes deal with specific epidemic or zoonotic diseases they are the proper preserve of the public sector. However, in recent years, many schemes associated with specific endemic diseases have been privatized. By doing so, a supply of breeding stock of certified health status becomes available to all farmers. The process also allows timely control or preventive action to be taken. An important aspect of these schemes is biosecurity; i.e. ensuring that once a disease is eliminated it is not reintroduced into the herd/flock. This is a painstaking and potentially expensive aspect of scheme membership. Biosecurity measures are valuable to scheme members and indicate the best way to allocate resources to biosecurity activities.

The costs of preserving health status may be greatly reduced if all farmers in a region are committed to an appropriate health scheme. This point can be exploited in remote areas of the country. However, as long as health schemes are voluntary, the problem of 'free-riders' makes it difficult to achieve eradication in more extensive regions. Nevertheless, some countries are committed to eradication of endemic cattle diseases such as BVD differentiation between countries in terms of animal health status could therefore arise and impede progress towards global free trade in livestock.

There is also the problem of number and diversity of health schemes in agriculture. Health schemes may exist to provide farm assurance, improve animal welfare, protect public health, reduce dependence on pharmaceuticals and facilitate administration as well as improve productivity or eliminate specific diseases. Given that the best interests of all stakeholders will not coincide there will be a need for some intervention to strike an appropriate balance.

A promising initiative that addresses some of the issues combines health planning and surveillance with disease eradication. It is a farmer-directed business that aims to create a pool of high health status herds for farms. The mandatory core of the programme involves annual veterinary inspections and associated health plans. A key element is an educational component for farmers to encourage uptake. This is centred on participating veterinary practices linked by computer network and e-mail to a central database. Details of farm visits are recorded on this database and made available for outside evaluation on a 'need to know' basis. These features ensure credibility through transparency and traceability. The next step is to link the whole system to other quality assurance programmes.

Risk Management

Although aetiology and disease management (preventive measures and monitoring programmes, etc.) is an important strategy, it is only part of an integrated approach. It follows that under increased world trade competition; preventive veterinary medicine is likely to be of increasing importance to farmers as part of a wider strategy for risk management.

The importance of disease in wider farm business risk management and the inherent risks associated with animal disease have led to the use of standard risk management techniques in animal health economics. Such techniques are often termed 'decision analysis'. Decision analysis often involves construction of a decision tree as a pictorial representation of the flow of events including both decisions (e.g. treatment options) and possible outcomes (e.g. mortality). The sum of probability weighted monetary values associated with each possible outcome is known as the expected value of the decision option. Decision options can be selected on the basis of their expected values. The approach is explicit, quantitative and prescriptive. It is flexible and easily understood. Although uncertainty often surrounds many of the quantitative assumptions, methods have been developed to elicit subjective values from the decision-maker. The aim is to make the best decision given the available information. This will not always be the right decision but the process can greatly improve the understanding of the decision-maker and his/her advisers. Greater understanding will improve subsequent decisions and raise awareness of key issues such as the relative impact of animal health on farm incomes and farm income risk. These features make decision analysis a useful basis for knowledge transfer in support of the animal health and welfare strategy. However, most recent applications in animal health economics have been aimed at decision-makers beyond the farm gate. While studies of farmer decision-making in this context suggest a more subjective approach.

Care is needed when using average costs of disease and standard measures of dispersion to support farm level decision-making under risk. This is because the distribution of such costs is often skewed.

ACCOUNTING FOR TIME IN ANIMAL HEALTH ECONOMICS

Decision-making at individual farm level is complicated by the cyclical nature of agricultural production systems. Fixed assets such as land and breeding livestock are 'harvested' repeatedly so that decisions in one production cycle must be taken with due consideration for their consequences in future cycles. This is particularly important in the case of animal disease where infection in one cycle often impairs performance in subsequent cycles, e.g. with mastitis. Susceptibility to disease in later cycles may also be affected by exposure in earlier cycles and in any case, tends to increase with age. Productivity on the other hand may initially rise with age and then decline. All these factors must be taken into account when dealing with the economics of animal health in breeding livestock.

Dynamic programming (DP) provides a framework for the economic analysis of multi-stage decision problems. It has frequently been applied to natural resource management problems including some in animal health economics. For example, optimal replacement of mastitic cows and the relative value of different mastitis control procedures. The technique has also provided a useful framework for establishing the economic weight of goal traits for use in dairy cattle breeding programmes where benefits accrue over long periods. Progress might be made without recourse to complex bio-economic simulation modelling at individual farm level.

Most estimates of average farm animal disease costs in the literature lack both economic and scientific rigour. Studies that quote the total cost of diseases rather than the avoidable loss exaggerate the benefits of investment in disease prevention and may thereby come to lack credibility with farmers. Even so, their implied value is small in comparison to normal variation in output prices for livestock. A different picture emerges from studies of animal disease as a source of risk to farm businesses. Animal disease may represent a significant proportion of the risk (variation in farm income) over which the livestock farmer has some control. There is also evidence that disease costs are positively skewed thus average costs could mask the effects of rare though potentially devastating epidemics. A knowledge transfer campaign based on risk management at whole-farm level and backed by research into the sources of variation in avoidable disease losses therefore holds promise.

A more holistic (systems) approach to animal health is also required in this context requiring an interdisciplinary research and development/extension effort. In particular, more epidemiological studies are needed to establish the effectiveness of alternative biosecurity strategies under different physical and financial circumstances. To be cost-effective, such strategies must provide proven protection against a wide range of diseases. It will also be important to include general farm management activities within the biosecurity strategy. For example, replacement policy for breeding livestock has considerable impact on animal health and on farm profits in the long-term. The management of fertility is also a crucial issue, closely associated with animal health and welfare as well as sustainability. By joining-up these disparate issues, it should be possible to demonstrate the full potential benefits of establishing and maintaining freedom from specific endemic diseases through membership of appropriate health schemes. The more farmers that join such schemes, the greater the benefit for all as the risks of breeches in biosecurity are reduced. Scheme members may also be able to pool knowledge and resources for mutual benefit.

A potential problem arises in the overlap between public and private goods/bads related to animal health at farm level. Also some of the endemic diseases have zoonotic potential thus creating a public interest in how farmers deal with them. Furthermore, how farmers deal with endemic disease may have consequences for animal welfare and the environment. These factors make it difficult to draw the distinctions between public and private interests. Farmers' perspective will be the necessary theme for knowledge transfer to encourage disease prevention in support of the strategy for animal health and welfare. However, a wider economic analysis will also be required to support the wider resource allocation decisions needed at national level to tackle issues of public concern that might otherwise arise such as zoonoses and animal welfare. Such decisions should consider possible use of funds. Some of the money saved due to decoupling subsidy from production could be spent on public concerns related to zoonoses, animal health and animal welfare via the cross-compliance mechanism.

Simulation modelling provides a vital basis for systems research in animal health. There are many epidemiological models but so far relatively few combine epidemiology with economics to identify optimal animal health establishment and maintenance strategies. Greater research effort in this area would help overcome the problem of lack of information that hinders the development of proper economic evaluations of animal disease. Such an approach makes the most of what information we have on the science of animal disease and helps to identify important gaps. By using mechanistic models where possible, adaptations can be made to reflect specific decision-making circumstances. This will become increasingly important in the more volatile markets that will follow liberalisation of trade in agricultural commodities. However, this does not mean that sophisticated simulation models and associated decision support systems will always be appropriate for use at farm level. Studies of knowledge transfer requirements in livestock agriculture suggest that many farmers require more traditional approaches. Carefully selected and sensitively communicated output from simulation studies, supported by appropriate local advice, training and information may therefore be the best approach.

CONCLUSIONS

i. In the present world, it is essential that we evaluate the economic feasibility of every animal rearing system. Proper animal health is a prime necessity for optimising the returns from the animals. A considerable part of the farm expenditure is for disease prevention/cure procedures. The farm study revealed that more expenses are incurred on anti-parasitic drugs, antibiotics and vitamin-mineral preparations. We have to look for minimizing the expenses on these, their indiscriminate use. The problems of antibiotic and anthelmintic resistance have to be considered. For using antibiotics, it would be better if the effective antibiotic is chosen with proper dosing and time schedule. Rotational grazing, using anthelmintics in cyclic order and burning of pastures may reduce the problem of anthelmintic resistance.

ii. Economic impact may be measured by measuring avoidable losses not total costs; using simulation methods to overcome lack of information and make best use of scientific knowledge; present uncertainty in cost estimates; express results relative to alternative investments farmers could make; adopt a systems approach at whole-farm level to take account of interactions between diseases and to incorporate farm management practices that indirectly affect animal health.

iii. Decision analysis techniques can reflect the contribution animal health can make to risk management, allow for variations over time in both biological and economic aspects of animal health systems.

Future needs: Reliable sources of epidemiological information have to be strengthened and the information has to be evaluated economically, the benefits of disease prevention (e.g. biosecurity) measures have to be analyzed, analyze the flow of goods (e.g. farm profits, animal welfare, public health, sustainability) from animal health and identify the appropriate veterinary services needed, examine the potential economies of scale, co-operation and integration for disease prevention schemes and explore the role for constantly acquiring knowledge in the development and delivery of animal health and welfare strategies.

20

Economic Appraisal of Animal Disease Control: Strategies in Livestock Entrepreneurship Development

HP Dwivedi, Mahesh Kumar

In early part of 20th century, the major emphasis of veterinarians was on the control of diseases that decimated animal population over large geographical area. Decision on whether to control these diseases could usually be made without aid of formal economic appraisal as generally the losses greatly exceeded control costs. However, in recent years trends have changed to typify animal production, particularly in those areas where intensive agricultural methods are practiced, resulting in knowledge of diseases and disease complexes that manifest themselves primarily through a decrease in productive efficiency and that in most cases area endemic becoming the most significant with respect to decrease in farm income. Since various intensities on control measures are often possible, it is necessary to determine the level of control strategy that makes economically optimal choice. The feature of disease control that makes it such a valuable investment is that it generally increases the efficiency of production process and hence it is unlike most other goods and service that farmer may generally to increase output without changing the nature of the process. That is why return on investments in disease control is usually high.

Today decision regarding animal health activities can rarely be made solely on biological rather a dynamic and integrated approach combining epidemiology and economic analysis is required to determine the nature and scope of health problem and implications if interventions. In general, economic analysis is to be regarded as a tool providing additional information on which to base a decision, rather than a definitive method on which to base the final policy decision. The advances in economic analysis of livestock diseases are to be described and compared with the traditional methods of simple loss measurement and cost/ benefit accounting. It is suggested that the traditional methods have restricted the development of economic applications in the field of animal disease. However, the developing framework of economic analysis of livestock disease requires further work to structure economic models, develop analytic methods and assemble the data necessary to feed them. It has been realized how economically important is animal disease and why, economic decision making in animal health management, basic methods of economic analysis and economic impact of common health and fertility problems should also be considered. The strength and credibility of animal disease economics analysis, and especially 'production economics,' stem from its clear links with identifiable technical processes and commonly confronted decisions about resource use. Despite its importance as a serious imperfections in livestock production, the phenomenon of disease has not been widely explored within this analytical framework. Animal disease is characterized as an economic problem and an economist's approach to what might otherwise be considered an essentially veterinary problem is explored. Some basic models, rotted in conventional production economics, are proposed to illuminate the economic costs of disease and the conceptual basis for optimal strategies in disease control. A number of areas for further methodological and empirical development are put forward.

ANIMAL DISEASE ECONOMICS

Animal health economics as a relatively new discipline divided the field into three inter-related aspects as quantifying the financial effects of animal disease, developing methods for optimizing decisions when individual animals, herds or population are affected and determining the costs and benefits of disease control measures. The four most common economic, modelling techniques (i.e. partial budgeting, cost-benefit analysis decision analysis, and systems simulation) are applied on three levels of veterinary decision-making: the animal herd, and national level.

Financial Evaluation

Financial evaluation has become a necessity in intensive livestock enterprises for the animal disease control at farm, national and international level. Economical justification is usually demanded by public sector funding agencies for long-term disease control programmes so as to harmonize the international trades of livestock products in developing countries like India, where livestock diseases are barrier to benefits.

Livestock production is a type of physical transformation process, where disease impairs this process and there is loss of efficiency posing both technical and economic problems. Technical efficiency loss occurs as to difference between the production function of healthy and diseased animals. Disease acts as a negative input and the relationship between input and output for given input is shifted downward. Recovery of planned output is possible only by utilizing veterinary and non-veterinary inputs in best possible least cost combination.

Assessing the Economic Cost of Disease

Total economic cost of disease can be measured as sum of output losses and control expenditure. Output losses refer to reduction in out put, i.e. it is benefit that is taken away (when milk of mastitic cow is totally discarded) or may be unrealized losses (decrease in economic traits of animal thus enhancing culling percentage). Expenditures are increased in input associated with disease control, i.e. veterinary interventions used therapeutically or prophylactically or increased use of manpower. Thus, economic costs are more than just sum of financial outlays. The outbreak of a highly infectious animal disease in a disease-free area is an ever-present risk. Recent epidemics in livestock populations in Europe suggest that the cost in terms of eradications, production losses and trade disruption may be high. The implications for meat and livestock industry, government policy and international trade rules are to be taken care of. The need for strict biosecurity and effective contingency plans needs to be stressed. Options such as private insurance, animal tracing systems and emergency vaccination are to be adhered to. Current measures for controlling animal disease epidemics raise various social and ethical issues that complicate the policy makers' task.

Though increase in level on control expenditure decreases out put losses but it is worth increasing the level of control expenditure to achieve incremental reduction in output losses. That combination of control expenditure and output losses which provide satisfactory level of disease control in least cost is best option using suitable allocation of resources available up to a point where the expenditure on the last unit of resource is just recouped by the additional returns. In a mastitis control campaign, regular use of test dipping and praying, dry-cow therapy and annual testing of milking machine with regular screening of herd are best measures with least total cost of disease providing the maximum decrease in incidence of mastitis.

Before implementation of any disease control strategy, it is necessary to consider how much variation in input to the animal production process influences the quality and quantity of output. If the intensity of control can be raised over a continuous spectrum so that a mathematical equation can be used to represent the data which can be interpreted as a production function and the optimum level of control is determined. Farmer should continue to increase production function until reaching the points where marginal (additional units) cost (expenses) equal marginal (additional units) benefits (revenue).

The animal health related sufficient information is always lacking to produce full production function due to greater involvement of intangibles and least concern of externalities and hence it is impossible to calculate values from it. So partial farm budget may be used, as it does not presuppose the estimation of continuous function and the knowledge of two or more and three discrete input-output relationship is sufficient. The economic arguments surrounding the use of foot and mouth disease (FMD) vaccination as an emergency, measure were analyzed. The trade arguments for disease-free status, the costs of an epidemic without vaccinations and the impact of emergency vaccination on costs were analyzed and it has been concluded that emergency vaccination would be rational within a wider radius of a detected farm, and that the earlier this can be done the more likely it is that disease spread and economic costs will be minimized.

Microeconomic vs. Macroeconomic Losses

In an epidemic, time series analysis of output and input data might reveal a sudden behavioural change in local farmers' activities thus allowing the measurement of the associated short run economic losses. The losses can be more easily associated with the particular disease under study. In the endemic setting, it would be perhaps possible to estimate differential economic behaviour attributed to animal disease if selected groups of farms with recurring outbreaks were contrasted with comparable disease-free producers in a time series analysis. Macroeconomic impact of improving livestock efficiency through better herd health. Using economic surplus analysis with pre-weaning mortality in swine as the example, they demonstrated the importance of improving livestock production efficiency in the face of international competition and how consumers gain from improved animal health should be adapted to other livestock commodities, variations in mortality levels, or production losses due to morbidity. Such analysis methods can be used to examine the appropriateness of expenditures on animal disease control programmes and animal health research.

Partial Farm Budgeting

It is simple description of financial consequences of particular change in farm management procedure of which disease control programme is a part. Partial indicate assessment is restricted to factors that are likely to change as a result of procedure changes. It is only aimed at disease problems that are assumed to occur on a farm with a high degree of certainty means study of endemic disease in individual farm bases, e.g. Bovine mastitis and internal parasitism. In these analyses, fixed costs are ignored and assess only small changes that do not affect total farm management or assess economic consequences of a change in farm procedure. It is beneficial since it permits realistic estimation of values to be made of the consequence of various actions without necessitating the keeping of complete financial records for the farms. But have arbitrary decisions are to be made, about which items to be included, and thereby any item that is affected may be included. Only comparisons can be made between the strategies to be tested but not necessarily provide optimum solution. Doubt counts usually create problem so these are not included.

In mastitis control campaign, the components that may be utilized for partial farm budgeting include *additional revenue realized from the changes*, r1, i.e. more sales of milk due to increased production after control programmer's implementation, *reduced costs stemming from change*, c1, i.e. reduced cost of treatment of mastitis further, *increased costs as a result of the change*, r2, i.e. cost of increased feed utilized due to increased production, and *costs of implementing the change*, c2, i.e. cost of strategy. Net return here is given by (r1+c1) – (r2+c2). If r1+c1 is greater than the proposed strategy is justified. A question arises whether net return or % return on marginal invested funds and marginal return most accurately reflect the profitable portion, if farmer has unlimited fund available to adopt any scheme than net return or % return on marginal investment is most profitable but if funds are limited, those available should be progressively invested in yielding highest and marginal return should be adopted. The main financial difference between different control strategies in farm is by mortality rate, if a group with no strategic treatment suffered an x% mortality compared to y% in uncritical scheme group. So mortality rate in no treatment group needed to be as low as y% before benefit from adopting critical scheme would be reduced to zero (Break even point).

Gross Margin Analysis

For judging benefits from an improvement in herd health, analysis may be carried out by means of partial farm budget (one problem under consideration) or by change in some economic index of performance within time. One such index gross margin analysis is expressed in relation to some unit of production. It is most practicable and widely accepted methods for assessing enterprise profitability and for comparing profitability of different enterprises on a farm and for estimating the effect of change (within limit) of fixed assets and other resources available to farmer, so with regard to animal health activities gross margin perhaps finds its greatest application in assessing the effectiveness of integrated health management programme. In gross margin analysis, all actual incomes from the enterprise in question are totaled and all variable costs directly attributed to operating that enterprise are subtracted. The outcome is enterprise gross margin or "profit before fixed costs".

Gross margin analysis is directly associated with the level of intensity of each activity. Many variable input costs determine the yield or level of output of activity as the level and type of feed, drenches and vaccine used may have a major effect on the animal production. Very little output would occur on farm unless money was spent on variable cost items. Fixed cost in short run is incurred regardless of the level of output.

SOCIAL BENEFIT-COST ANALYSIS

Early reports concerned with economic techniques reflected themselves primarily with estimating the cost of a particular disease to an individual producer or a nation but it incorrectly suggests that this amount of money is completely recoverable. So presently, the value of economic analysis lie on evaluations of the benefits of the control procedure, which is more accord with economic theory and positive orientation on information by drawing attention to benefits of action rather than the cost of inaction.

It also aids decision-making regarding limited resource allocation, hence it provides a basis for making rational choice from among alternative preventive or control action under various circumstances. Monetary values are used only as a common denominator for the value of particular resources in society. So, a complete economic analysis indicates the confidence in the monetary or utility ranking of the various strategies. Scientists estimated the losses and the benefits of theileriosis control by the infection and treatment methods of immunization using a computer spreadsheet models. The parameters of the models included national size and structure of cattle herds, the estimated impact of the disease in terms of incidence, case morbidity and case fatability rates, and the effect of immunization on the disease. It is suggested that when adequate data are available, the approach could be used to generate more accurate results for any study site, production system, country and the region as a whole.

As economic impact study of the anaplasmosis outbreak was commissioned to provide advice during the course of the outbreak and thorough economic evaluation of available control options. The study estimated that if anaplasmosis was not controlled and the disease established, the yearly losses to producers through death and sickness of animals, treatment and testing costs would be almost three times. The net present value and benefit-cost ratios were calculated for two possible control options. The results indicated that public control of anaplasmosis is questionably justified. The study went on to identify a number of steps, which could be taken to minimize the risk of future outbreaks or to minimize the size and cost of the outbreak. One important step is that authority be obtained under the Animal Disease and Protection Act to pay for treatment costs when it is feasible to use the test and treat option.

Points to Consider for Social Benefit-cost Analysis

The problem related to economic evaluation can be divided into either diseases loss at the producer level—essentially a matter for resource allocation from the private sector, or disease loss at the national and community level where large-scale public resources are required for disease control strategy and research and development programmes. Three development areas requiring more immediate priority are: (a) the development of analytical techniques for control and eradication programmes, (b) the creation of a community-wide data bank limited to those infectious diseases that are seen as community problems, and (c) the encouragement of health and production evaluations as a means of promoting greater efficiency at the producer level. The role of economists in the choices, which individuals and society at large make about exploiting various technical possibilities, has become inevitable.

Long-term animal disease control strategies require substantial investment and benefits gradually accumulate subsequently so necessity to weigh annual costs and benefits become more valuable than those occurring in future as in Rinderpest control in India and Swine fever eradication in Europe. Certain factors become more important to be considered while evaluating such large-scale control strategies:

- Society as a whole is to be benefited or not.
- Whether there is transfer of financial or non-financial benefits between sections of the community.
- Whether project should receive priority over other such projects.
- How heavily economic and social achievements of the project be weighted.

So economic evaluations in this situation require counting measurable costs and benefits with tabulation of non-financial consequences as well as raising necessity of social benefit cost analysis. A conceptual benefit-cost analysis framework model for the evaluation of economic usefulness of improved animal identification systems was designed to reduce the consequences of foreign animal diseases (FAD) such as production losses and contaminated animal foods. The aspects that need to be considered include: purpose of animal trace ability systems; strategies employed for the benefit-cost analysis of animal identification systems; and the background behind animal trace ability. The improved levels of animal identification in cattle may provide sufficient economic benefit in terms of reduced consequences of FAD.

Principle of Social Benefit-cost Analysis

The social benefit-cost analysis is attempted to quantify the social advantage/ disadvantage of a policy in term of common monetary value not as a financial analysis or simply accounting but as a true economic analysis. Some cost of benefits are expressed easily in pecuniary values other cost or benefits, however, are much more difficult to translate into monetary terms, i.e. intangibles. Only by using common denominator of money, it is possible to aggregate the gains and losses, which ultimately interest society as benefit and cost perceived in real terms. Consequently, it is important to quantify in monetary units all important factors as comprehensively as possible to make the problem area explicit although the value of intangibles are assessed somewhat subsequently.

The prefix social to benefit cost analysis is important, ad any organization involved to disease control programme should be aimed to maximize the net benefit to the society not it own purely private benefits. Economic appraisals are made of the benefits of research on vaccines for the control of Marek's disease, bovine parasitic bronchitis and enzootic abortion of ewes. Costs and benefits pertaining to brucellosis infection and its control and included a comparison of production and income levels for various herd situations were studied. Labour requirements and cost estimates for several disease control practices were compared and evaluated. Data were classified according to the geographic location of herd, herd size, and whether or not the herd was adult-vaccinated. Representative herd situations were developed to aid in the analysis. It was concluded that:

1. Brucellosis infection causes substantial losses in income to the individual cattleman, to the beef industry and to the state;
2. In the representative herd situations, losses due to brucellosis generally exceed costs of an intensive eradication programme, making the control programme an economically sound option;
3. The average beef herd would benefit from an effective brucellosis prevention programme;
4. Official certification of a herd as 'brucellosis-free' can and often does add value to that herd and
5. Complete herd depopulation may be the most economic solution to eradicating brucellosis in small, heavily infected herds.

Components of Social Benefit-cost Analysis

Social benefit-cost analysis comprises three components:

1. Estimation of benefits and costs.
2. Adjusting them to account for timing.
3. Strategy evaluations and comparison.

INTERNAL, EXTERNAL COSTS AND BENEFITS

Internalities (private cost and benefit) are those that accure directly to an investment project whereas costs and benefits accruing to others are termed externalities. Later are not reflected in the price mechanism so inadequate to guide correct investment decision from view of society so to protect social benefit internalization of externalities is required.

As in case of mastitis control campaign beside all cost and benefit of farm budget, the high use of antibiotics resulting in antibiotic in milk (externality) which causes side effect to consumers requires internalization of these external effects beside budget and legislation limiting the use of antibiotic. Dynamic programme to establish the optimum replacement policy for dairy herds, taking into account sub-clinical mastitis caused by the bacteria *Staphylococcus aureus* was beneficial. This particular pathogen is resistant to normal drug therapies and therefore, culling is the major method of control. Methods are described to account for output losses due to yield loss and a reduction in milk price caused by extra somatic cells secreted into the milk by infected cows. Extra culling was justified in both infected and control herds in order to reduce the level of infection in the herd. The method described allows replacement policy to be treated as control expenditure rather than an output loss in the economic analysis of farm animal disease. This approach will become even more important as consumers demand an alternative to the prophylactic use of antibiotics in agriculture without compromising food quality and safety.

Assessing costs: Costs usually relate resources consumed so all physical resources are requires to assign a monetary value to them. For any disease control programme, costs would include those of manpower, drugs, vaccines, quarantine building, compensations for slaughters, transportation, and training programme. Jactel (1987) analyzed losses due to mastitis and the cost/benefit of control measures after one and after three years in a model herd of 50 cows in different hypothetical situations. Gathura and Gathura (1991) evaluated the economic losses resulting from condemnation of cattle and small stock (sheep and goats) livers due to the presence of *Echinococcus granulosus* hydatids using meat inspection records.

Assessing Benefits: It is assessed by knowing effect of disease in absence of control and by estimating the likely consequences of control strategies. It is avoidance of losses or difference between losses experienced under no control and under current programme considering each alternative being investigated.

In FMD control programme, benefit may be avoidance of production losses, i.e. mortality, indirect and direct effects on meat and milk production, lameness in draught animals and from restriction on international trade.

Benefits

1. Readily quantifiable (live birth weight gain, production, etc.)
2. Benefits that exist but are not readily quantifiable in financial term as market prices are not clear or susceptible to accurate calculation (effect of brucellosis eradication in export price of beef).
3. Benefits not suitably evaluated economically (psychological benefits, etc.)

Costs and benefits related to each production unit with different control strategies are calculated and non-financial cost and benefits are tabulated to take in account while analyzing social benefit cost.

Adjustment of Values

The economic value of estimated costs and benefits needs to be adjusted to take account of time they occur. The adjusted values are referred as present values. Procedure used for adjustment is called as discounting where time movement is from future back to present. It is calculated by the formula:

$$PV = \frac{FVn}{(1+r)^n}$$ where, r is relevant annual discount rate.

Carpenter and Howitt (1982) described effect of subsidization of disease control programmes justified it as economically efficient, if social costs of early detection and control of diseases are considered as well as the private costs to the individual are taken into account. A method of analyzing the two sources of costs and the optimum investment in disease detection and control is developed. Subsidization of a diagnostic laboratory system can be shown to be efficient under this set of parameters. The distribution of the benefits from the increased surveillance level in the long and short run is shown to benefit both the producer and consumer.

EVALUATION AND STRATEGY COMPARISONS

One or more combination of following three measures of economic efficiency or investment may be adopted.

- Net present value
- Benefit-cost ratio
- Internal rate of return

Net present value (NPV): It represents present value of benefits less the present value of cost incurred. The positive value of NPV means highly feasible control strategy among all alternatives. It also gives idea of value of implementing the project.

Benefit-cost ratio (BCR): It is present value of benefits divided by present value of costs. The cost incurred and benefits received during each period of project are stated as present value and total is divided to get benefit-cost ratio. If ratio are greater than one, the strategy is assessed economically feasible.

Internal rate of return (IRR): It is return on investment in terms to an interest rate or discount rate. The rate of discount that makes the total of the discounted benefits equal to the total of discounted costs (NPV=0). Higher value of IRR refers most likely strategy.

Cost Effectiveness Analysis

This approach is appropriate where the benefits are difficult to quantity (monetary benefits of rabies control programme) or when production losses under each control strategy are equal. Under such circumstances, the requirement is for a method of analysis that determines how the desired results can be achieved at minimum (discounted) cost, what actually the cost effectiveness analysis does, cost-effective disease control on the dairy farm could enhance productivity and subsequently profitability. Previous economic studies on animal disease have focused on production losses and evaluation of disease eradication programmes and provided little guidance as to the optimal prevention action. The optimal strategy that minimizes total disease cost on the basis of farm survey results. The results emphasize the importance of introducing checks before new animal enter the herd and adequate vaccination protection as cost-effective control strategies. True extent of losses incurred is often not realized. Two new methods for evaluation are monitoring of productivity figures, and regular pathological assessments, such as cell counts in milk, worm eggs in faeces, liver or lung damage at slaughterhouse inspection, and so on. These monitoring systems may indicate the effects of any control programmes also.

21

Role of Banks for Development of Agriculture and Livestock Sector

Lal Ji Singh

Rural economy in India has been witnessing a dramatic and explosive growth, almost twice that of the urban economy and marketers of products and services are seized both of the opportunities and the challenges of rural marketing. It is apparent that transposing the urban mind-set to the rural context will not work and innovation and customization are the strategies to be adopted for reaching the rural markets.

The opportunities in rural markets are immense. Rural India is home to nearly 41% of the country's middle class and 58% of total disposable income as reported by National Council for Applied Economic Research (NCAER). The number of middle income and high income households in rural areas is expected to increase to 111 million by 2007. It is obvious that any organization, be it a manufacturer of goods or a service provider such as bank, has to effectively exploit this market segment for sustained future growth. However, to be able to succeed in tapping this huge rural consumer segment, it is necessary to understand the distinctive features of this economic class. A low per capita income, highly dispersed nature of the market, low literacy levels, widely variable incomes, inadequate infrastructure for storage, transportation and communication and strong cultural bias are the unique features of this market.

Thus, the nature of the products/services aimed for these markets have to be customized in size, packaging, appearance and price. The delivery/distribution channels too have to be suitable modified to cater to the dispersed and highly price sensitive rural markets. Promotion of products will have to be tailored though innovative and low-tech 2 rugged solutions to reach this target group. Development of a brand in these markets will have to rely more on symbols and colour-coding. Within this framework, marketers have to ensure that the consumer is assured of value for money. The widely varying income levels in the rural markets are both a challenge and an opportunity. Marketers have to address each income segment differently with customized products. The challenge in reaching these markets is to provide goods/services of the same quality as is available at urban outlets but at a lower cost which means the production costs have to be reworked and the efficiency of the entire system has to be vastly improved to bring down costs. Further, unlike in the urban market, where the growth in the economy creates demand for credit, in the nascent rural markets, a supply-leading approach has to be adopted whereby availability of credit will spur economic growth leading to increase in income and purchasing power.

Thus rural marketing involves designing innovative and context-related business models, which are low in cost, dynamic and responsive to local needs and provide value for the rural consumer. The role of technology in providing low cost solutions cannot be ignored. If the efficiencies of the urban market have to be provided in the highly dispersed rural markets, technology will have to be used innovatively to bring down costs. The emerging role of SHGs, in providing a sustainable delivery/distribution network is another initiative which needs to be fully explored.

BANKS' ROLE IN THE RURAL ECONOMY

State Bank of India was born out of a felt need for increasing the share of institutional credit in the rural economy, thereby mitigating the financial hardships of farmers who depended on credit obtained at usurious rates of interest. Much has been achieved in this direction but much more remains to be done to bring down the cost of credit in the rural economy by making available need based and timely credit at cheaper rates. The report dated 30th June, 2004, submitted by the Advisory Committee on flow of credit to Agriculture and related activities from the Banking System under the Chairmanship of Shri VS Vyas observed that the level of agricultural credit from commercial banks stood at Rs 85000 crores up to March 2004 and only 7 commercial banks met the target of 18% of the net credit outstandings to agriculture. This is despite the share of commercial banks in rural credit going up to 35% from 2% in 1970-71.

The report states that the pace of development of agriculture and allied activities needs to be accelerated for which credit is a critical facilitating agent. The risk in providing credit to the rural customers is higher due to various factors such as adverse weather conditions, insufficient water, poor quality of inputs and inadequate shortage and marketing mechanisms. The cost of risk mitigating systems such as insurance and pricing of credit cannot be fully passed on to the borrowers who are mostly in the small and marginal category barely subsisting on their incomes. The report suggests that this is a cost which needs to be borne by the state and central governments.

The recommendations of the Vyas Committee which have been accepted by RBI for implementation by commercial banks included the following:

1. Conversion of wasteland (24.5 mn Ha) and fallow land (16.6 mn Ha) into cultivable land through long-term development initiatives to be taken by the banks and the state governments.
2. Use of SHGs/NGOs and other voluntary bodies in rural areas as direct selling agents/local help to bridge the information gap.
3. Introduction of low cost ATMs in rural areas for cash transactions and use of IT in rural areas.
4. Proper appraisal of loan proposals and post-disbursement supervision will reduce the risk costs.

5. Contract farming is an emerging opportunity for assisting the small and marginal farmers in marketing their produce at remunerative prices.

Banks are required to support these initiatives. In addition to the above, the emerging opportunities in the rural sector provide ample scope for business development in the rural sector. The bank has recognized the extent of this business which is both necessary and profitable for the bank. An exclusive strategic business unit has been formed at the corporate centre for the purpose. A slew of products aimed at the agricultural sector for direct farming as well as for allied activities has been designed. These products include not only the traditional production (crop) loans but also investment credit for farm mechanization, minor irrigation and water management systems such as drip irrigation, rural godowns, transportation, cold storages, produce marketing loan, loans to commission agents, tissue-culture labs, horticulture, floriculture, dairy farming, poultry farming, hatcheries, agro-processing industries, agribusiness clinics, cyber-cafes (internet kiosks), etc. In short, the bank is involved in providing credit through the value chain from the farmer to the consumer.

On the staff, front agriculture graduates have been recruited as marketing and recovery officers to assist the rural branches in achieving the bank's goals in rural credit. Officials have been posted in regions exclusively to lead the marketing teams in their efforts. Finance is being provided to SHGs in a big way to accelerate the growth of rural credit. Thus, the bank is fully geared to fully exploit the business potential emerging in the rural sector and meet the targets set for the bank by the government.

OVERVIEW OF INDIAN AGRICULTURE

Agriculture in India has witnessed a gradual transformation from subsistence farming of early fifties to the present intensive agriculture contributing 22% of GDP (as on September 2005). "The Green Revolution" enabled transformation of the country from 'begging bowl' status (82 million tones in 1962-63) to that of 'self sufficient' (210 million tones production in 2003-04), warding off threat of famines and ushering an era of rural prosperity. This quantum jump became possible essentially due to introduction of new technology, willingness of the Indian farmer to take risks, and the development of extensive agriculture marketing infrastructure and thereby dramatic increase in the yields of input responsive high yielding varieties. The rail network, roads, assured marketing and remunerative prices for food grains-guaranteed by minimum support prices (MSP) played an important role in this development.

India is still predominantly an agricultural economy. Wheat and rice, two main crops responsible for the green revolution, have reached the highest production levels possible under the available technology, leading to stagnation in growth, if not decline, in few pockets of the country. This has led to a climate of despair among farmer families and policy makers, as still there exists a large gap between the productivity at the national level compared to those achieved at global level.

India's populace still faces widespread malnutrition and hunger even after 50 years of independence. UNO studies reveal that 5000 children die every day in

India because of malnutrition. The annual per-head availability of food grains in India is only 174 kg as against 304 kg in China. Statistics also indicate that India would be a net importer of food grains in future if we do not increase our productivity.

Agriculture Scenario in India

Population	1.1 billion plus
Cropped area	143 million hectares (net)
Cropping intensity	135%
Irrigated area	40% of cropped area
No. villages	0.63 million
Average farm holding	1.55 ha
Food grains production	>200 million tones
Average farm productivity	1.6 tones/ha
Fertilizer consumption	13 million tones
Fertilizer usage	98 kgs per ha.

67% of farmers depend on rain fed farming and 42% of food grains come from rain fed farming. India ranks high in area and production of many crops. However, productivity-wise (i.e. tones/ha) even now we are nowhere in the picture, as evident from the Table 21.1. India's position in production and productivity of major crops in the world is given in Table 21.1.

Table 21.1: Position of India in production and productivity of major crops in the world

Crops	India's share in the world				India's productivity (t/ha)	India's rank in the world in productivity
	Area		Production			
	%	Rank	%	Rank		
Wheat	11.2	2	11.4	2	2.5	32
Rice	28.5	1	21.4	2	2.8	35
Pulses	36.6	1	26.0	1	0.6	118
Groundnut	35.2	2	28.6	1	1.0	50
Sugarcane	20.0	2	22.6	2	65.9	34
Cotton	20.7	1	14.0	3	0.9	57

Farming is both a way of life and the principal means of livelihood to 65% of India's population of 110 crores. The average farm size is becoming smaller each year and the cost risk return structure of farming is becoming adverse with the result that the farmers are getting increasingly indebted. A farmers recent NSSO survey revealed that nearly 40% of farmers would like to quit farming, if they have an option to do so.

The support system needed by farmers like credit is in various stages of disarray. Thereby forcing small farmers to borrow money from moneylenders at high rate of interest, since less than 60% of the credit requirements of farmers is met by institutional sources. Farmers' several factors including debt to private money lenders at high rate of interest, soaring input cost, low output prices. The farmers need to be rescued from spirit of despair and doom.

DEVELOPMENT BANKER-ROLES REDEFINED

During the era of Green Revolution, as consequence to the legendary nationalization and branch expansion policies, banking system has successfully provided the much required credit flow to the agriculture sector to make the national mission a success. However, subsequently the flow of credit to this sector has acquired a routine nature lacking innovations. Despite the priority sector status, banks have been continuously lagging behind in achieving their national targets.

As the gap between demand and supply of rural credit is very large, Reserve Bank of India introduced an obligatory credit allocation by all commercial bank to priority sector (40%) which includes most of the lending to rural and small enterprises.

The time has come that the bankers think of agriculture finance not as mundane crop loan and development loans but as a profitable proposition through integration of agriculture industry and trade. The modern day agriculture banking should invest in capital intensive projects of controlled climate production technologies to produce desired quality produce, by post-harvest treatment facilities including grading, standardization, packing, value addition and branding for development of agri-retail chains and export oriented production and marketing. In the era of second green revolution, agriculture has to be renamed as agribusiness and for a banker it has become an integration of mass and class banking through quality lending approach by targeting creamy layer of priority sector like big farmers growing commercial crops. Some of such avenues that banker can look forward to are: Green house farming and controlled atmosphere cultivation for off season production of fruits and vegetables as well as production of market demand oriented specific quality produces. The activity commands heavy capital investment and is specifically market driven or export oriented and is therefore a profitable avenue for the bankers.

1. Biotechnology, embryo transfer, artificial seed production, micro-propagations, tissue culture of fruits/flowers/vegetables and horticulture nurseries at location where demand exists which in turn is the input for high-value crop cultivation and is a highly capital intensive activity with assured returns.
2. Scientific storage and transport facilities including establishment of rural godowns, gold storages, transport chains including the refrigerated vans and precooling centres for efficient quality management of the fruits and vegetables which has to act as support system for the market oriented production and needs a heavy investment requirement.
3. Value addition chains including food processing units catering export market or the domestic market are the result of change in food habits where the

perishability of the food products is overcome to have a regular and more hygienic supply of products to market. The value addition units are the integration of agriculture with industry and are the future of the agriculture postproduction management.

4. Commercial dairying including establishment of milk bulk chilling and processing units with more emphasis on the value added products of milk.

5. Agriculture retail chains are the upcoming concept of integrating agriculture with trade catering the upwardly affluent society with the choicest of agriculture commodities with or without branding at a premium prices.

6. Contract farming comes as an integral part of the value addition and agri-retailing wherein the farmer is contracted to plant the contractor's crop in his land harvest and deliver to the contractor, a quantum of produce, based upon anticipated yield and contracted acreage at a pre-agree price.

7. Contract farming is viable proposition for small and marginal farmers, who are otherwise left out in the market driven economy to get the benefits of the same. In addition to getting exposure to the latest production technologies, farmer is hedged against the price risk. Contract farming also provides a win-win situation for the banker who can mobilize bulk level of production credit to large number of farmers with assured repayments at lower follow-up costs.

Since ages, Indian economy has been an agricultural economy. Majority of our population are dependent on agriculture for their basic needs. At the time of independence, India was not self-reliant in cereal crops production and depended on imports and this condition continued till 1966-67 leading to crisis in foreign exchange reserves and balance of payments. The foreign debt increased manifold. The green revolution gave fillip to Indian agriculture from 1966-67 and consequently, Indian production of food grains, especially that of wheat and rice increased sharply.

In India, even after 56 years of independence 64% work force is engaged in agriculture, which contributes to about 24% of GDP. Total export of agricultural products (including marine products) during 1999-2000 has gone up to US $ 37.5 billion. However, India's share in world trade in agricultural commodities is less than 1%.

ROLE OF AGRICULTURE IN INDIAN ECONOMY

Agriculture is the largest sector of economic activity in India and has a crucial role to play in the countries economic development by providing food to people, raw material to industries, employment to very large population, capital for its own development and surplus for national economic development.

The distribution of national income shows that the share of various agricultural commodities, animal husbandry and ancillary activities has always been more than 40%. During eighties and subsequently during 1990-91, this has fallen to 33% and has further gone down to 24% in recent times. This trend of decling share of agriculture in national income is broadly in consonance with the conclusions derived by the development economies.

During last 70 years, the size of labour force dependent on agriculture had more than doubled and over the next decade it is projected to up by more than 25%. The occupational structure of the country has shown a lack of flexibility. Large proportion of increasing labour force has been absorbed in agriculture due to absence of any alternative employment opportunities and would only add further to the already low production and disguised unemployment.

Indian Agriculture at a Glance

India ranks no. 1 in the world in:

a. Irrigated area
b. Cattle population
c. Buffalo population
d. Milk production
e. Pulses production
f. Tea production and
g. Jute production.

And ranks no. 2 in respect of:

a. Paddy production
b. Wheat production
c. Groundnut production
d. Sugarcane production
e. Onion production
f. Fruits and vegetable production and
g. Tobacco production

India's total production of food grains increased from 50 million tonnes during 1950s to more than 200 million tonnes, a four-fold increase in food grains production after green revolution.

Green Revolution—Fatigue

- Food grains production cost in India is higher (Rice: Production cost in India is Rs 11.00/kg as against international cost of Rs 8.00 per kg.)
- Corbohydrate revolution—less focus on millets and pulses.
- Narrowing food basket.
- Poverty amidst plenty (Tonnes of food grains and millions of hungry stomachs.)
- More than 60% of country's labour force producing less than 26% of GDP.
- Higher unemployment and underemployment.

Even after 57 years of independence, the economic status of the farmers is not improving due to the following reasons:

- High input cost both fertilizers and pesticides and shortage of quality inputs.
- In adequate credit support.
- No market information/support.
- Uncertain monsoon.
- Low rate of mechanization.
- High cost of capital.

- Poor returns.
- Low social status of farmer.

Farmers' Need Assessment

A study conducted to assess the priority needs of the farmers reveal that, access to market, credit and information/advise are the top three important priorities for farmers. Other priorities are storage, crop insurance, quality inputs, agricultural implements, etc.

Market

Marketing of agricultural commodities face the problem of scale, problem of information (farmers do not know when to start planting, harvesting, selling, etc.).

Market inefficiency, price spread, too many players between producer and consumer, resulting in only 30% of what consumer pays is reaching the producer.

Govt. Extension Services

The farmers saw field level govt. extension officers more as suppliers of inputs than providers of technical services. Nowadays private extension is gaining momentum with a package of services like, technical advice, market information, credit and other support services at cost. The concept is gaining ground with the transformation of agriculture from a traditional activity to a commercial activity. Hitherto, the village fertilizer and pesticide dealers have become defacto extension specialists with their limited knowledge. The initiative of central government to establish agriclinics and agribusiness centres involving qualified agriculture and veterinary graduates with credit support from commercial banks is a welcome sign in this direction.

Central and state governments have established information kiosks (Kisan Call Centres) for transfer of information from laboratory to land. They need to be further strengthened with qualified staff to provide instant technical guidance to the farmers.

Indian agriculture is suffering with production by masses when compared with other developing/developed countries where mass production is achieved. One of the critical component of agricultural development is "credit". Even after 35 years of nationalisation, only 1.9 crores out of 12.7 crores farmers are able to access credit from banking sector leaving a huge gap of 10.5 crores farmers yet to be reached with credit by formal banking institutions. Apart from this crores of landless agricultural labourers are deprived of the institutional credit from banks, inspite of several initiatives of government for poverty alleviation.

Induction of Commercial Banks (CBs) into Rural Credit

As the gap between demand and supply of rural credit was very large so there was need to solicit support of the commercial banking sector for supplementing the government effort for providing credit access to rural people and with a view to ensure that the credit and development efforts are directed to the desired sectors of the economy, Government of India brought the social control over commercial banks in 1967. However, the voluntary control could not motivate commercial banks to the desired extent. The entry of commercial banks into rural lending was facilitated by nationalization of 20 major commercial banks in two phases. The move was further followed up by Reserve Bank of India (the central banking authority) with the introduction of obligatory credit allocation by all commercial banks to priority sector (40%) which include most of the lending to rural and small enterprises. The decentralized credit planning through Lead Bank Scheme was also introduced. Under these measures, banks were allowed to open large number of rural branches and recruit agricultural specialists to handle the volume of rural lending. All the 466 districts in the country are placed under one or other of the commercial banks called the District Lead Bank who spearhead the credit allocation **for Rural and Priority Sector Lending by all Formal Credit Agencies at the District Level**. Similarly, lead banks also were appointed at the state level to plan and monitor the credit flow to various sectors in the state.

Regional Rural Banks

Despite all these efforts, the credit access for the poorer sections of the society was limited when compared to richer clientele and the commercial banks were not tuned to the needs and requirements of the poor and small agriculturists. The co-operatives on the other hand had low resources to meet the expected demand. The solution was sought by establishing a separate banking structure, which would have the advantages of both the co-operatives (local presence) and commercial banks (business and resource base). With this background, the regional rural banks were started as a low cost commercial banks operating in rural areas and provide credit to rural poor. The RRBs are jointly owned by the Central Government, State Government and a Commercial Bank/State Cooperative Bank in the ratio of 50:15:35.

National Bank for Agriculture and Rural Development (NABARD)

A committee appointed by Government of India had reviewed the entire arrangement for institutional credit for agriculture and rural development and suggested that there is a need to provide undivided attention for development of rural credit system. Based on the recommendations, NABARD was set up in the year 1982 by integrating the rural credit functions of other agencies and Agricultural Credit Department of RBI to provide credit for the promotion of agriculture, cottage and village industries, handicrafts, other rural crafts and allied economic activities in rural areas in order to secure integrated rural development. Since its inception, NABARD is discharging its mandate through activities relating to credit planning, financial assistance, institutional development and promotional efforts.

Government of India and RBI jointly owned the equity of NABARD. NABARD raises its resources through re-deployment of surpluses, borrowings from multilateral and bilateral institutions, borrowing from the market, institutional deposits and contributions received from Reserve Bank of India.

National Agricultural Policy of Government (2002-2007)

The Agricultural Policy of the Government aims at achieving 4% growth every year in agriculture with a focus on: (a) Technology (b) Policy and (c) Institutions.

Technology and Globalisation

- To increase production at lease 4% per annum in all facets of agricultural sector.
- Investments to upgrade the information technology related to agriculture.
- Technology to link the farming community with local and global markets.
- Use of precision farming technologies that can serve national resources and agricultural inputs through appropriate policies.

Agricultural Policies and Globalisation

- To help enhancing agricultural trade.
- To increase export of agriculture and food products.
- To facilitate the process of integrating Indian agriculture with global economies.

Institutions and Globalisation

- Institutions to apply rules and policies to protect law and order and to ensure property rights.
- Institutions to attract capital inflows into agriculture.
- Improved domestic policies in financial sector by lending institutions for agriculture.
- Services to small and medium farmers via community-based savings instruments and credit for micro-enterprises that add value to agricultural commodities before they are exported/marketed.
- Social safety nets and investments in education and skills that equip farmers to diversify their income generating activities.

Emerging Areas in Agriculture

a. Export oriented production of horticultural crops, viz. fruits, vegetables, flowers, etc. by establishing of agriculture export zones in different parts of the country for area specific crops.
b. Contract farming for quality production and marketing with backward and forward integration for production of crops.
c. Organic farming by using biofertilizers and biopesticides.
d. Establishment of Kisan Call Centres for transfer of information to farmers from universities and research centres. Establishment of information "kiosks" by private persons.
e. Establishment of agriclinics and agribusiness centres.
f. Emphasis on processing, packing and transport of agricultural produce.
g. Biotechnology and tissue culture for better quality plant material.
h. Establishment of cold storages.
i. Establishment of rural godowns for storage.

j. Development of green houses for off season production of crops.

k. Broilers production under contract farming.

l. Dairy development.

Measures for Improving Flow of Credit to Agriculture—Special Agricultural Package announced by Government in 2004

Agriculture sector is given improved thrust by the government as it plays crucial role in the over all economic development of our country by contributing 24% to GDP. The Union Finance Minister on 18th June 2004 announced an action plan involving a package of measures aimed at alleviating the dept burden of drought hit agricultural borrowers and enhancing credit flow to Agriculture.

I. *Measures announced for Extending the Scope of Institutional Credit to Farmers*

- Doubling of credit to agriculture by commercial banks in a period of 3 years.
- 30% increase in agricultural credit over flow of credit to agriculture during 2003-04.
- Kisan Credit Cards—Every effort is made to enhance coverage of institutional credit including through KCCs.
- Outlets of bank branches will be energized to enhance flow of agricultural credit.
- Commercial banks will be advised to bring to their fold at least 100 new farmers and semi-urban branch during the current year (2004-05) with an aim to financing an additional number of farmers by banks.
- In every district, all commercial banks put together will finance 10 agriclinic during the current year (04-05).
- Each rural and semi-urban branch will take up at least two to three new investment projects in the areas of plantation and horticulture, fisheries, organic farming, agro-processing, livestock, micro-irrigation, watershed management, development of village ponds, etc.
- Loans to weaker section. Target of 10% to be achieved by banks. Public sector banks to lend more to small and marginal farmers.

II. *Measures announced for Alleviating the Debt Burden of Draught-hit Agricultural Borrowers*

The package contains an OTS scheme (one time settlement) for small and marginal farmers (to cover defaulters as on 31.03.2001) and includes introduction of the following new schemes.

1. Special scheme for distressed category of farmers who were affected by natural calamities and proposing rescheduling of loans with a scope for further lending.
2. Special scheme for farmers who have irregular loans and are not willful defaulters (i.e. those affected by other calamities) proposing reschedulement of loans with scope for further lending.
3. Special provision for relending to farmers who had settled their earlier loans through OTS/compromise, etc.
4. Relief measures for farmers indebted to non-institutional lenders (takeover of loans from money lenders).

Detailed guidelines were issued to all commercial banks during July 2004 for implementing the above packages.

Further, RBI has relaxed the guidelines of service area approach with a view to facilitate rural borrowers to have easy access to institutional credit from any bank of their choice at a competitive price and to provide banks, public and private with a level playing field.

State Bank of India has taken initiative to do away with scales of finance fixed for various crops by district technical committees to facilitate farmers to avail need-based production loans based on the improved package of practices followed by farmers for growing crops.

Bio-villages: A new development paradigm for rural development by M.S. Swaminathan Research Foundation, Chennai.

The concept of "Bio-village" involves concurrent attention to the conservation and enhancement of natural resources and poverty eradication. It is based on a pro-poor, pro-nature and pro-women orientation to technology development and dissemination, with emphasis on job led economic growth. Adding economic value to the time and labour of rural men and women living in poverty is the major pathway adopted for promoting sustainable lively hoods.

The name bio-village denotes human centred development where the health and happiness of rural families is the goal of development. The methods used to achieve the objectives are knowledge, skills, information and organizational empowerment of rural families.

Bio-village is a pro-poor, pro-women and pro-nature approach to economically feasible, ecologically viable and socially equitable sustainable development. It identifies various alternatives in the sustainable management of natural resources through forward-backward linkages for providing lively hood security. Bio-village model of development focus on the following:

- Enabling the community to understand the potentials of sustainable natural resource management and introduce various livelihood opportunities in farm and non-farm sector.
- Strengthening the human resource development through skill and knowledge empowerment and building grass root institutions such as self-help groups to take up the development initiatives under the framework of bio-village.
- Enhance the social status of rural poor by improving their skill, knowledge and fostering confidence among them to strive for social change.

EMERGING AREA IN LIVESTOCK PRODUCTION AND ALLIED ACTIVITIES

India ranks no. 1 in the world in cattle population, buffalo population, milk production. White revolution played an important role in envisaging high yield genes, cross-bred, artificial insemination and other improved technological development. As the population is increasing fast land holding gets shrinking and it is being smaller and smaller. Under this environment, we have to focus more on non-farm activities which will need lesser land holding. Increased income, employment generation in rural areas and also providing a healthy generation to the country. Bank has approved various bankable schemes for dairy development, poultry development for egg production, hatcheries, broiler production, duck-rearing, piggeries, sheep and goat rearing, etc. Salient features of some of the schemes are as under:

Agriclinic and Agribusiness Centres

Purpose: To provide self-employment opportunities to technically trained persons and strengthen transfer of technology and extension of services.

Eligibility: Agricultural graduates/graduates in subject allied to agriculture like horticulture, animal husbandry, forestry, dairy, veterinary, poultry, pisciculture and other activities.

Project cost: Individual activity: Rs 10 lacs.

Group activity: Rs 50 lacs (group = individuals of which 1 management graduate).

Interest: As applicable to direct agricultural advances.

Margin and security

Slab	Margin	Security
Up to Rs 5 lacs	NIL	Primary: Hypothecation of assets created Collateral: NIL
Above Rs 5 lacs	15 to 25%	Primary: Hypothecation of assets created. Collateral: Mortgage of land or third party guarantee with the permission of controller.

Repayment: 5 to 10 years with grace period of maximum 2 years.

TECHNICAL ASPECTS TO BE CONSIDERED WHILE FINANCING DIFFERENT ACTIVITIES UNDER ANIMAL HUSBANDRY

Dairy Farming

1. The expertise of the beneficiary in relation to the size of the proposed dairy should be ascertained. Marketing facilities available should also be studied carefully.
2. With the help of bank's technical officer, veterinary/animal husbandry officer only healthy animals in the early stage of lactation should be purchased.
3. It is better to purchase freshly calved animals in their second/third lactation.
4. Loan should be provided for the purchase of at least 2 milch animals unless the beneficiary already owns at least one animal (one animal purchased initially and the second one after an interval of 6 to 8 months).
5. It should be ascertained that the borrower has necessary accommodation for keeping the animals. Space requirement for different types of animals is as follows:

   - Cow   60 sq feet
   - Calf   20 sq feet
   - Heifer   30 sq feet

Minimum height of shed and side walls should be 10–12' and 5–7' respectively. Floor must be impervious with a slope of 2.5%.

6. Green fodder must be cultivated in the own field, i.e. for larger units having more than 10 animals the individual should own 1 acre of land for every 5 animals financed.
7. Availability of health cover and breeding facility should be within 5 km distance from the farm.
8. The animals should be vaccinated against deadly diseases like anthrax, haemorrhagic septicemia, rinderpest, black quarter and food and mouth disease.
9. Good quality water, concentrate and other feed materials must be available locally.
10. The animals must be ensured under master policy. Insurance premium is @ 4.5% in case of cross-bred cows and 4% in case of others.

Financing for Dairying

A banker should take the following factors into consideration before financing a dairy unit.

  i. A minimum grazing area of 1 acre is required for every 5 cattle.
 ii. Minimum clean drinking water requirement of cattle is 130 to 150 litres/day.
iii. The cattle shed should be constructed on high elevation with pucca and non-slippery floor, away from water logging area and near to road and market.
 iv. The minimum height of the shed should be 10 to 12' and of side walls should be 5 to 7'.
  v. Space requirement for each type of animal is as follows:

  * Cow   60 sq feet
  * Calf   20 sq feet
  * Heifer 30 sq feet

 vi. Feed requirement of the cattle is as follows:

Animals	During L.P./D.P.	Green fodder (kg)	Dry fodder (kg)	Concentrates (kg)
Buffaloes	L.P.	25–30	4–5	3.5–4
7–8 litres of milk/day	D.P.	20–25	7–8	0.5–1

vii. Certificate of health and age should be obtained from the veterinary doctor.
viii. Important indicators of various types of animals.

	Buffalo	Cow (Indian)	Cow (cross-bred)
Age of maturity	3 to 4 yrs	3 to 4 yrs	9 to 12 months
Sexual cycle	21 days	21 days	21 days

Contd.

	Buffalo	**Cow (Indian)**	**Cow (cross-bred)**
Gestation period	10 months + 10 days	9 months + 9 days	9 months + 9 days
Age at 1st calving	3-1/2 to 4-1/2 yrs	3-1/2 to 4-1/2 yrs	1-1/2 to 2-1/2 yrs

ix. The animals and cattle shed should be insured. Insurance premium is 4.5% of the cost in case of cross-bred cows and 4% in case of others. It may change from time to time.

Package of Practices

To run the dairy enterprise on profitable lines, the following packages of practices should be adhered to:

i. Cows and buffaloes yielding on an average 3500 litres and 2100 litres of milk, respectively, must be purchased.

ii. A minimum of 20 kg of green fodder along with dry fodder (straw) and some concentrates should be given to cattle.

iii. A mineral mixture @ 20 gm/kg of concentrate mixture can also be added to make up mineral deficiencies.

iv. Feed heifer and cows in the late pregnancy @ 1 kg concentrate mixture daily in last two months.

v. Cull and male calves at birth in cattle and buffaloes calves should be weaned as soon as possible after calving.

vi. The sheds can economically constructed by using cement asbestos sheets supported on angle iron and hollow iron pillars or small brick pillars.

vii. While using artificial insemination techniques care should be exercised to see that the exotic inheritance of the herd is limited to between 50 to 62.50%.

viii. A teaser bull can be added to the herd to combat the problem of heat detection.

ix. To avoid losses due to mortality and reducing the expenditure on treatment, animals should be vaccinated at proper time and as per schedule.

x. Defective and low yielding animals should be culled as early as possible.

xi. Insurance cover should be provided to all the animals in the herd.

xii. Proper market for the milk should be explored to avoid risk and losses.

Model Scheme for Financing a Dairy Unit of 10 Cross-bred Cows

Economics of 10 Cross-bred Cows Unit

	Amount in Rs
A. Capital cost	
i. Cost of 10 C.B. cows giving average daily milk yield of 10 lit. in a lactation period of 280 days (i.e. 14 days per day at the time of purchase) @ Rs 10000 per cow including transportation cost	1,00,000/-

ii. Cow shed @ 60 sq ft/cow and Rs 60/sq ft.	36,000/-
iii. Calf cum heifer pens @ 25 sq ft/calf and Rs 60/sq ft	15,000/-
iv. Store cum heifer pen (200 sq ft @ Rs 100/sq ft)	20,000/-
v. Equipments @ Rs 200/animal	2,000/-
vi. Chaff cutter	5,000/-
vii. Insurance cost @ 4.5% of cost of animal for 1 year	4,500/-
viii. Concentrate feed for three months @ 3 kg/cow/day and @ Rs 5/kg	13,500/-
ix. Miscellaneous	4,000/-

B. Total scheme cost   2,00,000/-

Less margin @ 15%   30,000/-

Bank's finance   1,70,000/-

C. Annual lactation days and dry days: Considering 280 days as lactation period followed by 120 days of dry period. (Details given at milk flow chart depicted at the end for 2 cows cycle).

Days	1st year	2nd year	3rd year	4th year	5th year
Lactation days	2150	2600	2600	2550	2400
Dry days	550	1000	1000	1050	1200

D. Feeding cost during lactation period (L.P.) and dry period (D.P.) per cow per day

Items	L.P. (Rs)	D.P. (Rs)
a. Green fodder @ 25 kg during lactation 20 kg during dry period (@ Rs 40/q)	10	08
b. Dry fodder @ 10kg. (@ Rs 100/q)	10	.10
c. Concentrate feeds @ 3 kg and 1 kg during L.P. and D.P. resp. (@ Rs 5/kg)	15	05
Total	**35**	**23**

Poultry Farming

i. The agro-climatic conditions must be suitable for rearing birds in the area.

ii. It should be ascertained that the applicant has knowledge/experience in raising poultry.

iii. Selected site should be away from main roads and free from water logging conditions.

iv. The poultry shed should be adequate to accommodate the number of birds to be raised. The poultry house should be according to standard requirements and should give protection to birds from sun, rain, wind and predators.

v. Suitable arrangements should be made for purchase of high quality one day old chicks or layers from reputed sellers at reasonable prices.

vi. Sufficient clean water should be available for birds. It should also be ascertained that the poultry feed is available from close proximity at reasonable price.

vii. Proper veterinary services must be available near the farm for treating the birds. Birds should be vaccinated against poultry diseases.

viii. Firm arrangements must be made for marketing of eggs/broilers/culled birds.

ix. Arrangements should be made for insurance of birds and the insurance policy should be made in favour of the bank. Layers @ Rs 4.23% birds, broilers @ Rs 0.71/birds, building and equipments @ 0.40% of cost.

x. Proper records of all purchases and sales should be maintained.

Financing for Poultry Units

i. The site should be dry, without water logging, well drained and properly accessible. It should be 500 meters away from the existing farm.

ii. Distance between brooder shed, grower shed and layer shed should be 100 feet from each other.

iii. Distance between two layer sheds should be 70 feet.

iv. The shed should have East West orientation.

v. Height of shed should 16 to 22 feet with a maximum width of 35 feet and a length of 100 to 400 feet.

vi. Feed mixing unit should be minimum 300 feet away from sheds.

vii. Floor space norms

S. No.	Civil structure	Layers sheds (sq. ft.)		Broilers	
		Deep litter system	Cage system	Deep litter system	Cage system
1.	Brooder shed (0–8 weeks)	0.5	0.40	–	–
2.	Grower shed (9–20 weeks)	1.0	0.70	–	–
3.	Layer shed (21–72 weeks)	2.0	0.80	–	–
4.	Broiler shed (0–8 weeks)	–	–	1.00	0.60

viii. Feed and feed requirement

S. No.	Type of bird	Age in weeks	Type of feed	Requirement (in kg)	
				Deep litter system	Cage system
1.	Layers (chicks)	0–8	Chick mash	2.0	2.0
2.	Layers (growers)	9–20	Grower mash	6.0	5.0
3.	Layers (adults)	21–72	Layer mash	40–42	37–39
4.	Broilers	0–4	Starter mash	3.75–4.00	–
5.	Broilers	5–8	Finish mash	3.75–4.00	–

ix. Vaccination schedule for layers and broilers as suggested by poultry experts should be strictly followed. All vaccinations should be completed before 15 to 16 weeks of age.

x. The birds should be insured. The premium rates of insurance of birds, equipment and building, etc. are:

Birds	Building and equipment
Layers @ Rs 4.23/bird	@ 0.40% of cost
Broilers @ Rs 0.71/bird	

xi. The total flock is brought in batches depending on the availability of sheds. Interval between introductions of batches should be 12 weeks.

xii. The economic size is 50000 birds for a layer unit in traditional area. For broilers, the unit size can be determined primarily based on the market potential in the area.

All the initiatives discussed above need massive financial support both from government and banks. The financial institutions should look at agriculture as a viable commercial activity rather than a traditional one and thus play a major role in changing the face of rural economy. It is all the more essential in the present day that all the institutions connected with agriculture and rural development should work with the sprit of partnership to give boost to the rural economy as per the policy initiatives of the government.

22

Insurance Schemes for Livestock Sector

VK Bhasin

CATTLE INSURANCE

Cattle insurance was governed under Market Agreement as devised by GIC and the rates, terms, conditions, etc. all were applicable to all the four insurance companies. However, w.e.f. May 2003, it is no longer under Market Agreement.

This policy covers indigenous cross-bred and exotic cattle owned by private owners, various financial institutions, dairy farms, cooperatives, corporate dairies, etc. The word cattle include milch, cows and buffaloes calves and heifers, stud bulls, bullocks and he-buffaloes and mithuns. Age group is specified for all the animals. The evaluation of the animal is done by a veterinarian.

SCOPE OF COVER/INSURANCE COVERAGE

The policy shall give indemnity only for death of cattle due to:

i. Accident (inclusive of flood, cyclone, famine) or any other fortuitous circumstances (fortuitous means accidental in origin).
ii. Diseases (inclusive of rinderpest, blackquarter, haemorrhagic septicemia, foot and mouth disease subject to vaccination against each).
iii. Surgical operations.
iv. Strike riot and civil commotion and terrorism.
v. Earthquake.

Policy is subject to certain standard and general exclusions. Animals are identified by way of ear tagging. The policy covers both scheme and non-scheme animals. Scheme animals are those animals, which are sponsored by the government agencies and are financed by some financial institutions, which may or may not involve any subsidy. Master policy arrangements are usually done with DRDA, bank, and cooperative societies, etc. There is a provision of long-term policies also.

Note: All cattle of individual insured or dairy farm should be insured. No selection is allowed.

Foetus (Unborn Calf) Insurance Scheme

This scheme covers the risk of death of embryo/foetus due to:

a. Accident (Inclusive of flood, cyclone, famine) or any other. Fortuitous circumstances (fortuitous means accidental in origin).
b. Diseases (Inclusive of rinderpest, blackquarter, haemorrhagic septicemia, foot and mouth disease subject to vaccination against each.
c. Surgical operations.
d. Strike riot and civil commotion and terrorism.
e. Earthquake.

The scheme is applicable to both the embryo transferred from a selected donor to the synchronized recipient or frozen embryo transferred to the recipient and also the embryo/foetus developed by artificial insemination technique. This can be covered as a separate policy in addition to cattle insurance policy covering the recipient mother cow/buffalo.

The cover operates from the 60th day of the transfer of live quality embryo/successful insemination and terminates from 220 +/–5 days for cow from the date of confirmation of pregnancy or from the date of calving whichever is earlier. It is not an annual policy. The perils covered are stillbirth, abortion of all kinds except malafied or induced once. Accidental risk, include abortion under veterinary advice to save the mother in conditions like downer's cow syndrome, prolapse of uterus, portion of uterus, fracture of limb, etc. The sum insured is fixed and depends on the age of the embryo.

Calf Heifer Rearing Insurance Scheme

The coverage under this policy is meant for calves/heifers from one day to 32 months. The valuation depends upon the age of the cow and is fixed according to the age of the calf. All terms and conditions applicable to cattle are applicable here also. Minimum coverage is taken from 12 months, however, this is not an annual policy.

Sheep and Goat Insurance

This scheme is also governed under Market Agreement. Policy provides indemnity to indigenous cross-bred and exotic sheep and goat against death due to accident (including fire, lightening, flood, cyclone, famine, strike, riot and civil commotion) and disease. Earthquake and landslide covers are also provided. Standard and common exclusions apply as per cattle policy. Animals are identified by means of small brass buttons ear tags. Animals under scheme category enjoy certain benefits in premium rate and claim procedure.

Camel Insurance

The camels are covered against death due to accident or disease as per standard cattle insurance policy. The maximum SI is restricted to Rs 3000/-.

Pig Insurance

All indigenous, cross-bred and exotic pigs are covered, however, under scheme category exotic animals are not covered. The age group is from 4 months to 3 years. The coverage is against death due to accident or disease. Exclusions as per cattle policy apply here also. Permanent total disablement, breeding and furrowing risks are not covered. Vaccination in applicable diseases is compulsory. Evaluation depends upon the age of the animal. Animals are identified by means of small brass buttons ear tags.

Horse, Mule, Donkey, Pony, Yak Insurance

The coverage is as per standard cattle policy. However, the age group is restricted to 2 to 8 years.

Poultry Insurance

This is also governed by Market Agreement, amongst all the four subsidiary companies. The policy shall provide indemnity against death of birds due to accident (including fire, lightning, flood, cyclone, strike, riot and civil commotion and terrorism) or diseases contracted or occurring during the period of insurance. The word poultry includes layers, broilers and hatchery birds, which are exotic and cross-bred. Indigenous and non-descript birds will not be insured. All birds in a farm should be covered. The scheme is applicable to poultry farms consisting of minimum 100 birds under scheme category and 500 birds under non-scheme category. In general, it is 100 broilers per batch, 500 layers per batch and 2000 hatchery birds per batch. For layers, the cover is provided from 1 day to 20 weeks, 21 to 72 weeks or 1 day to 72 weeks. Broilers are covered from 1 day to 6 weeks or 8 weeks. Hatchery birds are covered from 1 day to 72 weeks. The value of the bird is fixed according to the age. The cover is provided against death of the birds due to accident or disease. All applicable cases, vaccination is a must. The valuation of the birds is arrived by a multiplying factor with the age in weeks. The multiplier is applied to the prevailing feed cost and the day old chick cost is added to arrive at weekwise valuation. Certain common and standard exclusions applied. Since all the birds are covered, there is no need for identification. The poultry farmer is expected to maintain all the relevant records like feed register, flock record on day to day basis, daily stock register, mortality, culling, vaccination, feed consumption, production, de-beaking, and incidents of diseases, sales and purchase.

Duck Insurance

Applicability

i. All types of migratory and non-migratory birds in India.
ii. Duck farms consisting of minimum of 100 ducks for non-IRDP and 50 ducks for IRDP and other government subsidized schemes.

   Note: All birds in duckery farm should be insured.

Duck Insurance Scheme shall provide indemnity against death of ducks due to accident including lightning, flood, cyclone, famine, riot and strike, civil commotion or diseases contracted or occurring during the period of insurance.

This insurance is akin to poultry insurance except the age group, which is grouped into three.

   i. Day old to 52 weeks.
  ii. 53 to 104 weeks.
 iii. 105 to 120 weeks.

Cattle Insurance

Heifer rearing insurance scheme for scheme/non-scheme beneficiaries.

1. The companies may implement this scheme with caution and separate statistics may be maintained for review of the scheme.
2. The sum insured is only indicative and depending on local market conditions, it can be altered. Proportionate premium amount may be charged using the method given below.
3. The minimum period of coverage should not be less than 12 months.
4. In case of non-scheme animals, the premium rate would be @ of 4% and accordingly, the premium amount should be computed. The premium rate for scheme animals would be @ 2.25%.
5. The premium amount is computed from 1 day to 32 months. For example, in respect of scheme animals, the premium is Rs 207 for 32 months and in respect of non-scheme animals, the premium is Rs 368 for 32 months (valuation table enclosed).
6. The formula adopted for calculation of premium is as under:

The aggregate sum insured	Scheme animals	Non-scheme animals
From 1 day to 32 months	Rs 1,10,450.00	1,10,450.00
Average sum insured	Rs 3,451.60	3,451.60
for 32 months	or 3,452.00	3,452.00
Apply premium rate	Rs 3,452 × @ 2.25%	3,452 × @ 4.00%
on average amount	= Rs 77.67	= 138.08
Average for one month	Rs 77.67/12	138.08/12
	= Rs 6.47	= 11.50
Premium for 32 months	Rs 6.47 × 32	11.50 × 32
	Rs 207.00	368.00

If the cover is given from 6 months onwards, the sum insured for earlier months is excluded from aggrl: gale sum insured while calculating the premium.

7. The scope of cover and executions are as per Standard Cattle Insurance Policy.
8. The claim procedure will be same as under Cattle Insurance Policy.

As far as buffalo calves are concerned, there is an existing scheme and no charges have been made.

23

Financial Credit and Financial Management

Shubha Johri, Richa Bahadur

Project appraisal is a tool with lending financial institution and banks to make an independent and objective assessment of various aspects of an investment proposal. It determines viability of a project. Viability of a project is assessed in terms of inter-relationship of its economic, technical, financial, social and managerial aspects, e.g. demand from market determines plant capacity and production process, which in turn would determine means of financing.

Project appraisal aims at identifying strengths and weaknesses in the projects. The main objective is to minimize the risk of lending by improving quality of the project

In other words, it is the process of assessing and questioning proposals before resources are committed. Project appraisal is a requirement of regeneration of the funding programme.

One basic question remains here what can project appraisal deliver?

Project appraisal delivers benefits in terms of assisting in decision-making to the partners of the project as well as guides banks and financial institution for extending loans to these projects.

Project appraisal helps a partnership:
- to be consistent in choosing projects.
- to make sure that its programme benefits all sections of the community.
- to provide documentation to meet financial and audit requirements.

Appraisal justifies spending money on a project: Appraisal asks fundamental questions about whether funding is required and whether a project offers good value for money. It can give confidence that public money is being put to good use, and help identify other funding to support a project.

Appraisal is an important decision-making tool: Appraisal involves the comprehensive analysis of a wide range of data, judgments and assumptions, all of which need adequate evidence.

It ensures that projects will be properly managed, by ensuring that appropriate financial and monitoring systems are in place, that there are contingency plans to deal with risk situations.

PROCESS OF PROJECT APPRAISAL

It follows a specific pattern because it requires multidimensional analysis of various inter-related aspects.

Analyzing Economic Aspect

Here appraisal determines economic value of cost and benefit. Economic analysis is required to assess whether the project benefits are greater than project costs to justify investment. Various economic benefit may increase output of goods or services leading to increase in wages or employment, larger government revenues, high return on investment to owners capital.

The economic impact of project implementation is analyzed with specific indicators, which can be static or dynamic. Static indicators use non-discounting methods where time is not involved in the analysis while with dynamic indicators length of time is considered. Four major dynamic indicators are used for both financial and economic evaluations of the projects.

Net Present Value (NPV)

It is the present value (PV), of net benefits of the project. It is obtained by discounting the stream of the net benefits produced by the project over its lifetime back to its value in the chosen base period, usually the present.

Internal Rate of Return (IRR)

A discount rate that equates the present value of future cash flows with the initial investment.

In other words, IRR is the discount rate if used to discount the projects net present value equals to zero.

As per the general practice in investment projects, if IRR is greater than some target rate of return or cost of capital then accept the project, if IRR is less than the appropriate cost capital, it should not be accepted.

Payback Period

Length of time to recover initial cash out flows on the projects. According to the payback method, the shorter the payback period, the more desirable the project.

Benefit Cost Ratio (BCR)

It is simply the ratio of the sum of the projects discounted benefits to the sum of its discounted investment and operating costs.

A project should be accepted if its BCR is greater than or equal to one.

Analyzing Technical Aspect

Technical appraisal of the project involves a critical study of the following:-

Location

There are a number of factors that influence industrial location.

Raw material supplies: There are some industries located near to the source of raw materials particularly industries with high material index. For example, iron and steel mills, sugar mills, timber industry.

Industries using perishable materials also tend to be located close to the raw material sources.

Proximity of markets: Certain types of industries tend to be located near the market mostly final output is bulky or fragile or perishable like milk, meat, etc.

Transportation Facilities

Transportation cost plays a major role while deciding mode of transportation. The companies do generally not prefer places with high transportation cost.

Infrastructure Facilities

It includes power, fuel supply, electricity, water supply, and roads, etc. Technical feasibility study should consider the adequacy and suitability of the plant layout, the equipment and their specification apart from above-mentioned factors.

Analyzing Financial Aspect

Purpose of financial analysis is to ascertain the revenue producing nature of the project. It should ensure that satisfactory accounts are maintained for effective control of expenditure. Also, since banks finance only a part of investment cost of a project, it is necessary to ensure that funds from other sources are available on acceptable terms.

Projects are Appraised in following Financial Aspects

Cost Analysis

A proper cost analysis should be worked out to decide cost of production.

Pricing

Price must be fixed very judiciously because price is the cause of demand.

Financing

It is concerned with raising the funds and making their efficient use.

Income and Expenditure

This analysis helps in ascertaining the cost involved and profit expected from the project.

Financial analysis helps in identifying financial soundness of the project in terms of efficient operations, cost of production, return on investment, profitability, pricing, budgeting and effective control.

Commercial or Market Aspect Analysis

An intensive scanning and analysis of the proposed environment in which industrial unit has to function should form the basis for analyzing market opportunities are expressed in terms of demand forecasts, market share, etc.

Political and Labour Aspect Analysis

Financial institution pays attention to political environment and labour conditions of the area where the project is to be located.

The lending institution appraises the project to examine its viability on technical, economic, commercial and financing grounds. If the appraised report is found satisfactory, the loan application will be considered favourably.

Project Report

Once the project is identified project report is formulated after examining various relevant aspects.

An expert prepares a project report after detailed study and analysis of the various aspects of a project. It provides a comprehensive analysis of the inputs and outputs of the project.

Importance of the Project Report

Project report is very important requirement for implementing the project. It communicates the practicality of a project in terms of different factors like economy, finance, technology, and social responsibility. It is needed by the entrepreneur for carrying out expansion or starting production. Financial corporations and banks for granting loans need it, to check how production should be organized to yield maximum returns.

Contents of a Project Report

Project report has following contents:

- Objective and scope of the report.
- Product characteristics (specifications, product uses and application, standards and quality).
- Installed capacity, anticipated demand, and price structure.
- Price, sources and properties of raw materials.
- Process of manufacturing, production schedule, production technique.
- Plant and machinery (essential infrastructure).
- Land and building (land area, construction schedule).
- Financial implications (working capital requirement, cost profitability).
- Marketing strategies and trading practices.
- Requirement of staff, labour, expenses on wage payment.

An entrepreneur can himself prepare the report or take assistance from experts like small industries development organization and some times even state government helps in matters of financial assistance.

Role of Development Banks in Project Appraisal

Development banks are supposed to play a significant role in the establishment of industrial projects, besides the conventional role of supplying term capital. The management of development bank carries out two tasks simultaneously. As a financial agency, development bank provides term loans. Secondly, it is concerned with profitability and safety aspects of the investment.

The task of project appraisal in a development bank is often very difficult. It evaluates a project from various angles like technical, economic, financial and market/commercial. If a project is found suitable from all the four angles, assistance is granted by development bank.

After assistance has been granted for a project, the development bank must keep a close watch on its progress with a view to ensure that assistance is utilized for the purpose for which it was sanctioned, and to assess whether the project will be completed within the original estimates of capital cost and to evaluate production performance and working results against the original expectations.

The bank may exercise an effective control over the affairs of the assisted company by nominating its own representatives in the board of the directors of the company.

Process of Project Evaluation by Development Bank

In considering loan application for financing a project, development banks in India take into account the following factors:

TECHNICAL APPRAISAL

The technical appraisal involves a critical examination of:

- Suitability of the technical process.
- Locational aspect, i.e. nearness to the sources of raw material, availability of utilities—water, power, transport facilities, availability of skilled and unskilled labour and market for the product.
- Plant layout equipment and production flow.
- Utilization of by products and disposal of factory wastes.
- Construction and installation schedule.

FINANCIAL APPRAISAL

Projects showing earnings sufficient to cover fixed cost, operational and maintenance costs giving an adequate return on total investment are considered to be financial sound.

Following financial aspects are analyzed:

Cost Estimates

- Cost of land, conveyance, building.
- Plant and machinery cost and other taxes.
- Miscellaneous fixed assets—furniture, office equipments, tools.
- Startup costs, including the cost of raw materials, direct wages, salaries, etc.

Financing Pattern

- Share capital.
- Long-term loans from financial institutions.
- Public deposits.

Besides examining financing pattern with the help of debt equity ratio, banks look at other important ratios also to evaluate the financial and operational cost of the project. These ratios are:

- Current ratio.
- Return on equity.
- Net profit ratio.
- Gross profit ratio.

Banks evaluate projected profitability and cash flow in terms of the three important indicators like:

- Debt service coverage ratio.
- Interest services coverage ratio.
- Internal rate of return.

In the evaluation of project, different viewpoints are analyzed. In the management view, the crucial ratio is return on investment, from the shareholder's view the earning per share, from the lender's view debt service coverage ratio is considered as important.

ECONOMIC APPRAISAL

- Contribution of the project to the economy.
- Employment potential.
- Prospects of exports.
- A study of pricing policy in relation to demand.

Finally in order to ensure satisfactory progress of the project and proper utilization of money sanctioned, the development bank should see that experienced technical and managerial personnels are engaged by assisted units.

CAPITAL EXPENDITURE DECISIONS

Long life and smooth functioning of an organization of any nature demand consumption of certain resources like machinery, raw material, etc. These resources are called assets in organization.

Amount spent by an organization for acquiring these resources can be classified into:

- Revenue expenditure.
- Capital expenditure.

Revenue expenditure is defined as expenditure incurred on day-to-day running of business like rent of the factory, salaries of employees, consumable supplies, raw material, etc.

Capital expenditure is defined as expenditure creating future benefits.

Capital expenditures are incurred to acquire or upgrade a physical asset such as land, building, tractor, machinery and equipment by an organization.

Capital Expenditure Means

- Acquiring assets like tractor, machinery, etc.
- Making them ready for use.
- Legal cost of buying the assets.
- Transportation cost.
- Any cost incurred in making the asset like tractor, machinery ready for use.

Capital expenditure is the most important decision to be made by management of an organization because:

- It involves a huge sum of money to be invested.
- Reversal of decision means bringing loss as the organization has to sell the purchased asset at a lesser price than its original cost.
- Company's growth and development depends upon these capital expenditure decisions as they affect the productivity of the organization.

For example: Buying a tractor is a capital expenditure decision for agriculture firm and it is important because it involves huge sum of money and company's growth and development depend upon the decision of buying a tractor because tractor will affect the productivity of the firm.

Capital expenditure decision involves the decision of allocation of funds (money) to long-term assets like plant, machinery, building, etc. that would yield benefits in future. That is why these capital expenditure decisions are also called investment decisions of any firm.

For example: Plant, building and machinery are there in an organization and will continue to give their services to the organization till their life, i.e. yielding benefits in future.

CAPITAL BUDGETING

The technique used to measure the verifiability of worthiness of capital expenditure decisions is called capital budgeting.

Capital budgeting measure the worthiness of capital expenditure decision by critically evaluating cash inflows and cash outflows.

Capital budgeting is referred as strategic allocation of the firm's funds.

On the basis of time value of money, capital budgeting can be divided into two categories:

Non-discounting method: This method does not consider time value of money. It is divided into:

- Pay back period (PBP).
- Accounting rate of return (ARR).

Discounting method: This method is based on time value of money. It means that this method discounts the cash flows on the basis of time value of money. It is divided into:

- Net present value (NPV).
- Benefit cost ratio or profitability index (BCR or PI).
- Internal rate of return (IRR).

Few Terminologies of Capital Budgeting

Cash flow: It is the movement of money or cash of an organisation. It is divided into two types:

Cash outflow or initial outlay: It is defined as the amount of money or cash going out of organisation. It is represented generally by CO.

For example: If ABC organisation has purchased a thresher of Rs 100000/- than in this case the cash of Rs 100000/- is going out of the organization so cash outflow (CO) is Rs 100000/-.

Cash inflow: It is defined as the amount of money or cash coming in the organisation. It is generally represented by C.

For example: If we go with the same example than being the capital expenditure decision of ABC will increase the productivity because of this more money or cash will come to the organisation if in the first year after it purchased the able to bring Rs 5000/- in the organisation and in second year again Rs 4000/-. So cash inflow in C_1 is Rs 5000/ (Here 1 is representing first year) and C_2 is Rs 4000/ (Again 2 is representing second year). So C_1 and C_2 are cash inflows of two years of an organisation.

Difference between Cash Flow and Profit

Cash flow includes only the cash or money whereas profit includes both the cash and the sources from where the money will be coming to the organisation, i.e. non-cash items.

It is important to understand the differentiation as in capital decisions every-thing is based on cash flows and not on profit.

Time Value of Money

It means the value of a unit of money is different in different time periods. For example, the value of one rupee is more in 1960 and 1970 as compared to today.

Cost of Capital

Capital expenditure decision involves huge sum of money. The companies are required to arrange for this huge money so they take loan from banks or from any other financial institutions. The interest rate on which these organizations take loans for capital expenditure decision is called cost of capital. It is represented by k.

For example: Agriculture firm needs to buy a machinery costing Rs 4500000. So for buying this machinery if this agriculture firm has taken a loan from SBI bank at interest rate of 12%. Then this 12% is cost of capital.

Cost of capital is defined as the minimum rate of return required to be invested in the project or rate that equates present value with future value of cash flows. It is also called opportunity cost of capital, discount rate, hurdle rate and rate of return.

Present value: What is the value of money today?

Future value: What will be the value of money in future?

Non-discounting Method

This method does not consider time value of money. It is divided into:

Pay Back Period (PBP)

Pay back period means the number of year required to recover the initial outlay invested in capital expenditure project decisions.

If the project generates constant annual cash inflows. PBP can be calculated by dividing initial outlay by annual cash inflow.

$$PBP = \frac{\text{Initial outlay or initial investment or cash outflow}}{\text{Annual cash inflow}} = \frac{CO}{C}$$

For example: Suppose a capital expenditure project requires an initial outlay of Rs 60000/- and yields annual cash inflows of Rs 12000/- for 7 years.

$$\text{Pay back period} = \frac{60000}{12000} = 5 \text{ years}$$

If the project generates uneven annual cash inflows, PBP can be calculated by adding up the annual cash inflows until the total is equal to initial outlay.

For example: Suppose a capital expenditure of tractor for an agricultural firm requires a cash outflow of Rs 20000/- and generates Rs 8000, Rs 5000, Rs 4000, Rs 3000 and Rs 3000/- during next 5 years.

$$PBP = C_1 + C_2 + C_3 + C_4$$
$$PBP = 8000 + 5000 + 4000 + 3000$$

PBP = 4 years because the by adding the cash inflows of four years the total is equal to cash outflow.

Advantages of PBP: Many firms set standard pay back period and start ranking the pay back period of different alternatives on the basis of standard pay back period. Alternative with shortest pay back period is selected.

- It is simple to understand and easy to calculate.
- It involves less cost so it is cost-effective in nature and commonly used by small organization.

Disadvantages of PBP

- It ignores the time value of money and time value of money plays a very important role in running a business for a longer period of time.
- All capital expenditure decisions are for a longer period of time.
- It ignores cash inflows after the pay back period.
- It measures only the recovery of initial outlay and not whether the capital expenditure will generate profit to the organisation.

The disadvantage of ignoring the time value can be solved by discounted pay back period (DPBP). DPBP first discount the cash flows and then calculate the amount of period required to recover the initial outlay.

Accounting Rate of Return (ARR)

ARR also called as return on investment (ROI) and average rate of return (ARR).

It uses accounting information like profit of the organisation revealed in the financial statements, i.e. balance sheet, profit and loss account to measure the worthiness of capital expenditure decision. It is defined as the ratio of average profit after tax or average income and average investment.

$$ARR = \frac{\text{Average profit after tax or average income} \times 100}{\text{Average investment}}$$

$$\text{Average} = \frac{\text{Opening value of investment} + \text{Closing value of investment}}{\text{Investment}} = 2$$

For example: The following are the details of a pharmaceutical company/firm and assume tax rate to be 50%.

Particulars	1st year	2nd year	3rd year
Initial investment 90000			
Sales	120000	100000	80000
Expenses	60000	50000	40000
Profit before depreciation and tax	60000	50000	40000
Depreciation	30000	30000	30000
Profit before tax	30000	20000	10000
Tax (50%)	15000	10000	5000
Profit after tax	15000	10000	5000

$$\text{Average investment} = \frac{90000 + 0}{2} = 45000$$

$$\text{Average profit after tax or average income} = \frac{15000 + 10000 + 5000}{3} = 10000$$

$$ARR = \frac{\text{Average profit after tax or average income} \times 100}{\text{Average investment}}$$

$$ARR = \frac{10000 \times 100}{45000} = 22.22\%$$

Acceptance criteria: This method will accept all those projects whose ARR is higher than the minimum rate established by the management of an organization and reject those projects which have ARR less than the minimum rate.

For example: If in the above example the minimum rate established by the management of pharmaceutical firm is 18%. So as per acceptance criteria the above project will be accepted because ARR is higher than minimum rate of 18% set up by management.

Advantages of ARR

- It is simple to understand and to use. It does not involve complicated calculations.
- It takes into consideration accounting profits of all the years in comparison to PBP which ignores cash inflows after the pay back period.

Disadvantages of ARR

- ARR uses accounting profit not cash flows in appraising the projects. Accounting profit is based on arbitrary assumptions and choices and also includes non-cash items, so it is not advisable to use ARR for measuring the worthiness or project.
- It ignores the time value of money and time value of money plays a very important role in running a business for a longer period of time.

All capital expenditure decisions are for a longer period of time.

Commonly practised by small and medium sized enterprises. ARR is best method for measuring the performance and for controlling but it should be an undesirable method for find out the worthiness of a capital expenditure decision as it may lead to unprofitable allocation of capital there by bringing loss to the firm in their investment.

Discounting Method

This method is based on time value of money. It is divided into **net present value (NPV)** and **internal rate of return (IRR)**.

Net Present Value (NPV)

It equates the present value of cash outflows with inflows. It is defined as the sum of the present values of all the cash flows.

Cash outflow means money going out of the organisation. So it is represented by minus sign, i.e. –CO.

Cash inflows means money coming inside the organisation. So it is represented by plus sign, i.e. + C_I or C_1

Formula for calculating NPV

$$NPV = CO + \frac{C_1}{(1+k)^1} + \frac{C_2}{(1+k)^2} + \frac{C_3}{(1+k)^3} + \cdots\cdots\cdots \frac{C_n}{(1+k)^n}$$

CO = Cash outflow

$C_1, C_2, C_3 \text{------} C_n$ = Cash inflows

k = Cost of capital, discount rate, hurdle rate, rate of return

Steps in NPV

- Cash flows of the capital expenditure decisions should be forecasted based on realistic assumptions.
- Select an appropriate cost of capital of the project.

Acceptance criteria

- Accept the project when NPV is positive, i.e. NPV>O.
- Reject the project when NPV is negative, i.e. NPV<O.
- May accept the project when NPV is Zero, i.e. NPV=O.

For example: Project X cost Rs 2500 now and is expected to generate annual cash inflow of Rs 900/-, Rs 800/-, Rs 700/-, Rs 600/- and Rs 500/- for 5 years. Cost of capital is Rs 1 0%. Compute NPV.

$$NPV = -2500 + \frac{900}{(1+10\%)^1} + \frac{800}{(1+10\%)^2} + \frac{700}{(1+10\%)^3} + \frac{600}{(1+10\%)^4} + \frac{500}{(1+10\%)^5}$$

NPV= -2500 + 818 + 661 + 526 + 410 + 310

NPV= 226

Project will be accepted as NPV positive, i.e. NPV>O

Advantages of NPV

- It takes into consideration the time value of money and the time value of money plays a vital role in measuring the verifiability of the capital expenditure decisions.
- It is consistent with the main objective of organisation, i.e. to increase the wealth of the firm.
- It considers all the cash flows of the project.

Disadvantages of NPV

- In NPV, elements of uncertainty exist because it is based on realistic assumption that is why it is difficult to calculate cash flows and cost of capital.
- NPV is biased towards long-term project because as it does not consider the life of project.
- It is not commonly used as it involves huge amount of money and it is a difficult process.

Capital Rationing

It means allocation of capital on the basis of scarcity. NPV cannot be used if the firm is facing capital rationing problem. So, to overcome the problem of capital rationing discounting method named benefit cost ratio (BCR) or profitability index (PI) is used.

It is defined as present value of future cash inflows divided by initial investment or initial outlay or cash outflow.

$$BCR \text{ or } PI = \frac{\text{Present value of future cash inflows}}{\text{Initial investment or initial outlay}}$$

Acceptance criteria

- If greater than 1 accept the project.
- If less than 1 reject the project.

Advantages of BCR or PI: It measures the present value per rupee of initial investment or initial outlay or cash outflow.

Disadvantages of BCR or PI

- If the initial investment is spread over more than one year than BCR or PI cannot be used.
- It cannot be used individually, it has to be used in combination with NPV to measure the verifiability of the project.

Internal Rate of Return (IRR)

It is discounting method which provides the information about the rate of return the project will generate, i.e. it provides the information of the rate at which the benefits will be generated from the project.

Formula to calculate IRR: IRR is calculated by trial and error method.

For example: The following are the details of a project with a cost of capital 14%.

Year	0	1	2	3	4
Cash outflow	100000				
Cash inflows		30000	30000	40000	45000

$$CO = \frac{C_1}{(1+r)^1} + \frac{C_2}{(1+r)^2} + \cdots\cdots\cdots \frac{C_n}{(1+r)^n}$$

CO = 100000

$C_1 = 30000$, $C_2 = 30000$, $C_3 = 40000$, $C_4 = 45000$

k = 14%

$$100000 = \frac{30000}{(1+r)^1} + \frac{30000}{(1+r)^2} + \frac{40000}{(1+r)^3} + \frac{45000}{(1+r)^4}$$

Calculation of *r* involves trial and error method. We have to try different value of *r* till we find that right hand side is equal to left hand side. So, for trying the value of *r* we have to proceed with value closure to cost of capital.

So with right hand side we will first proceed with 15%.

$$\frac{30000}{(1+15\%)^1} + \frac{30000}{(1+15\%)^2} + \frac{40000}{(1+15\%)^3} + \frac{45000}{(1+15\%)^4} = 100802$$

The value being slightly higher than our target value of Rs 100000 (value of right hand side). So this will increase the value of r so now we will try with 16%

$$\frac{30000}{(1+16\%)^1} + \frac{30000}{(1+16\%)^2} + \frac{40000}{(1+16\%)^3} + \frac{45000}{(1+16\%)^4} = 98641$$

This value is lower than 100000, we can conclude that the value of r lies between 15% and 16%.

Now we will calculate NPV separately for 15% and 16%

At 15% = 802

At 16% = 1359

Sum 802 + 1359 = 2161

And again to calculate r

$$\frac{802}{2161} = 0.37$$

So r will be 15 + 0.37 = 15.37%

Since the cost of capital is 14% and the project will generate 15.37% as rate of return. If in a project r is higher than k, project will be accepted.

Acceptance criteria: Accept the project if internal rate of return is greater than cost of capital, i.e. $(r>k)$.

Reject the project if internal rate of return is less than cost of capital, i.e. $(r<k)$.

Advantages of IRR

- It takes into consideration the time value of money and the time value of money plays a vital role in measuring the verifiability of the capital expenditure decisions.
- It is consistent with the main objective of organisation, i.e. to increase the wealth of the firm.
- It is the only method which gives accurate information about the rate of return that the project will generate.

Disadvantages of IRR: If cash outflow occur at regular intervals than IRR cannot be used.

Thus we look at capital budgeting technique all the methods have their own advantages and disadvantages. So the organisation must go with that method for finding out the verifiability of capital expenditure decisions which best suits their organisation and fulfils their need and requirement.

EXAMPLE OF CAPITAL EXPENDITURE DECISION

Mr. Rahul Singh (M.D.) of M/s RK Pvt. Ltd. (dealing into agricultural products) has been considering problem of replacement of thresher, after discussing with Mohan Kumar his accountant he was able to find three possible alternatives.

Apparently three possible alternatives are as follows:

a. To order nearly same as present thresher machine, and from same Indian supplier.
b. To order a new thresher machine from a supplier of France.
c. To order a new thresher machine from a supplier of America.

After evaluating the alternatives, cash outflows or cash inflows of the three alternatives are as follows:

Items		A	B	C
Cash outflows	Rs	10000	10000	10000
Cash inflows	Year			
	1	3000	6000	5000
	2	3000	4000	4000
	3	4000	5000	4000
	4	4000	3000	4000
	5	4000	2000	3000
	6	4400	2000	2000
Total		**22400**	**22000**	**22000**

The company decided to use pay back non-discounting method to measure the verifiability or worthiness of the alternatives.

Pay Back

This method aims to calculate the time period in which project cash inflow is equal to cash outflow.

So pay back periods for the three alternatives are as follows:

Alternatives	Pay back period
A	3 yrs
B	2 yrs
C	2 yrs 3 months

As per pay back, the company should go with B alternative—To order a new thresher machine from a supplier of France because B alternatives is taking the least time to make cash in flows equal to cash outflow. Lesser time taken to recover the expenses more the profit is to a company.

Now if the same company decides to use net present value discounting.

Method to measure the verifiability or worthiness of the alternatives with the same cash inflows and cash outflow.

Cost of capital is 10%.

For alternative A

$CO=10000$, $C_1=3000$, $C_2= 3000$, $C_3=4000$, $C_4=4000$, $C_5=4000$, $C_6=4400$

$$-10000+\frac{3000}{(1+10\%)^1}+\frac{3000}{(1+10\%)^2}+\frac{4000}{(1+10\%)^3}+\frac{4000}{(1+10\%)^4}\frac{4000}{(1+10\%)^5}+\frac{4400}{(1+10\%)^6}$$

$10000 + 2727.27 + 1363.64 + 1212.12 + 909.09 + 727.27 + 666.67$

-2393.94

For alternative B

$CO=10000$, $C_1=6000$, $C_2=4000$, $C_3=5000$, $C_4=3000$, $C_5=2000$, $C_6=2000$

$$10000 +\frac{6000}{(1+10\%)^1}+\frac{4000}{(1+10\%)^2}+\frac{5000}{(1+10\%)^3}+\frac{3000}{(1+10\%)^4}\frac{2000}{(1+10\%)^5}+\frac{2000}{(1+10\%)^6}$$

$10000 + 5454.55 + 1818.18 + 1515.15 + 681.82 + 363.64 + 303.03$

136.36

For alternative C

$CO=10000$, $C_1=5000$, $C_2=4000$, $C_3=4000$, $C_4=4000$, $C_5=3000$, $C_6=2000$

$$10000+\frac{5000}{(1+10\%)^1}+\frac{4000}{(1+10\%)^2}+\frac{4000}{(1+10\%)^3}+\frac{4000}{(1+10\%)^4}\frac{3000}{(1+10\%)^5}+\frac{2000}{(1+10\%)^6}$$

$10000 + 4545.45 + 1818.18 + 1212.12 + 909.09 + 545.45 + 303.03$

-666.67

As per NPV, the company should go with B alternative—To order a new thresher machine from a supplier of France because the acceptance criteria of NPV says those alternative, are beneficial for the company whose resultant is greater than zero.

GENERAL PRINCIPLE AND PRACTICES

Capital Expenditure Project Decision in Public Sector

In public sector units, capital expenditure project appraisal and management consist of four stages.

Ist Stage—Appraisal

Appraisal involves sponsoring agency and the sanctioning authority.

Both the parties should be clear about the objectives/a capital expenditure project aims to meet and considerations of all the possible alternatives to achieve the given objectives.

Sponsoring agency: It has the overall responsibility for proper planning and management of projects. It must obtain the necessary approvals from sanctioning authority and ensure that the project proceeds as per lines approved by sanctioning authority.

Sponsoring agency may be a government department, local authority, health board or other state body or agency.

Sanctioning authority: It should evaluate all the alternatives on the basis of costs and benefits and make recommendation on the most cost effective solution. Where possible, recommendations should be quantified so as to facilitate comparison.

Capital expenditure project requires sanctioning at different level. So it is important to identify an appropriate sanctioning authority for a particular proposal.

Sanctioning authority can be government, department of finance, a local or regional authority or its management, board or manager of state or regional bodies and agencies. It depends upon the size of proposal, complexity of issues, whether to change the existing policy or not and experience and expertise of the department.

Preliminary appraisal: Sponsoring agency does preliminary appraisal. It involves detailed description of the nature and objectives of the project and other relevant information of social, economical and legal basis.

Format of preliminary appraisal: A preliminary appraisal should include a clear statement of the need for which a project is designed to meet and the degree to which it would aim to meet. It should identify all the possible alternatives including the alternative of doing nothing and quantify the key elements of all alternatives. They should choose the best alternative and must support their judgment on cost benefit basis.

On the basis of preliminary appraisal, sponsoring agency gives recommendation whether conducting detailed appraisal of the project is worthwhile or to drop the project. The recommendation should clearly state the terms of reference and if detailed appraisal are required more staff and other cost, prior approval from sanctioning authority must be taken.

Detailed appraisal: Detailed appraisal serves four very important functions:

- It provides the sponsoring agency with a basis for taking a decision to proceed further with project.
- It provides the sanctioning authority with a basis for deciding whether to approve or reject the proposal.
- It serves as the reference document to assess the effects of changes that may occur during the development of the project.
- It serves as the reference document to ensure evaluation of the project after completion.

Detailed appraisal checklist

- Define clearly the needs the project should meet and its objective why there is a need of project and what are the requirements on which needs will be met.
- List the alternatives—maximum possible ways through which the objective can be achieved including the alternative of doing nothing.
- List the constraints—there will invariably be constraints in reaching objectives. Constraints can be financial, technological, legal, environmental, physical, social, etc. Constraints must be explored and should be taken account because they will limit the range of possible alternatives which are feasible or acceptable.
- Quantify cost and specify the sources of funding—cost quantification should cover cost and benefits generated by the use of asset as well as cost involved in their establishment.
- Analysis of alternatives—analysis include financial analysis, cost-benefit analysis, cost-effective analysis and cash flow analysis.
  - *Financial analysis* includes projection of profit and loss account and balance sheet.
  - *Cost benefit analysis* helps to assess whether or not the social and economic benefits associated with a project are greater than social and economic costs.
  - *Cost-effective analysis* helps to compare the costs of all possible alternatives of achieving a particular objective so that best choice can be made.
  - *Cash flow analysis* should be done with discounting and non-discounting techniques to analyze cash inflows and cash outflow of all possible alternatives so has to choose the best one.
- Identify the risk associated with each alternative and if possible suggest a strategy to deal with the risk.
- Choose best alternative and draw a plan of action for final execution.
- Sponsoring agency should give recommendation for the alternative which according to them is the best for the final approval and should be ready for any change in their choice by sanctioning authority.

IInd Stage—Planning

This stage involves detailed planning and costing of the project. It consists of seven steps.

1. Establishment of project management structure.
   It involves the following steps:
   - Kind of management structure suitable for the project.
   - Accountability for various aspects of the project.
   - Kind of reporting system.
2. Preparation of a design brief: The design brief is a detailed description of the project alternative which has been approved finally, describing about the objectives and the parameters to be taken in account by planning professionals.

3. Detailed planning and design: On the basis of parameters given in design brief detailed planning and designing in terms of cost for final implementation of the project is done.
4. Review of proposal by using information provided by planning process.
5. Obtaining approval of the sanctioning authority.
6. Calling tenders.
7. Review of proposal—using tender prices for the review.

IIIrd Stage—Implementation

The critical task of implementation stage is to manage and monitor the project to ensure that it is executed satisfactorily within the budget and on time.

IVth Stage—Post-project Review

This aims to draw lessons for the future.

It includes the following:

- Whether the basis on which a capital expenditure project was undertaken proved correct.
- Whether the planned outcome is matching with actual outcome.
- Whether the appraisal and management procedure adopted proved to be satisfactory.

24

Managing Finance in Livestock Sector

Rajendra P Bharti

All businesses whether big or small are carried out for earning profits in the short run and for creating and maximizing the investor's wealth in the long run. Profit is measured in terms of money and wealth is measured in terms of potential, assets and other resources to generate more profits with increased rate and on sustainable basis. Business is all about taking risk because the human efforts, money and other inputs are committed first and the revenues in terms of realization of sales proceeds or the service charges are received afterwards. Starting a business therefore requires entrepreneurial skills and attitude. It is very important that before deciding to invest the entrepreneur has ensured that he has positive answers for following vital questions.

Are Goals Well Defined?

This question is to be answered on minimum four parameters which are:

- Personal aspirations of the entrepreneur
- Size of business
- Prospects and potential of sustaining the business
- Entrepreneur's ability to tolerate risk

Does the Entrepreneur have Right Strategy?

Strategy can be normally evaluated on following parameters:

- Clear definition and conceptualization of the factors of business
- Long-term sustainability
- Expected rate of growth

Whether the Entrepreneur has Competence to Execute the Strategy?

The positive answers to this question depend on:

- How passionate the founder/entrepreneur is about the execution of the project?
- What are the available resources? Are they adequate?
- Whether necessary infrastructure is available or can be managed?

- There is tremendous scope for starting new ventures of allied agricultural activities such as: dairy farming, fisheries, poultry farming, sheep and goat breeding, bee-keeping, horticulture, sericulture and floriculture, etc.

Those who have knowledge (not necessarily formal qualifications), skills and a strong will to create and run a business of their own can test themselves on above entrepreneurial competence and think of a project which has best synchronization with:

i. The entrepreneur himself/herself
ii. The current and emerging environment
iii. Market demand
iv. Infrastructure and
v. Means of financing

Normally, as soon as a person starts thinking about a business, howsoever small, the further process of thought is blocked by a big question; do I have enough money to finance the venture? And in many cases where the money resources are not available, the business idea is not conceived at all. This is a myopic view about business and particularly small businesses that have good potential in rural and semi-urban areas. The studies have suggested that in our country, the potential of businesses dependent on live-stock has not been fully exploited. On analysing the impediments for this sector's less than desirable contribution, we find that finance is a big concern.

This chapter, therefore, attempts to provide a basic understanding of finance that can help the entrepreneurs manage finance for their ventures including those which are carried out with the help of livestock.

Once a business idea has been conceptualised and found to be prima-facie compatible with the entrepreneur, he has to think about the sources of money for buying inputs and for accessing services. In all businesses, certain assets; physical, technological, intellectual or livestock, etc. are required to be acquired. These assets when used skillfully with some more inputs produce items of goods or types of services which are sold or offered in exchange of money. The success of business endeavour is measured in terms of excess of revenue generated by sale or provision of services over all costs of inputs. This excess is termed as profit.

FINANCIAL MANAGEMENT

Financial management has emerged to acquire the greatest importance in almost every business enterprise; big, medium or small. Traditionally, the objective of financial management was considered to be the maximization of profit. But eventually, it has been established that the main objective of financial management is to maximise the wealth of the investors and create long-term value for the enterprise. As a matter of fact, financial management serves the firm in realizing its vision and mission and the success of business strategy normally depends on effective management of finances.

In the context of entrepreneurs starting business dependent of livestock in rural or semi-urban areas, the firms are generally individual ownership or small partnership firms. They do not have access to capital markets. They primarily rely on trade credit, bank finance, lease financing and in many cases local lender. Efficient management of finance cannot only help in earning more profit but can also strengthen the enterprise in becoming financially self-dependent and capable of leveraging high future growth.

After selecting the project, the firm needs to conduct the technical analysis that studies the practical feasibility and when combined with financial analysis it leads to manage the finances in such a way that profitability is increased. The relationship between these activities can be better understood by Fig. 24.1.

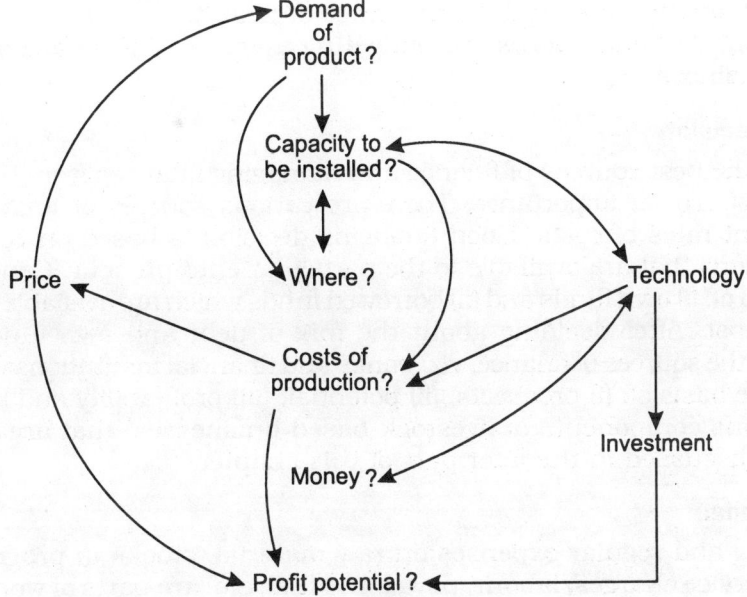

Fig. 24.1: Technical analysis

Financial analysis will always be in the context of the entrepreneur's capabilities and resources and will involve broadly following sequences of estimations:

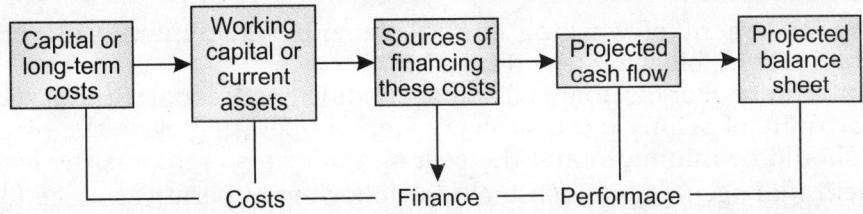

Having done the above analysis, the process of financial management starts. This is about making following major four groups of decisions:

1. Capital budgeting and investment decision.
2. Financing decision.

3. Working capital management.
4. Management of profit: Retention or withdrawl by investor.

In small firms, the first three are of greater significance since profit is normally used for consumption and investment in growth.

Capital Budgeting and Investment Decision

Capital budgeting includes estimation of all costs that are to be incurred in buying and creating long-term and short-term assets. In case of a livestock based business, it will be about purchase cost of livestock and day-to-day routine expenses of shelter, food and maintenance of health.

Investment decision follows the budgeting exercise. This is a commitment of funds to business.

Financing Decision

Identifying the best sources of finance and managing finances from those sources are issues of crucial importance. There are various sources of finance available with different rates of costs. Good financing decision is based on comparison of various options that are available to the particular entrepreneur. Generally, it is a combination of: (i) own funds and (ii) borrowed funds which are available at minimum combined cost. After deciding about the mix of debt and own funds, the firm approaches the sources of finance, viz. banks and financial institutions which extend credit on the basis of: (i) prospects, (ii) potential, (iii) profitability and (iv) people.

The various components of livestock-based businesses, that are financed by banks are discussed in the later part of this chapter.

Working Capital

The running and regular expenses on raw material, stocks in progress, stores, storages, service charges, labour, power and fuel, etc. are parts of working capital requirement. While in industries, working capital is a very big issue, it is important in small enterprises related to livestock also. It includes efficient management of:
  i. Cash.
 ii. Inventories of various stocks of consumables and other utilities of routine business operations.
iii. Credit or finance.

The management of working capital depends on dynamic movement of operating cycle in following way (Fig. 24.2).

The entrepreneur or his financial manager has to ensure that without sacrificing on opportunity of selling more, at every step of operating cycle the blockage of money should be minimum and the cost of money also remains the least.

Efficient management of cash includes following imperatives since (i) money has a cost and (ii) its purchasing power goes down with passage of time:
  i. No idle cash but adequate availability for reasonable contingencies.
 ii. While borrowing, on minimum effective rate of interest and borrowing to be done only when internal rate of return is higher than borrowing costs.
iii. Realising proceeds of credit-sales as early as possible.

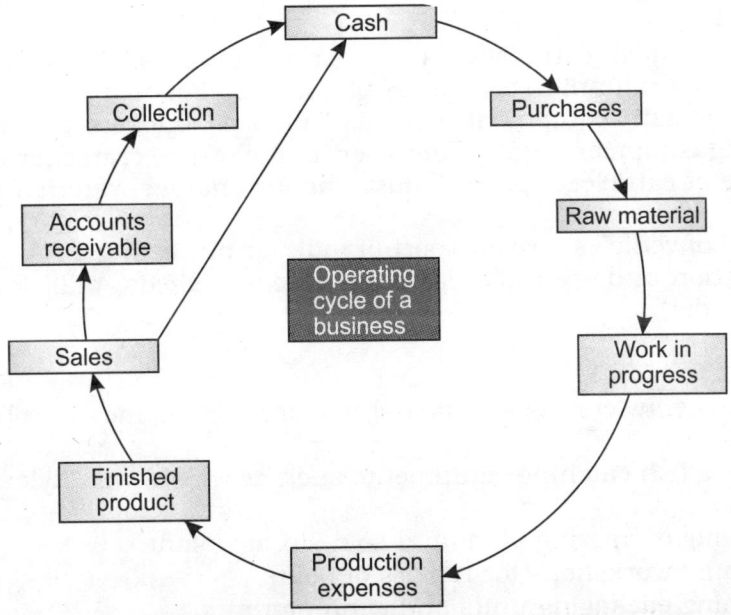

Fig. 24.2: Operating cycle

Inventory management aims at reducing total costs of inventory including ordering costs, storage costs, purchase costs and insurance, etc. while ensuring that production is optimized to meet largest portion of demand.

Extending credit is a crucial decision. Normally, goods should be sold on credit to those who are strong on 4 Cs model, i.e. character, capital and capability and capacity. Realising dues of credit sales require strategic recovery measures.

FINANCING OF LIVESTOCK-BASED BUSINESS

After nationalisation of banks and more importantly after initiation of reform process, micro-finance has emerged as a strong support. Apart from commercial, cooperative and rural banks, some strong development financial institutions like NABARD are extending credit for businesses based on livestocks. Of late, banks have simplified procedures and credit delivery system has been made more efficient. However to take finance, the entrepreneur should ensure that he is ready with:

- Assessment of costs and expected cash flows.
- The business plan including economics of scheme.
- Particulars of assets and liabilities.
- Certificates of training/know-how if required.
- Quotation of costs.
- Documents of assets.
- Personal guarantees.

In livestock dependent businesses, finance from banks is available for:

Dairy Farming

a. Purchase of milch cattle such as cows and buffaloes.
b. Purchase of draft animals such as bullocks.
c. Purchase of dairy equipments such as milk cans, buckets, cream separators, fat testing equipment, butter churner, milk bottles, crates for milk bottles.
d. Purchase of cattlefeed, green fodder, labour charges, veterinary medicines, etc.
e. Purchase of vehicles for transport of milk for marketing.
f. Construction of dairy buildings such as cattle sheds, milk sheds, pits for silage (fodder).

Fisheries

a. Purchasing trawlers (fishing boats) and marine engines (mechanization of trawlers).
b. Purchasing fish catching equipments such as winch, wire nylon and fishing material.
c. Establishing of freezing plant and cold storage plant.
d. Establishing workshops for repairs of boats.
e. Establishing packaging units and canning units.
f. Paying expenses in connection with purchase of ice, arranging storage of ice and fish in the boats, packing boxes, lubricants, etc.

Poultry Farming

a. Purchase of day-old chicks.
b. Purchase of poultry equipments viz. chick feeder, layer feeder, water pans, layer nets, etc.
c. Purchase of feeds and medicines during growing period.
d. Payment of labour charges and other overheads inclusive of eggs.
e. Construction of poultry sheds and storage rooms.

Sheep and Goat Breeding

a. Purchase of breeding stock and kids.
b. Purchase of feed.
c. Purchase of equipments.
d. Payment of rental charges for grazing yards, and labour charges for shearing, milking and grazing.
e. Construction of yards, etc.

The success of financial management will largely be driven by:

i. Sensitivity with environment
ii. Constant monitoring of all assets and liabilities for ensuring the best matching of maturity between the two
iii. Efficient negotiation of credit and buying terms
iv. Excellent maintenance of assets including livestock, and
v. Change management skills.

25

Latest Issues of WTO in Agriculture and Livestock Sector

MC Sharma, Chinmay Joshi, Rupasi Tiwari

FORMATION OF GATT/WTO

General Agreement on Trade and Tariffs **(GATT)** was started in **1947** with the aim of reducing inequality and even distribution of the international wealth and to ensure financial security and stability. **A treaty now known as GATT** came into being initially with **23 countries including India**. Currently, it has got **149 countries** as its **members**, which account for **93% of the International Trade**. The very essence of this treaty is that all the member countries give other member countries the most favoured nation status. **In Marrakesh round on 15th April 1994 lead to the formation of WTO**, which came into **being on 1st January 1995** and has **the status of International Monetary Fund and World Bank**. It has its **headquarters at Geneva, Switzerland**.

Under WTO obligations, each member country must provide for a minimum prescribed level of protection to intellectual property rights (IPRs). The idea behind such a commitment is to facilitate cross-border enforcement of such rights. The member countries may provide for higher standards of protection as they deem fit. However, the Agreement on Trade-Related Aspects of Intellectual Property Rights (TRIPs) lays down the minimum standards to be adopted by the member countries for protection of IPRs

The following are the IPRs which are sought to be protected under WTO obligations:

1. Copyrights and related rights
2. Trademarks
3. Geographical indications
4. Industrial designs
5. Patents
6. Layout of designs of integrated circuits
7. Protection of undisclosed information and trade secrets

A transition period of 5 years (which expired on 1.1.2000) was provided to all developing countries to give effect to the provisions of the TRIPs agreement. As per current requirements, member countries which did not provide product patents in certain areas of technology as on 1.1.1995, can delay the grant of product patents in those areas up to 1.1.2005. India falls under this category since Indian Patent laws do not provide for the grant of product patents.

A country which did not make available patent protection for pharmaceutical and agricultural chemical products as on 1.1.1995 has to provide a means for accepting applications for such inventions (mailbox), apply applicable priority rights and provide exclusive marketing rights (EMRs) for such products.

For grant of EMRs in India, all the following conditions must be satisfied:

1. A patent application must have been filed after 1.1.1995 in any WTO member country.
2. Patent and marketing approval must have been granted in that member country.
3. An application has been filed in the mailbox in India.
4. Marketing approval has been obtained in India.

EMRs are available for 5 years from grant or till the patent is granted or rejected, whichever is earlier. In India, the Patent (Amendment) Act, 1999 was passed in March 1999 to provide for mailbox and EMR facility in accordance with the WTO obligations.

Given below is India's position *vis-à-vis* its obligations under the TRIPs agreement.

Copyrights and Related Rights

The TRIPs agreement requires member countries to comply with the substantive provisions of the Berne Convention in respect of copyrights and related rights. Computer programmes are to be protected as literary works. The term of protection for copyrights and right of performers and producers of phonograms is to be no less than 50 years. In case of broadcasting organizations, the term of protection is to be at least 20 years. India is a signatory to the Berne Convention and Indian Copyright laws conform to the all WTO requirements. In fact, Indian Copyrights Laws provide for greater protection to Copyrights than is required under WTO obligations in some matters such as period of copyright protection (60 years in India). The law was amended in December 1999 to grant a 25 years term of protection for neighbouring rights.

Trademarks

WTO obligations required member countries to give equal protection to service marks as to trade marks. Accordingly, the Trade Marks Act, 1999 was passed for providing equal protection to service marks. Indian Trade Mark laws conform to WTO requirements.

Geographical Indications

This issue has been of particular interest to India, especially after a patent was obtained for basmati rice in the United States by Ricetec Inc. Under the TRIPs agreement, each member country must provide for legislation to prevent the use of any means in the designation or presentation of a good that indicates or suggests that the good in question originates in a geographical area other than the true place of origin of the good. India has a great interest in this area since there have been reports that Nigerian and Sri Lankan Tea growers have been passing off their tea as Darjeeling Premium Tea (which commands the highest price in the market). Untill recently, protection from such misuse was granted through passing off action in courts or through certification marks. However, in order to provide better protection to geographical indications, the Geographical Indication of Goods (Registration and Protection) Act, 1999 has been enacted in India.

Industrial Designs

Under WTO obligations, member countries must provide for protection to independently created new or original industrial designs. Member countries, however, have an option to exclude from protection, designs dictated by technical or functional consideration, as against aesthetic consideration, constituting the coverage of industrial designs. Accordingly, Industrial Design Act, 2000 was enacted to make Indian laws compliant with WTO obligations in this respect.

Patents

This is one area where Indian laws do not comply with WTO obligations. Under the TRIPs agreement, member countries must provide for both product as well as process patents. However, currently, Indian patent laws do not provide for product patents. Under WTO obligations, inventions in all fields of technology, whether products or processes shall be patentable if they meet the tests of being novel, involving an inventive step and being capable of industrial application. In addition to the general security exception, which applies to the entire TRIPs Agreement, specific exclusions are permissible from the scope of patentability. These exclusions are in respect of inventions whose commercial exploitation is to be prevented to protect public order or is found to be against morality or against human, animal plant life or health or to avoid serious prejudice to the environment. In addition, exclusions from patentability are available in respect of diagnostic, therapeutic and surgical methods for the treatment of human and animals, plants and animals other than microorganisms, and essentially biological processes for the production of plants and animals other than non-biological and microbiological processes. In respect of plant varieties, there is an obligation to provide for protection either by:

 i. Patents or
 ii. An effective *sui generis* system or
 iii. By any combination of the above 2 methods

The TRIPs agreement does not give the details of an effective sui generis system. It has been left to each member country to define an effective sui generis system and to determine its elements.

The Patents (Second Amendment) Bill, 1999 is before the Joint Committee of the Houses for discussion. Similarly, in respect of the sui generis plant protection system, a draft bill has been prepared and is before the Joint Committee of the Houses of the Parliament for discussion.

Layout of Designs of Integrated Circuits

Basically, WTO obligations in this respect require member countries to comply with the international agreement administered by WIPO (more commonly known as the "Washington Treaty") with some enhancements. WTO obligations require granting protection to IPRs in respect of lay-out designs which are original in the sense of being the result of their creator's own intellectual efforts. Equal national treatment to foreign right holders must be given and a term of protection for 10 years has been prescribed. India is a signatory to the Washington Treaty and by and large complies with the WTO obligations in this matter.

Protection of Undisclosed Information

WTO obligations require member countries to protect trade secrets. The WTO obligations require that suitable legislations are in place which enable persons to prevent information lawfully within their control from being disclosed to, acquired by or used by others without their consent in a manner contrary to honest commercial practices. In India, there is no separate law for this purpose. Such complaints are dealt under the Contracts Act. The common law on the subject is constantly evolving and courts have provided relief where allegations of wrongful disclosure have been proven.

It is clear that India affords suitable protection to IPRs in all matters except product patents. There is a fear that granting product patents will make medicines very expensive in India and therefore there is lack of political consensus on the issue. However, there are other issues involved also. Most multinational drug companies do not introduce their latest drugs in India fearing patent violation. This may deprive the Indian people of the latest medicines available. Besides, lack of adequate product patent protection also hinders research and development in India. India has a pool of skilled knowledge workers. This valuable resource may go down the drain if adequate patent protection is not made available. In any case, since India is a signatory to the TRIPs agreement, sooner than later, India will have to amend its patent laws to make them compliant with WTO obligations.

SOME IMPORTANT ISSUES IN WTO NEGOTIATIONS ON AGRICULTURE

The original General Agreement on Tariffs and Trade (GATT) 1947 applied to trade in agriculture also, but it allowed various exceptions to the rules on non-tariff measures and subsidies, which led to severe distortions in world agricultural trade. For instance, the GATT 1947 allowed countries to use export subsidies on agricultural primary products whereas export subsidies on industrial products were prohibited. The GATT rules also allowed countries to resort to import restrictions (e.g. import quotas) in the agriculture sector under certain conditions, notably when these restrictions were necessary to enforce measures to effectively limit domestic production. The result of all this was a proliferation of impediments to world agricultural trade, including by means of import bans, quotas setting the maximum level of imports, minimum import prices, non-tariff measures maintained by state-trading enterprises, etc.

This insulation of domestic markets was in part due to the fact that in the aftermath of the Second World War many governments were concerned primarily with increasing domestic agricultural production so as to feed their growing populations. Import access barriers, particularly in the developed world, ensured that domestic production could continue to be sold. At the same time, export subsidies were increasingly used by them to dump their surpluses on to the world market, depressing world market prices. This factor and low world food prices reduced the incentive for farmers in developing countries to increase or even maintain their agricultural production levels. To get into the roots of this disarray in world agriculture, it was felt that the disciplines of GATT, which traditionally focussed only on import access problems, should be extended to measures affecting trade in agriculture, including domestic agricultural policies and the subsidisation of agricultural exports.

Six years after the conclusion of the Tokyo Round of Negotiations (conducted between 1973 and 1979), GATT member governments decided to prepare for a new round of multilateral trade negotiations. By the time, the GATT members met in Punta del Este in 1986 to launch the Uruguay Round of Trade Negotiations, consensus had been reached that it was necessary to reform agricultural policies in order to achieve trade liberalisation in agriculture. The idea was to progressively reduce trade distorting subsidies, improve import access and curb export subsidies in agriculture. These negotiating ideas were further developed in subsequent consultations till some broad agreement was hammered out. The Agreement on Agriculture (AoA) as its stands today has formed part of the Final Act of the Uruguay Round of Multilateral Trade Negotiations (1986-1993) and it was signed as part of the Uruguay Round Agreement by the member countries in April 1994 at Marrakesh in Morocco. It came into force on 1 January, 1995.

The Agreement known as the Final Act of the Uruguay Round, representing the outcome of the seven-year long multilateral trade negotiations, was signed by the then Minister of Commerce at the Ministerial level meeting held at Marrakesh on 15 April, 1994. A *suo moto* statement was subsequently made by the Commerce Minister in the Lok Sabha on 19 April, 1994. The statement, inter-alia, stated, "There was endorsement of the results of the Uruguay Round as a whole from all countries, developing and developed".

SANITARY AND PHYTOSANITARY (SPS) MEASURES

The SPS Agreement encourages Governments to establish national SPS measures consistent with international standards, guidelines and recommendations developed by International Organizations. The WTO itself does not have any standards. The standards developed by leading scientists in the field and governmental experts on health protection and are subject to international scrutiny and review.

According to the definition of an SPS measure, the agreement applies to measures taken which are given in Table 25.1.

Table 25.1: SPS measures

To protect	From
Human or animal life	Risks arising from additives, contaminants, toxins or disease-causing organisms in their food, beverages, feed, stuffs;
Human Life	Plant- or animal-carried diseases (zoonoses);
Animal or plant life	Pests, diseases or disease-causing organisms;
A country	Damage caused by the entry establishment or spread of pests.

International standards provide the legal framework as well as the basis for international trade. They define the identity of the products and describe its basic composition, quality and safety required for the international trade. The agreement on TBT attempts to bring about harmonization in technical regulations and standards including packaging, marking and labelling requirements for smooth flow of trade.

The Agreement on the Application of Sanitary and Phytosanitary Measures has a twofold objective. It aims to both:

i. Recognise the sovereign right of members to provide the level of health protection they deem appropriate; and

ii. Ensure that SPS measures do not represent unnecessary, arbitrary, scientifically unjustifiable, or disguised restrictions on international trade.

The important dates leading to the SPS regime are given in Table 25.2.

Table 25.2: Important dates leading to SPS measures

Year		Landmark
1924	:	Establishment of Office International des Epizooties (OIE).
1945	:	Formation of World Bank and International Monetary Fund.
1947	:	Birth of General Agreement on Tariff and Trade (GATT).
1962	:	Establishment of Codex Alimentarius.
1974-79	:	Inclusion of SPS concern for food safety and health on humans, animals plant in TBT and agreement on SPS measures.
1947-85	:	Seven rounds of trade negotiations.
1986	:	Call for SPS measures in agricultural trade.
1988	:	Identification of priority areas related to SPS measures—Harmonization-Transparency and Improvement.
1991	:	Dunkel Draft on IPR.
1993	:	Establishment of Secretariat of International Plant Protection Convention (IPPC)—start of standard setting process related to SPS measures.
1993	:	Eight round of Uruguay negotiations bringing agriculture under GATT regime.

Table 25.2: Important dates leading to SPS measures.*(Contd.)*

Year		Landmark
1994	:	GATT Agreement paving way for WTO.
1995	:	Formation of WTO and Dispute settlement Body (DSB).
2000	:	Preparation of draft guidelines on risk consistency by SPS regime.
2001	:	The Doha Summit of subsidies.

INTERNATIONAL STANDARDS

Article 3 of the SPS Agreement envisages application of the International Standards as the basis for SPS regulations of the member countries. Any divergence of standards and regulation adds to the cost of the international trade. At the same time, divergences arising from legitimate differences in the societal preferences, technical developments environmental and health conditions may be justified. In such conditions, mutual recognition of standards is a desirable option. **Articles 3, 4 and 5 of the SPS** agreement encourages governments to harmonize or base their national measure on the International standards, guidelines and recommendation developed by WTO member governments in International organization. These organizations include food safety, the Joint FAO/WHO Codex Alimentarius Commission (CAC), for animal health, the Office International des Epizooties (OIE) and for the plant health the FAO International Plant Protection Convention (IPPC).

Codex Alimentarius Commission (CAC)

It has the **membership of over 160 countries** and it has developed Codex Alimentarius, which is **a collection of International food standards for all the food product**s. It includes almost **5000 standards** aimed at protecting the health of the consumers. **India is the member of CAC and Ministry of Health is the nodal agency** but it does have any process for developing international standards. There is an urgent need to develop net work of laboratories to certify that the products meet national and international standards. **The key issues are the agricultural and industrial chemicals, pesticides, residues limit, hazard analysis critical control point (HACCP) system and detection of food-borne pathogens, mycotoxins, veterinary drug residues and heavy metals.**

International Des Epizooties (OIE)

It was **established in 1924 with 28 members** countries and **presently has 145 member countries**. The OIE provides current **information on disease occurrence, coordinate studies on disease surveillance and control and harmonizes regulation for trade in animals and animal products**. The OIEs specialist commission **coordinates with 110 OIE reference laboratories and 06 collaborating centres**. In scientific and technical matters concerning diagnostic tests and vaccine, standards commission collaborates with other International organizations such as FAO, WHO, IICA and PAHO to promote harmonization at international level. **It is expected that the WTO members**

would complete the process of harmonization latest by the year 2004. But there are several contentious issues, which have to be sorted out. These include: right of the WTO members to maintain standards which are stricter than the international standards, the decision-making process by a single majority vote vis-a-vis a consensus-based approach, subjectivity in quantitative risk assessment, validity of assumption for risk assessment, etc.

The Standard Setting Process

The procedures for formulating standards vary among various countries, the harmonization as per **3 Article of SPS Agreement** required for a coherent transparent and effective system of International standards.

Article 4.2 encourages member countries to develop **Mutual Recognition Agreements (MRAs)**. The MRAs play an important role in building confidence, reduces costs by avoiding duplicative testing and eliminating delays.

Article 6 of the SPS Agreement deals with the adaptation to regional condition like recognition of pest or disease free areas or areas of low pest or diseases prevalence. To benefit from this clause, the country should identify and maintain areas free of animal diseases.

Article 7 of the SPS measure requires for establishing credibility as the basis for promoting trade, for which transparency is important.

Article 9 of the SPS measure envisages that members shall accept the SPS measure of the other members as equivalent even if these differ from their own or from those used by the other members trading in the same product.

The Present Reform Programme

Up to 1995, GATT rules were largely ineffective in disciplining key aspects of agricultural trade. In particular, export and domestic subsidies came to dominate many areas of world agricultural trade, while the stricter disciplines on import restrictions were often flouted. The 1986-1994 Uruguay Round negotiations went a long way towards changing all that.

Numerical Targets for Cutting Subsidies and Protection

The reductions in agricultural subsidies and protection agreed in the Uruguay Round (Table 25.3).

Table 25.3: Reduction in agricultural subsidies and protection in Uruguay Round

Attribute	Developed countries 6 years: 1995-2000	Developing countries 10 years: 1995-2004
Tariffs		
Average cut for all agricultural products	–36%	–24%
Minimum cut per product	–15%	–10%

Table 25.3: Reduction in agricultural subsidies and protection in Uruguay Round *(Contd.)*

Attribute	Developed countries 6 years: 1995-2000	Developing countries 10 years: 1995-2004
Domestic support		
Cuts in total ("AMS") support for the sector	–20%	–13%
Exports		
Value of subsidies (outlays)	–36%	–24%
Subsidized quantities	–21%	–14%

Notes: Least-developed countries do not have to reduce tariffs or subsidies. The base level for tariff cuts was the bound rate before 1 January 1995; or, for unbound tariffs, the actual rate charged in September 1986 when the Uruguay Round began.

Only the figures for cutting export subsidies appear in the agreement. The other figures were targets used to calculate countries' legally binding "schedules" of commitments. Each country's specific commitments vary according to the outcome of negotiations. As a result of those negotiations, several developing countries chose to set fixed bound tariff ceilings that do not decline over the years.

Agriculture trade is now firmly within the multilateral trading system. The WTO Agriculture Agreement, together with individual countries' commitments to reduce export subsidies, domestic support and import duties on agricultural products were a significant first step towards reforming agricultural trade. The reform strikes a balance between agricultural trade liberalization and governments' desire to pursue legitimate agricultural policy goals, including non-trade concerns. It has brought all agricultural products (as listed in the agreement) under more effective multilateral rules and commitments, including "tariff bindings" — WTO members have bound themselves to maximum tariffs on nearly all agricultural products, while many industrial tariffs remain unbound. For the first time, member governments are committed to reducing agricultural export subsidies and trade-distorting domestic support. They have agreed to prohibit subsidies that exceed negotiated limits for specific products. The commitments to reduce domestic support are a major innovation and are unique to the agricultural sector.

THE CURRENT NEGOTIATIONS

The Uruguay Round agreement set up a framework of rules and started reductions in protection and trade-distorting support. But this was only the first phase of the reform. Article 20 of the Agriculture Agreement committed members to start negotiations on continuing the reform at the end of 1999 (or beginning of 2000). Those negotiations are now well underway. They began using Article 20 as their basis. The November 2001 Doha Ministerial Declaration sets a new mandate by making the objectives more explicit, building on the work carried out so far, and setting deadlines.

The negotiations are difficult because of the wide range of views and interests among member governments. They aim to contribute to further liberalization of agricultural trade. This will benefit those countries which can compete on quality and price rather than on the size of their subsidies. That is particularly the case for many developing countries whose economies depend on an increasingly diverse range of primary and processed agricultural products, exported to an increasing variety of markets, including to other developing countries. The following issues are among those that have been raised in the negotiations:

The Objective: Continuing Reductions and Other Issues

Further substantial reductions in tariffs, domestic support and export subsidies are prominent issues in the negotiations. In addition, some countries say an important objective of the new negotiations should be to bring agricultural trade under the same rules and disciplines as trade in other goods. Some others, reject the idea for a number of reasons.

Sometimes, it is translated into conceptual differences, reflecting the importance that members attach to the major issues in the negotiations. Some countries have described the mandate given by Article 20 as a "tripod" whose three legs are export subsidies, domestic support, and market access (these are more commonly called "the three pillars" of agricultural trade reform). Non-trade concerns and special and differential treatment for developing countries would be taken into account as appropriate. Others say it is a "pentangle" whose five sides also include non-trade concerns and special and differential treatment for developing countries as separate issues in their own right. So far, these differences of approach have not delayed the discussions.

The negotiations are now in their 5th year, but under a reformulated mandate—the **Doha Declaration that ministers issued in Doha, Qatar, in November 2001**. Negotiators missed the 31 March 2003 deadline for producing numerical targets, formulas and other "modalities" for countries' commitments. A revised draft "modalities" paper was put on the negotiating table in March 2003 and although it was not agreed, it was used to discuss technical details in subsequent months. A number of "framework" proposals dealing with main points of the modalities were submitted and discussed before and during the **Fifth Ministerial Conference in Cancún, Mexico, September 2003**, but it was not until 1 August 2004 that a "framework" was agreed. The next stage is to agree on full "modalities", which will in turn be used to work out the final agreement on revised rules, and individual countries' commitments. Some members have suggested the negotiations might unofficially aim to complete the "modalities" by the **Hong Kong Ministerial Conference in December 2005**, but without making a formal commitment. The Doha Declaration had envisaged that countries would submit comprehensive draft commitments, based on the "modalities", by the Cancún Ministerial Conference — but without modalities, this target was not met either. Meanwhile, the final deadline for completing the negotiations, 1 January 2005, was officially postponed on 1 August 2004, without a new date set.

Phases 1 and 2: 2000-2002

The negotiations began under Article 20 of the Agriculture Agreement. This says WTO members had to negotiate to continue the reform of agricultural trade.

Article 20 of the Agriculture Agreement: Recognizing that the long-term objective of substantial progressive reductions in support and protection resulting in fundamental reform is an ongoing process, Members agree that negotiations for continuing the process will be initiated one year before the end of the implementation period, taking into account:

a. The experience to that date from implementing the reduction commitments;

b. The effects of the reduction commitments on world trade in agriculture;

c. Non-trade concerns, special and differential treatment to developing-country members, and the objective to establish a fair and market-oriented agricultural trading system, and the other objectives and concerns mentioned in the preamble to this agreement;

d. What further commitments are necessary to achieve the above mentioned long-term objectives.

Phase 1: 2000-01

The first phase began in early 2000 and ended with a stock-taking meeting on 26-27 March 2001. Altogether, 126 member governments (89% of the 142 members) submitted 45 proposals and three technical documents. Six negotiating meetings (officially called "Special Sessions" of the Agriculture Committee) were held: in March, June, September and November 2000, and February, March 2001. This first phase consisted of countries submitting proposals containing their starting positions for the negotiations. The meetings discussed each of these proposal in turn. The proposals received in the first phase covered all major areas of the agriculture negotiations and a few new ones.

Phase 2: 2001-02

The work programme was decided at the March 2001 stock-taking meeting. It set a time table of six informal meetings in May, July, September and December 2001, and February 2002. In this phase, the discussions were by topic, and included more technical details. This was needed in order to find a way to allow members to develop specific proposals and ultimately reach a consensus agreement on changes to rules and commitments in agriculture. Papers presented were not official WTO documents, but usually off-the-record "non-papers". Despite the increased complexity, developing countries continued to participate actively.

THE DOHA DECLARATION

In November 2001, the 4th WTO Ministerial Conference was held in Doha, Qatar. The declaration issued on 14 November launched new negotiations on a range of subjects, and included the negotiations already underway in agriculture (and services).

The declaration builds on the work already undertaken in the agriculture negotiations, confirms and elaborates the objectives, and sets a time table. Agriculture is now part of the single undertaking in which all the linked negotiations are to end by 1 January 2005 (except some "early harvest" subjects which have earlier deadlines).

The declaration reconfirms the long-term objective already agreed in Article 20: to establish a fair and market-oriented trading system through a programme of fundamental reform. The programme encompasses strengthened rules, and specific commitments on government support and protection for agriculture. The purpose is to correct and prevent restrictions and distortions in world agricultural markets.

The Doha Mandate

We recognize the work already undertaken in the negotiations initiated in early 2000 under Article 20 of the Agreement on Agriculture, including the large number of negotiating proposals submitted on behalf of a total of 121 members. We recall the long-term objective referred to in the Agreement to establish a fair and market-oriented trading system through a programme of fundamental reform encompassing strengthened rules and specific commitments on support and protection in order to correct and prevent restrictions and distortions in world agricultural markets. We reconfirm our commitment to this programme. Building on the work carried out to date and without prejudging the outcome of the negotiations we commit ourselves to comprehensive negotiations aimed at: substantial improvements in market access; reductions of, with a view to phasing out, all forms of export subsidies; and substantial reductions in trade-distorting domestic support. We agree that special and differential treatment for developing countries shall be an integral part of all elements of the negotiations and shall be embodied in the schedules of concessions and commitments and as appropriate in the rules and disciplines to be negotiated, so as to be operationally effective and to enable developing countries to effectively take account of their development needs, including food security and rural development. We take note of the non-trade concerns reflected in the negotiating proposals submitted by Members and confirm that non-trade concerns will be taken into account in the negotiations as provided for in the Agreement on Agriculture. Modalities for the further commitments, including provisions for special and differential treatment, shall be established no later than 31 March 2003. Participants shall submit their comprehensive draft Schedules based on these modalities no later than the date of the Fifth Session of the Ministerial Conference. The negotiations, including with respect to rules and disciplines and related legal texts, shall be concluded as part and at the date of conclusion of the negotiating agenda as a whole.

Without prejudging the outcome, member governments commit themselves to comprehensive negotiations aimed at:

- Market access: substantial reductions
- Export subsidies: reductions of, with a view to phasing out, all forms of these
- Domestic support: substantial reductions for supports that distort trade

The declaration makes special and differential treatment for developing countries integral throughout the negotiations, both in countries' new commitments and in any relevant new or revised rules and disciplines. It says the outcome should be effective in practice and should enable developing countries to meet their needs, in particular in food security and rural development. The ministers also take note of the non-trade concerns (such as environmental protection, food security, rural development, etc.) reflected in the negotiating proposals already submitted. They confirm that the negotiations will take these into account, as provided for in the Agriculture Agreement.

Modalities

Originally, a 12-month programme, this phase deals with one of the most critical stages of the agriculture negotiations. It aims to set "modalities" or targets (including numerical targets) for achieving the objectives set out in the Doha Ministerial Declaration: "substantial improvements in market access; reductions of, with a view to phasing out, all forms of export subsidies; and substantial reductions in trade-distorting domestic support". It will also include some rule making. This stage will therefore determine the shape of the negotiations' final outcome.

The "modalities" will be used for members to produce their first offers or "comprehensive draft commitments". The Doha Ministerial Declaration said this had to be done by the Fifth Ministerial Conference in Cancún, Mexico, 10-14 September 2003, a few months after the 31 March 2003 deadline for modalities. As it turned out, members failed to meet the March 2003 deadline for agreeing "modalities" and then turned their attention to an outline or "framework" of the modalities, which was eventually agreed on 1 August 2004. The periods involved can therefore be described as: "preparations for modalities" (March 2002-July 2003), "Cancún and the framework phase" (August 2003-August 2004), and "the modalities phase" (September 2004).

The preparations for "modalities" began with technical work on detailed possibilities for each of the three main areas (or "pillars") of the Agriculture Agreement, viz:

- Export subsidies/competition;
- Market access; and
- Domestic support.

Special treatment for developing countries is treated as an integral part of all of these, and non-trade concerns are taken into account.

The first set of meetings covered the **export** side: subsidies, competition, taxes, and restrictions.

The 31 March deadline came and went, but positions remained wide apart and there was no consensus on the draft or on how to modify it. Some countries, notably some of those seeking more moderate reforms, said they could not accept it as basis for negotiation unless it were altered.

After the missed 31 March 2003 deadline, negotiators busied themselves sorting out a number of important and complex technical issues that are a necessary part of the package. Among them are: the domestic support categories (various "boxes"), tariffs, tariff quotas (including their administration), export credits, food aid, various provisions for developing countries, provisions for countries that recently joined the WTO, trade preferences, how to measure domestic consumption (a proposed reference for several provisions), and so on.

CANCÚN DEADLOCK: SEPTEMBER 2003

The preparations in Geneva for the 11-14 September 2003 Cancún Ministerial Conference brought agriculture and the other Doha Agenda issues together, in meetings and consultations of the General Council and other bodies.

The US and EU chose to work on a "framework" of key issues, rather than the entire "modalities". This had the advantage of focusing on a smaller number of major points, which would be more manageable for ministers in the few days of the Cancún conference. Even as a "framework", it contained a number of gaps. For much of the paper, the US and EU deliberately avoided including numbers, such as percentages or coefficients for tariff reductions. They also left open the question of special treatment for developing countries, saying they ran out of time and in any case it would be more appropriate for the developing countries to make their own proposals.

Consultations in Geneva and around the world after Cancún confirmed members' desire to build on the work done before and during the ministerial conference. As 2004 began, the favoured approach seemed to be to tackle the "frameworks" first, and then to complete the "modalities".

THE NEGOTIATIONS IN GENEVA: MARCH 2004

Meanwhile, in Geneva the first "agriculture week" after Cancún was 22-26 March 2004, and it marked a new approach. Of the three "pillars" (export subsidies and competition, domestic support and market access), many identified market access as technically the most difficult.

Many commented on the "blended" formula. Under this approach, tariffs would be divided into three groups. One group would be made duty-free, the tariffs in another group would be reduced by a simple average with a minimum reduction per product (the Uruguay Round approach), and in the third they would be reduced by the "Swiss formula" (a harmonizing formula that reduces higher tariffs by greater amounts and simultaneously sets a maximum final tariff rate.

The Cairns Group said it was unconvinced by the blended formula. What was important is to ensure substantial improvements in market access for products, and not numbers that are an illusion of improved market access, the group said.

The G-10 argued that the blended formula did not provide enough flexibility. This group also stressed that it opposed setting ceilings for tariff rates and having to expand all tariff quotas. The EU said the blended approach provided enough flexibility to cover all issues, including non-trade concerns and special treatment for developing countries, and with appropriate numbers to offer a high level of ambition as well. The US also said the picture would be clearer when the numbers were inserted, but after the framework stage was over.

Some groups' priority concerns were accepted in principle by others. For example, most speakers agreed that developing countries should be allowed to give special treatment to a category of special products. Differences remained about the conditions that would apply. The EU accepted a call from China and other new members that they were already undergoing reforms and had low tariff rates and therefore should not have to face the same scale of reductions as older members.

India said it accepted that all members will have to contribute to reform, but others will have to accept that some countries are unable to contribute as much because of developmental constraints.

FRAMEWORK FOR ESTABLISHING MODALITIES IN AGRICULTURE

1. The starting point for the current phase of the agriculture negotiations has been the mandate set out in Paragraph 13 of the Doha Ministerial Declaration. This in turn built on the long-term objective of the Agreement on Agriculture to establish a fair and market-oriented trading system through a programme of fundamental reform. The elements below offer the additional precision required at this stage of the negotiations and thus the basis for the negotiations of full modalities in the next phase. The level of ambition set by the Doha mandate will continue to be the basis for the negotiations on agriculture.

2. The final balance will be found only at the conclusion of these subsequent negotiations and within the Single Undertaking. To achieve this balance, the modalities to be developed will need to incorporate operationally effective and meaningful provisions for special and differential treatment for developing country members. Agriculture is of critical importance to the economic development of developing country members and they must be able to pursue agricultural policies that are supportive of their development goals, poverty reduction strategies, food security and livelihood concerns. Non-trade concerns, as referred to in Paragraph 13 of the Doha Declaration, will be taken into account.

3. The reforms in all three pillars form an interconnected hole and must be approached in a balanced and equitable manner.

4. The General Council recognizes the importance of cotton for a certain number of countries and its vital importance for developing countries, especially LDCs. It will be addressed ambitiously, expeditiously, and specifically, within the agriculture negotiations. The provisions of this framework provide a basis for this approach, as does the sectoral initiative on cotton. The Special Session of the Committee on Agriculture shall ensure appropriate prioritization of the cotton issue independently from other sectoral initiatives. A subcommittee on cotton will meet periodically and report to the Special Session of the Committee on Agriculture to review progress. Work shall encompass all trade-distorting policies affecting the sector in all three pillars of market access, domestic support, and export competition, as specified in the Doha text and this Framework text.

5. Coherence between trade and development aspects of the cotton issue will be pursued as set out in paragraph 1.b of the text to which this Framework is annexed.

Domestic Support

6. The Doha Ministerial Declaration calls for "substantial reductions in trade-distorting domestic support". With a view to achieving these substantial reductions, the negotiations in this pillar will ensure the following:

   - Special and differential treatment remains an integral component of domestic support. Modalities to be developed will include longer implementation periods and lower reduction coefficients for all types of trade-distorting domestic support and continued access to the provisions under Article 6.2.
   - There will be a strong element of harmonisation in the reductions made by developed Members. Specifically, higher levels of permitted trade-distorting domestic support will be subject to deeper cuts.
   - Each such Member will make a substantial reduction in the overall level of its trade-distorting support from bound levels.
   - As well as this overall commitment, Final Bound Total AMS and permitted *de minimis* levels will be subject to substantial reductions and, in the case of the Blue Box, will be capped as specified in Paragraph 15 in order to ensure results that are coherent with the long-term reform objective. Any clarification or development of rules and conditions to govern trade distorting support will take this into account.

Overall Reduction: A Tiered Formula

7. The overall base level of all trade-distorting domestic support, as measured by the Final Bound Total AMS plus permitted *de minimis* level and the level agreed in Paragraph 8 below for Blue Box payments, will be reduced according to a tiered formula. Under this formula, members having higher levels of trade-distorting domestic support will make greater overall reductions in order to achieve a harmonizing result. As the first instalment of the overall cut, in the first year and throughout the implementation period, the sum of all trade-distorting support will not exceed 80% of the sum of Final Bound Total AMS plus permitted *de minimis* plus the Blue Box at the level determined in Paragraph 15.

8. The following parameters will guide the further negotiation of this tiered formula:

   - This commitment will apply as a minimum overall commitment. It will not be applied as a ceiling on reductions of overall trade-distorting domestic support, should the separate and complementary formulae to be developed for Total AMS, *de minimis* and Blue Box payments imply, when taken together, a deeper cut in overall trade-distorting domestic support for an individual member.
   - The base for measuring the Blue Box component will be the higher of existing Blue Box payments during a recent representative period to be agreed and the cap established.

Final Bound Total AMS: A Tiered Formula

9. To achieve reductions with a harmonizing effect:
   - Final Bound Total AMS will be reduced substantially, using a tiered approach.
   - Members having higher Total AMS will make greater reductions.
   - To prevent circumvention of the objective of the Agreement through transfers of unchanged domestic support between different support categories, product-specific AMSs will be capped at their respective average levels according to a methodology to be agreed.
   - Substantial reductions in Final Bound Total AMS will result in reductions of some product-specific support.

10. Members may make greater than formula reductions in order to achieve the required level of cut in overall trade-distorting domestic support.

De Minimis

11. Reductions in *de minimis* will be negotiated taking into account the principle of special and differential treatment. Developing countries that allocate almost all *de minimis* support for subsistence and resource-poor farmers will be exempt.

12. Members may make greater than formula reductions in order to achieve the required level of cut in overall trade-distorting domestic support.

Blue Box

13. Members recognize the role of the Blue Box in promoting agricultural reforms. In this light, Article 6.5 will be reviewed so that members may have recourse to the following measures:
    - Direct payments under production-limiting programmes if:
      - Such payments are based on fixed and unchanging areas and yields; or
      - Such payments are made on 85% or less of a fixed and unchanging base level of production; or
      - Livestock payments are made on a fixed and unchanging number of head; or
    - Direct payments that do not require production if:
      - Such payments are based on fixed and unchanging bases and yields; or
      - Livestock payments made on a fixed and unchanging number of head; and
      - Such payments are made on 85% or less of a fixed and unchanging base level of production.

14. The above criteria, along with additional criteria will be negotiated. Any such criteria will ensure that Blue Box payments are less trade-distorting than AMS measures, it being understood that:

- Any new criteria would need to take account of the balance of WTO rights and obligations.
- Any new criteria to be agreed will not have the perverse effect of undoing ongoing reforms.

15. Blue Box support will not exceed 5% of a member's average total value of agricultural production during an historical period. The historical period will be established in the negotiations. This ceiling will apply to any actual or potential Blue Box user from the beginning of the implementation period. In cases where a member has placed an exceptionally large percentage of its trade-distorting support in the Blue Box, some flexibility will be provided on a basis to be agreed to ensure that such a member is not called upon to make a wholly disproportionate cut.

Green Box

16. Green Box criteria will be reviewed and clarified with a view to ensuring that Green Box measures have no, or at most minimal, trade-distorting effects or effects on production. Such a review and clarification will need to ensure that the basic concepts, principles and effectiveness of the Green Box remain and take due account of non-trade concerns. The improved obligations for monitoring and surveillance of all new disciplines foreshadowed in Paragraph 48 below will be particularly important with respect to the Green Box.

Export Competition

17. The Doha Ministerial Declaration calls for "reduction of, with a view to phasing out, all forms of export subsidies". As an outcome of the negotiations, members agree to establish detailed modalities ensuring the parallel elimination of all forms of export subsidies and disciplines on all export measures with equivalent effect by a credible end date.

End Point

18. The following will be eliminated by the end date to be agreed:
- Export subsidies as scheduled.
- Export credits, export credit guarantees or insurance programmes with repayment periods beyond 180 days.
- Terms and conditions relating to export credits, export credit guarantees or insurance programmes with repayment periods of 180 days and below which are not in accordance with disciplines to be agreed. These disciplines will cover, inter-alia, payment of interest, minimum interest rates, minimum premium requirements, and other elements which can constitute subsidies or otherwise distort trade.
- Trade distorting practices with respect to exporting STEs including eliminating export subsidies provided to or by them, government financing, and the underwriting of losses. The issue of the future use of monopoly powers will be subject to further negotiation.

- Provision of food aid that is not in conformity with operationally effective disciplines to be agreed. The objective of such disciplines will be to prevent commercial displacement. The role of international organizations as regards the provision of food aid by members, including related humanitarian and developmental issues, will be addressed in the negotiations. The question of providing food aid exclusively in fully grant form will also be addressed in the negotiations.

19. Effective transparency provisions for Paragraph 18 will be established. Such provisions, in accordance with standard WTO practice, will be consistent with commercial confidentiality considerations.

Implementation

20. Commitments and disciplines in Paragraph 18 will be implemented according to a schedule and modalities to be agreed. Commitments will be implemented by annual instalments. Their phasing will take into account the need for some coherence with internal reform steps of members.

21. The negotiation of the elements in Paragraph 18 and their implementation will ensure equivalent and parallel commitments by members.

Special and Differential Treatment

22. Developing country members will benefit from longer implementation periods for the phasing out of all forms of export subsidies.

23. Developing countries will continue to benefit from special and differential treatment under the provisions of Article 9.4 of the Agreement on Agriculture for a reasonable period, to be negotiated, after the phasing out of all forms of export subsidies and implementation of all disciplines identified above are completed.

24. Members will ensure that the disciplines on export credits, export credit guarantees or insurance programmes to be agreed will make appropriate provision for differential treatment in favour of least-developed and net food-importing developing countries as provided for in Paragraph 4 of the Decision on Measures Concerning the Possible Negative Effects of the Reform Programme on Least-Developed and Net Food-Importing Developing Countries. Improved obligations for monitoring and surveillance of all new disciplines as foreshadowed in Paragraph 48 will be critically important in this regard. Provisions to be agreed in this respect must not undermine the commitments undertaken by members under the obligations in Paragraph 18.

25. STEs in developing country members which enjoy special privileges to preserve domestic consumer price stability and to ensure food security will receive special consideration for maintaining monopoly status.

Special Circumstances

26. In exceptional circumstances, which cannot be adequately covered by food aid, commercial export credits or preferential international financing

facilities, ad hoc temporary financing arrangements relating to exports to developing countries may be agreed by members. Such agreements must not have the effect of undermining commitments undertaken by members in Paragraph 18 above, and will be based on criteria and consultation procedures to be established.

Market Access

27. The Doha Ministerial Declaration calls for "substantial improvements in market access". Members also agreed that special and differential treatment for developing members would be an integral part of all elements in the negotiations.

The Single Approach: A Tiered Formula

28. To ensure that a single approach for developed and developing country members meets all the objectives of the Doha mandate, tariff reductions will be made through a tiered formula that takes into account their different tariff structures.

29. To ensure that such a formula will lead to substantial trade expansion, the following principles will guide its further negotiation:

   - Tariff reductions will be made from bound rates. Substantial overall tariff reductions will be achieved as a final result from negotiations.
   - Each member (other than LDCs) will make a contribution. Operationally, effective special and differential provisions for developing country members will be an integral part of all elements.
   - Progressivity in tariff reductions will be achieved through deeper cuts in higher tariffs with flexibilities for sensitive products. Substantial improvements in market access will be achieved for all products.

30. The number of bands, the thresholds for defining the bands and the type of tariff reduction in each band remain under negotiation. The role of a tariff cap in a tiered formula with distinct treatment for sensitive products will be further evaluated.

Sensitive Products

Selection

31. Without undermining the overall objective of the tiered approach, members may designate an appropriate number, to be negotiated, of tariff lines to be treated as sensitive, taking account of existing commitments for these products.

Treatment

32. The principle of 'substantial improvement' will apply to each product.

33. 'Substantial improvement' will be achieved through combinations of tariff quota commitments and tariff reductions applying to each product. However, balance in this negotiation will be found only if the final negotiated result also reflects the sensitivity of the product concerned.

34. Some MFN-based tariff quota expansion will be required for all such products. A base for such an expansion will be established, taking account of coherent and equitable criteria to be developed in the negotiations. In order not to undermine the objective of the tiered approach, for all such products, MFN-based tariff quota expansion will be provided under specific rules to be negotiated taking into account deviations from the tariff formula.

Other Elements

35. Other elements that will give the flexibility required to reach a final balanced result include reduction or elimination of in-quota tariff rates, and operationally effective improvements in tariff quota administration for existing tariff quotas so as to enable members, and particularly developing country members, to fully benefit from the market access opportunities under tariff rate quotas.
36. Tariff escalation will be addressed through a formula to be agreed.
37. The issue of tariff simplification remains under negotiation.
38. The question of the special agricultural safeguard (SSG) remains under negotiation.

Special and Differential Treatment

39. Having regard to their rural development, food security and/or livelihood security needs, special and differential treatment for developing countries will be an integral part of all elements of the negotiation, including the tariff reduction formula, the number and treatment of sensitive products, expansion of tariff rate quotas, and implementation period.
40. Proportionality will be achieved by requiring lesser tariff reduction commitments or tariff quota expansion commitments from developing country members.
41. Developing country members will have the flexibility to designate an appropriate number of products as special products, based on criteria of food security, livelihood security and rural development needs. These products will be eligible for more flexible treatment. The criteria and treatment of these products will be further specified during the negotiation phase and will recognize the fundamental importance of special products to developing countries.
42. A special safeguard mechanism (SSM) will be established for use by developing country members.
43. Full implementation of the long-standing commitment to achieve the fullest liberalisation of trade in tropical agricultural products and for products of particular importance to the diversification of production from the growing of illicit narcotic crops is overdue and will be addressed effectively in the market access negotiations.
44. The importance of long-standing preferences is fully recognised. The issue of preference erosion will be addressed. For the further consideration in this regard, Paragraph 16 and other relevant provisions of TN/AG/W/1/ Rev.1 will be used as a reference.

Least Developed Countries

45. Least developed countries, which will have full access to all special and differential treatment provisions above, are not required to undertake reduction commitments. Developed members, and developing country members in a position to do so, should provide duty-free and quota-free market access for products originating from least developed countries.

46. Work on cotton under all the pillars will reflect the vital importance of this sector to certain LDC members and we will work to achieve ambitious results expeditiously.

Recently Acceded Members

47. The particular concerns of recently acceded members will be effectively addressed through specific flexibility provisions.

Monitoring and Surveillance

48. Article 18 of the Agreement on Agriculture will be amended with a view to enhancing monitoring so as to effectively ensure full transparency, including through timely and complete notifications with respect to the commitments in market access, domestic support and export competition. The particular concerns of developing countries in this regard will be addressed.

This technical phase started with discussions of: converting specific duties to ad valorem equivalents; exporting state trading enterprises; subsidized food aid; disciplines for subsidized export credit, guarantees and insurance, for 180 days or less; review and clarification of Green Box domestic supports; tariff quota administration; the base for tariff quota expansion; tropical products and goods produced as substitutes for narcotics; the method for setting caps on Amber Box supports for specific products; and the base period for commitments on domestic support.

EXPORT SUBSIDIES AND COMPETITION

As the negotiations develop, the discussion on export subsidies and competition shifts from broader over-arching principles to details under specific headings.

Export Subsidies: Phase 2

In phase 1, the discussion on export subsidies and competition spans several sub-headings. After that, as the talks go into greater detail, these are separated. On export subsidies, one proposal in Phase 2 involves a 50% reduction as an immediate downpayment, followed by eliminating subsidies completely in 3 years (for developed countries) or 6 years (for developing countries).

Another proposal is similar but with more emphasis on flexibilities for developing countries. It includes expanding the types of export subsidies that developing countries are currently allowed under Article 9.4 of the Agriculture Agreement. This group's proposed formula would continue reductions at the same pace as under the present agreement while negotiations continue, followed by complete elimination within 3 years of the negotiations' end or 2006, whichever is earlier—with a longer deadline for developing countries.

These proposals receive some support, and some opposition, particularly over the complete elimination of export subsidies.

An alternative proposal includes "rebalancing" or "modulation"—more moderate reductions on some products in return for steeper reductions on other products, with the possibility of raised ceilings—without eliminating export subsidies. Again, this idea has received both support and opposition, some countries predicting that with rebalancing, the products they most need to export will face competition from the highest subsidies.

Some countries emphasize matching measures on imports with those on exports. Subsidy reductions would be gradual and not lead to elimination. To match the concept of bound tariffs, export subsidies would be bound per unit (e.g. per ton).

Many countries say other forms of export subsidies (such as food aid, subsidized export credit and insurance, trading by state enterprises) should be disciplined, and say they will elaborate on this later. Even among the countries that agree on the need to tackle these, there is a difference of opinion as to whether these other forms are as serious as direct export subsidies.

Some smaller developing countries argue that export subsidies should be eliminated but over a longer period of time to help them adjust to higher food import bills. They call for stronger measures to help net food-importing developing countries and least developed countries adjust.

Food Aid: Phase 2

All agree that food aid for humanitarian purposes is essential. Most of the discussion has been about how best to ensure that the aid goes to those really in need, does not harm domestic production in countries receiving aid, does not distort trade (in particular jeopardize exports from competing suppliers), responds genuinely to demand, does not amount to the disposal of surpluses in subsidizing countries, and does not allow countries to get around their export subsidy commitments.

Most countries argue that aid should only be in the form of grants, i.e. not on credit. But some warn that this could be too rigid and prevent food aid from promptly reaching those who need it.

Many developing countries are calling for binding commitments from donor countries on the amounts they supply, with rising amounts of food at times of high prices, aid supplies in response to demand, technical and financial assistance to help countries develop domestic production instead of relying on food aid, and increased transparency through notifications to the WTO Agriculture Committee. Some developed countries also endorse some of these ideas.

Food Aid: Preparations for 'Modalities'

Most countries say aid is not a problem if it is given in response to an appeal from a relevant international organization (such as the World Food Program, Food and Agriculture Organization, etc. or if the organization declares an emergency).

But what if the aid is given bilaterally or through other institutions? Some countries would suspect that this is an attempt to offload surpluses, although some delegations point out that individual governments can respond to an emergency faster than international organizations. There are also differences about whether aid should only be in grant form, or whether price discounts and credit should be disciplined under export subsidy disciplines.

The Revised First Draft 'Modalities' on Food Aid

The draft deals with this in Attachment 6, which is a proposed replacement for Article 10.4 of the Agriculture Agreement. The technical details include proposed criteria for determining whether there is a genuine need for food aid (such as appeals from recognized international organizations) and whether the food is being given on specific terms—for example only aid given in grant form would qualify. Other aid would have to be included in export subsidy reduction commitments or be banned. (Food aid has been a subject discussed in technical consultations since the draft was issued, with some progress on the details.)

End Point and Implementation

The negotiated date will mark the end of export subsidies as listed in members' reduction commitments ("scheduled"); all export credits, export credit guarantees or insurance programmes with repayment periods beyond 180 days; those with shorter repayment periods but failing to conform with disciplines that are to be negotiated; trade-distorting practices of state trading enterprises that are considered to be subsidized ("the issue of the future use of monopoly powers will be subject to further negotiation"); and food aid that does not conform with various disciplines, which will also be negotiated.

The reductions will be by annual instalments, and with parallel treatment for the different forms of export subsidy, although the details still have to be negotiated. Some leeway in the reduction steps is allowed for "coherence" with members' "internal reform steps".

The small print balances the need for transparency, providing information with respect to commercial confidentiality.

Special and Differential Treatment

Again, developing countries are allowed more lenient terms. Elimination can take longer time. They can continue to subsidize transportation and marketing (Article 9.4 of the Agriculture Agreement) "for a reasonable period, to be negotiated", beyond the date for ending the main subsidies. At the same time, when members get rid of subsidized components of credit and insurance, they have to be able to avoid harming the interests of least-developed and net food-importing developing countries. And special consideration is given to poorer countries' state trading enterprises whose monopoly privileges aim to keep domestic prices stable for consumers and to ensure food security.

Special Circumstances

"Ad hoc temporary financing arrangements" that would normally be disciplined should be possible in exceptional circumstances and under strict conditions for exports to developing countries, so long as these arrangements do not undermine the commitments that members will make. Details are to be negotiated.

Market Access: Tariffs and Tariff Quotas

Nowadays, among WTO members, agricultural products are protected only by tariffs. All non-tariff barriers had to be eliminated or converted to tariffs as a result of the Uruguay Round (the conversion was known as "tariffication"). In some cases, the calculated equivalent tariffs—like the original measures that were tariffied—were too high to allow any real opportunity for imports. So a system of tariff-rate quotas was created to maintain existing import access levels, and to provide minimum access opportunities. This means lower tariffs within the quotas, and higher rates for quantities outside the quotas.

The discussion since the Uruguay Round has focused broadly on two issues: the high levels of tariffs outside the quotas (with some countries pressing for larger cuts on the higher tariffs), and the quotas themselves—their size, the way they have been administered, and the tariffs charged on imports within the quotas.

By the time of the 2002-2003 preparations for "modalities", the discussions cover six headings: tariffs; tariff quotas; tariff quota administration; special safeguards; importing state trading enterprises, and other issues. Within each heading, are a list of subheadings such as: general comments; scope/definitions/ product coverage; stages/time tables; transparency and notification; and so on. Special and differential treatment for developing countries and non-trade concerns are discussed under all of them, and again members differ as to whether the Doha declaration treats these as equals or whether non-trade concerns have a lesser priority.

During the discussion, new members and transition economies repeatedly argue for special and differential treatment for countries in their position, because of the state of their economies and because the new members are still implementing market-access commitments under their membership agreements.

Again, some important players have not proposed specific numbers, and this has led to criticism from others.

Market Access: Special Agricultural Safeguards (SSGs)

Safeguards are contingency restrictions on imports taken temporarily to deal with special circumstances such as a sudden surge in imports. They normally come under the Safeguards Agreement, but the Agriculture Agreement has special provisions (Article 5) on safeguards.

The special safeguards provisions for agriculture differ from normal safeguards. In agriculture, unlike with normal safeguards:

- Higher safeguards duties can be triggered automatically when import volumes rise above a certain level, or if prices fall below a certain level.
- It is not necessary to demonstrate that serious injury is being caused to the domestic industry.

The special agricultural safeguard can only be used on products that were tariffied—which amount to less than 20% of all agricultural products (as defined by "tariff lines"). But they cannot be used on imports within the tariff quotas, and they can only be used if the government reserved the right to do so in its schedule of commitments on agriculture. In practice, the special agricultural safeguard has been used in relatively few cases.

Food Safety: Phase 2

One proposal: This needs to be tackled as part of liberalization talks in order to avoid critics who accuse the WTO of requiring governments to force their consumers to accept unsafe food. The proposal is for a written "Understanding" agreed among WTO members. It would do no more than endorse dispute panel and Appellate Body interpretations of sanitary and phytosanitary (SPS) provisions on precaution. (Some other members question whether this is appropriate as part of the agriculture negotiations rather than under SPS).

Another proposal: Developments in food safety issues since the end of the Uruguay Round negotiations mean the current talks need to deal with food safety. Examples include: new consumer concerns about genetically modified organisms; recent disease outbreaks such as BSE; and toxic substances such as dioxin. These are being examined in other organizations such as the OECD and Codex, and the WTO should coordinate with these other efforts, according to this view.

The discussion: This is the first time this topic has been discussed in the negotiations. All agree that consumers must be protected. All also agree on the need to avoid protectionism in disguise. The discussion is about whether the SPS Agreement (specially Article 5.7, which deals with risk and precaution) is clear enough to maintain that balance appropriately. Some countries support clarifying it through an understanding that would also send the right signals to consumers. Others say this should be discussed in the SPS and Technical Barriers to Trade committees, and not in the agriculture negotiations.

Food Safety

Advocates of including this in the negotiations say members should not rely on dispute rulings, but use the negotiations to clarify essential elements, taking Appellate Body and dispute panel reports into account. In particular: measures should be proportionate to the food safety target; they should not discriminate; they should be applied consistently; costs and benefits of alternative measures should be compared; scientific data should be re-evaluated as new information emerges; measures should be based on science. Others counter that this is a sanitary and phytosanitary measures (SPS) issue and not one for the agriculture negotiations. Some complain that in general, SPS measures are already replacing tariffs as unwelcome trade barriers.

Consumer Information and Labelling

Advocates argue that voluntary or mandatory labelling would be a way to deal with some non-trade concerns—such as animal welfare or information on genetically modified organisms—without distorting trade. It could help consumers make their choices on such things as animal welfare and sustainable production of plants, and by giving consumers confidence in labelled products it would also improve market access, they say.

Some advocates say they are pursuing this subject in the Technical Barriers to Trade (TBT) Committee. They link progress in the TBT Committee with progress in the agriculture negotiations, a point several other members object too.

A number of other countries say this is not a subject for the agriculture negotiations, but one for the TBT Committee, and in the case of food safety, other bodies such as the WTO SPS Committee and the food labelling committee of Codex Alimentarius. Several also object to mandatory labelling.

Specifically on animal welfare, one proposal envisages dealing with this non-trade concern through a combination of labelling and Green Box domestic support criteria—the latter to compensate for effects on costs or production as a result of complying with animal welfare standards. Some countries counter that animal welfare is mainly a concern in wealthy nations and better welfare can sometimes be achieved without subsidies.

Geographical Indications and Food Quality

A geographical indication is a term used to describe both the origin and characteristics of a product. In the WTO, geographical indications are discussed under three headings, only one of these being directly part of the agriculture negotiations. (In the Intellectual Property-TRIPS-Council, members are negotiating a multilateral register for geographical indications for wines and spirits. They are also debating whether the "higher" level of protection currently given to wines and spirits could be extended to other products—including whether there is a mandate to discuss this. Some countries link the extension under TRIPS with the agriculture negotiations, an idea some others staunchly reject.)

In the agriculture negotiations, a third aspect of this subject has been developed. It deals with negotiating over specific terms that are currently used elsewhere and in at least some cases may have become generic, so that they would be reclaimed for use only by producers in the original geographical area. As a related issue, there have also been proposals on labelling.

In the negotiations, the subject issue has been controversial. A number of members say geographical indications should be addressed in the agriculture negotiations. Some others strongly oppose this, arguing that they should be discussed in the TRIPS Council and Technical Barriers to Trade Committee (which deals with issues such as labelling).

DOMESTIC SUPPORT: AMBER, BLUE AND GREEN BOXES

In WTO terminology, subsidies in general are identified by "Boxes" which are given the colours of traffic lights: green (permitted), amber (slow down, i.e. be reduced), red (forbidden). In agriculture, things are, as usual, more complicated. The Agriculture Agreement has no Red Box, although domestic support exceeding the reduction commitment levels in the Amber Box is prohibited; and there is a Blue Box for subsidies that are tied to programmes that limit production. There are also exemptions for developing countries (sometimes called an "S and D Box"). By the time of the preparations for "modalities", each heading contains a list of subheadings such as: general comments; scope/definitions; base period points; reduction/expansion formulas; transparency and notification; and so on. Some countries raise "other" domestic support issues such as animal welfare. There are over 200 interventions in the 23-25 September 2003 session.

During the discussion, developing countries, new members and transition economies repeatedly argue for special and differential treatment.

For the new members that are transition economies, the call is based on the state of their economies and because the new members are still implementing commitments under their membership agreements. Some call for special and differential treatment to be based on "objective criteria" such as the level of development and per capita income, arguing that some "developing countries" are richer and have more developed agriculture sectors than some transition economies.

Amber Box: Who Can Use It?

34 WTO members have commitments to reduce their trade-distorting domestic supports in the Amber Box (i.e. to reduce the "total aggregate measurement of support" or AMS). Members without these commitments have to keep within 5% of the value of production (i.e. the "de minimis" level) — 10% in the case of developing countries.

Some developing countries repeatedly stress their argument that small vulnerable economies need special treatment, including trade preferences and longer times to adjust.

The 'Amber Box'

From the broad ideas of the first phase, greater detail is developed in the second phase. Some countries propose steeper cuts on higher levels of support, with some disaggregation according to products (current Amber Box reductions are aggregates over all products). Some countries want Amber Box subsidies to eventually be eliminated completely.

Some of the discussion is linked to the two other categories of domestic supports, the "Blue" and "Green" boxes: whether the concepts should be retained, whether the Blue Box should be restricted or eliminated, whether some Green Box subsidies should be moved into the Amber Box because they distort trade. Some speak of overall caps covering subsidies in all categories.

Amber box details: There has been some discussion of the idea (not accepted by everyone) that some domestic supports have the same effect as export subsidies because the supports vary according to market prices (rising when prices fall, and vice versa), and large proportions of production are exported. Opinions also differed on whether commitments to reduce Amber Box subsidies should be disaggregated according to product, or stay at total AMS (aggregate measurement of support).

"De minimis" levels: (subsidies that fall within small limits). There is a general willingness to look at de minimis levels for developing countries and possibly transition economies (most of these countries are bound by de minimis levels rather than AMS reduction commitments). Proposals include: no change; higher levels for developing countries and/or transition economies; lower levels or abolition for developed countries, etc.

Inflation: Some countries say their AMS commitments have been eroded by inflation. They propose that inflation should be built into the commitments. Others disagree.

The 'Green Box'

In order to qualify for the "Green Box", a subsidy must not distort trade, or at most cause minimal distortion. These subsidies have to be government-funded (not by charging consumers higher prices) and must not involve price support. They tend to be programmes that are not directed at particular products, and include direct income supports for farmers that are not related to (are "decoupled" from) current production levels or prices. "Green box" subsidies are therefore allowed without limits, provided they comply with relevant criteria. They also include environmental protection and regional development programmes. Canada has proposed setting limits on all "boxes" combined, which would mean limits on Green Box subsidies as well.

Some countries say they would like to review the domestic subsidies listed in the Green Box because they believe that some of these, in certain circumstances, could have an influence on production or prices. Some others have said that the Green Box should not be changed because it is already satisfactory. Some say the Green Box should be expanded to cover additional types of subsidies.

One proposal would maintain the Green Box as a set of measures that do not distort trade or are minimally distorting. Among the additions would be programmes that reimburse additional costs arising from the protection of animal welfare, and special flexibility for developing countries tackling food security and poverty alleviation.

Another proposal envisages retaining the Green Box but updating the base periods for "decoupled" income supports, changing threshold levels for income insurance and safety net programmes, and similar adjustments on relief from natural disasters.

Several developing countries propose additional flexibility for their needs, including a "development box" added to the Green Box.

Some countries are more critical of the Green Box as it stands, arguing that despite its objectives it does distort trade by encouraging more production and lowering world prices. One country proposes: a quantitative means of measuring whether a policy is "non-distorting"; removing direct payments, decoupled income support, and subsidized income insurance and safety nets; revising criteria for structural adjustment programmes that include factor "retirement"; notification and evaluation criteria for disaster relief, investment aids, environmental programmes, and regional assistance; transparency for food security measures and food aid; and limits on Green Box spending.

A number of critics of the Green Box say this proposal is interesting, but would like to examine it further. A number of other members object to capping the Green Box, arguing that Green Box measures meet the fundamental criteria of non or minimal distortion.

One of the themes taken up, particularly by developing countries, is the view that while individual Green Box programmes may appear to be non-distorting, the cumulative effect of the large amounts spent does distort for a number of reasons.

More countries have reservations about proposals on the Green Box. Proposed are: greater flexibility for developing countries under this box, i.e. developing countries would be allowed to use certain measures without restriction by putting them in the Green Box; and some definition for determining whether measures really are minimally trade distorting.

These were based partly on the argument that the large amounts that are being spent under the Green Box and through switching from the Amber and Blue Boxes do have an effect on wealth and income that can significantly distort production and trade.

Some members argue that the Green Box subsidies are defined as those that cause no or minimal distortion. Therefore, they say, any shift in support to the Green Box should be welcomed. Some also opposed putting some of the measures in the Green Box.

Animal Welfare and the Green Box

The discussion on animal welfare includes the ideas of compensating farmers for the extra costs they bear when they are required to meet higher standards of animal welfare. Under the proposal, these payments would be in the Green Box of permitted domestic support. The debate has partly been about whether this would be at the expense of human welfare, particularly in poorer countries.

The 'Blue Box'

The Blue Box is an exemption from the general rule that all subsidies linked to production must be reduced or kept within defined minimal (*de minimis*) levels. It covers payments directly linked to acreage or animal numbers, but under schemes which also limit production by imposing production quotas or requiring farmers to set aside part of their land. Countries using these subsidies—and there are only a handful—say they distort trade less than alternative Amber Box subsidies. Currently, the only members notifying the WTO that they are using or have used the Blue Box are: the EU, Iceland, Norway, Japan, the Slovak Republic, Slovenia, and the US (now no longer using the box).

At the moment, the Blue Box is a permanent provision of the agreement. Some countries want it scrapped because the payments are only partly decoupled from production, or they are proposing commitments to reduce the use of these subsidies. Others say the Blue Box is an important tool for supporting and reforming agriculture, and for achieving certain "non-trade" objectives, and argue that it should not be restricted as it distorts trade less than other types of support. The EU says it is ready to negotiate additional reductions in Amber Box support so long as the concepts of the Blue and Green Boxes are maintained. A number of developed and developing countries favour getting rid of the Blue Box (moving it into the Amber Box). They propose additional disciplines while it is being phased out. These countries see the Blue Box as an interim or transitional measure to help subsidizing countries move away from Amber Box subsidies. The counter argument is that the Blue Box should be preserved—although some members are prepared to discuss modifications—arguing that it distorts less than the Amber Box and helps make reforms easier to undertake.

AUGUST 2004 FRAMEWORK: DOMESTIC SUPPORT

All developed countries will make substantial reductions in distorting supports, and those with higher levels are to make deeper cuts from "bound" rates (the actual levels of support could be lower than the bound levels). The way to achieve this will include reductions both in overall current ceilings ("bound levels"), and in two components—Amber Box and de minimis supports. The third component, Blue Box supports, will be capped; at the moment the Blue Box has no limits. The fine print contains a number of details but also stresses that these have to meet the long-term objective of "substantial reductions".

All of these reduction commitments and caps will apply. However, the new ceiling at the end of the implementation period (mathematicians would say "the binding constraint") will be the lower of the value of trade-distorting support resulting from (i) the overall cut and (ii) the sum of the reductions/caps of the three components. In other words, countries would have to make the required reductions in Amber Box and de minimis support, and be within the capped limit of the Blue Box. Then, if they are still above the overall limit, they will have to make additional cuts in at least one of the three components in order to match the ceiling set by the overall cut.

Developing countries will be allowed gentler cuts over longer periods, and will continue to be allowed exemptions under Article 6.2 of the Agriculture Agreement (they can give investment and input subsidies that are generally available and are integral parts of development programmes, and provide domestic support to help farmers shift away from producing illicit crops).

Overall: Tiered Formula with Down payment

For the overall level of support (Amber Box, de minimis and Blue Box combined), a "tiered formula" will be used. This will be designed so that higher levels of support (those in higher "tiers") will have steeper cuts. On top of that, in the first year, each country's ceiling of permitted overall support will be cut by 20%. Details include how to measure the Blue Box component for the overall cut ("the higher of existing Blue Box payments during a recent representative period to be agreed and the cap established in Paragraph 15", which will be 5% of a country's agricultural production during a yet-to-be-specified period).

Amber Box: Tiered Formula with Caps on Specific Products

Amber Box ("final bound total AMS") supports will also be cut using a tiered formula, so that higher supports have steeper cuts. There will be limits on supports for specific products—"product-specific AMSs will be capped"—in order to avoid shifting support between different products. Since the tiered formula applies to the total of support on all products, the text also says that the result will be cuts in support specified for some products.

De Minimis

Currently developed countries are allowed a minimal amount of Amber Box support ("de minimis"). For support that is not given to specific products, this is defined as 5% of the value of total agricultural production. For support given to a specific product, the limit is 5% of production of that product. Developing countries are allowed up to 10% of these. The framework says de minimis will be reduced by an amount to be negotiated, with special treatment for developing countries, which will be exempt if they "allocate almost all de minimis support for subsistence and resource-poor farmers".

Blue Box

Blue Box supports, currently unlimited, are to be capped at no more than 5% of the value of a country's agricultural production over a period that still has to be negotiated. Some flexibility will be allowed for countries whose Blue Box supports are an exceptionally large proportion of their trade distorting subsidies.

The framework endorses a point made by countries that defend the use of the Blue Box. They have argued repeatedly that they need to be able to switch from the more trade-distorting Amber Box subsidies to the less distorting Blue Box supports in order to make reform less painful and more feasible. The text therefore says "members recognize the role of the Blue Box in promoting agricultural reforms".

The definition of the Blue Box will be changed to include direct payments that do not require any production, provided the payments are based on certain fixed production conditions (related to acreages, yields, numbers of livestock, or historical production levels). But new criteria will also be negotiated to ensure the Blue Box really is less trade-distorting than Amber Box measures.

Green Box

Criteria for defining supports as "Green Box" will be reviewed and clarified to ensure that the supports really do not distort trade, or do so minimally. At the same time, the exercise will preserve the basic concepts, principles and effectiveness of the Green Box, and take account of non-trade concerns such as environmental protection and rural development.

DEVELOPING COUNTRIES

Broadly, the discussion about developing countries boils down to three main questions: Should developing countries be given a large amount of special treatment or should the negotiations avoid setting separate rules for separate groups? Should the agricultural deal accept that there are distinctly different subcategories of countries within the developing country category? And should special and differential treatment allow developing countries to protect themselves against trade from other developing countries?

Phase 1

Developing countries are active in agriculture negotiations and several groups have put their names to negotiating proposals. In general, they reflect a diverse range of interests in the debate, and the distinctions are not always clear.

For example, the Cairns Group — which favours much greater liberalization in agricultural trade — is an alliance that cuts across the developed-developing country boundaries. Fourteen of its 17 members are developing countries. Like most WTO members, the Cairns Group would also like to see developing countries given some kind of "special and differential" treatment to take account of their needs. Several developing countries have submitted proposals that would lead to clearly separate rules for developed and developing countries. Some countries say WTO arrangements should be more flexible so that developing countries can support and protect their agricultural and rural development and ensure the livelihoods of their large agrarian populations whose farming is quite different from the scale and methods in developing countries. They argue, e.g. that subsidies and protection are needed to ensure food security, to support small scale farming, to make up for a lack of capital, or to prevent the rural poor from migrating into already over-congested cities. India's and Nigeria's proposals are among those that emphasize food security issues for developing countries. At the same time, some developing countries make a clear distinction between their needs and what they consider to be the desire of much richer countries to spend large amounts subsidizing agriculture at the expense of poorer countries.

Many developing countries complain that their exports still face high tariffs and other barriers in developed countries' markets and that their attempts to develop processing industries are hampered by tariff escalation (higher import duties on processed products compared to raw materials). They want to see substantial cuts in these barriers.

On the other hand, some smaller developing countries have expressed concerns about import barriers in developed countries falling too fast. They say that they depend on a few basic commodities that currently need preferential treatment (such as duty-free trade) in order to preserve the value of their access to richer countries' markets. If normal tariffs fall too fast, their preferential treatment is eroded, they say. Some developing countries see this situation as almost permanent. Others, view it as a transition, and are calling for binding commitments on technical and financial assistance to help them adjust, including the creation of a technical assistance fund for the purpose.

Some developed and developing countries have argued that all developing countries should participate in liberalization and integration into world markets, even if the terms are more relaxed. (In the 1986-94 Uruguay Round negotiations, participants agreed that the rules and disciplines to be negotiated would be equally applied to all member governments.)

WTO statistics show that developing countries as a whole have seen a significant increase in agricultural exports. Agricultural trade rose globally by nearly $100bn between 1993 and 1998. Of this, developing countries' exports rose by around $47bn— from $120 to $167bn in the period. Their share of world agricultural exports increased from 40.1 to 42.4%. But within the group, some individual developing countries have seen their agricultural trade balance deteriorate—their imports have risen faster than their exports.

DEVELOPMENT BOX, SINGLE COMMODITY PRODUCERS, SMALL ISLAND DEVELOPING STATES, SPECIAL AND DIFFERENTIAL TREATMENT

Broadly speaking, the debate is about how to treat developing countries' problems in the negotiations' outcome. Two or three strands feature in the discussion:

Market orientation vs. protection: Whether special protection and support (e.g. exempting certain products from all commitments) should be allowed for developing countries to address their particular situations, or whether liberalization with some flexibility is more effective.

Unique vs. shared concerns for developing and developed countries: Whether issues such as food security and rural development should be handled uniquely for developing countries, or whether others such as transition economies and developed countries should also be covered.

Unique vs. shared weaknesses among developing countries: Whether provisions should apply generally to all developing countries, or whether specific groups of developing countries need extra provisions. Underlying this discussion is the question of whether a liberal trade regime would favour some developing countries with inherent advantages in agriculture, or whether other developing countries would be hurt by more liberal trade.

The debate develops into a discussion about whether the "enabling clause" might be revised. The enabling clause is officially the "decision on differential and more favourable treatment, reciprocity and fuller participation of developing countries". It was adopted under GATT in 1979 and enables developed members to give differential and more favourable treatment to developing countries. Although it allows flexibility, including additional special treatment for least developed countries, the clause interpreted to require preferential treatment to be generally available to all developing countries.

Development Box Details

One proposal envisages provisions that would only apply to developing countries, and would consist of broad flexibilities rather than specific prescribed policies. The emphasis is on targeting low-income farmers lacking resources, and on secure supplies of staple foods. The means would be exemptions from commitments on these staples, the possibility of negotiating higher tariffs, allowing developing countries to use simple safeguards to protect staples, a ban on developed countries "dumping" agricultural products, an international food security fund, and so on. Another agrees with the idea of flexibilities for developing countries, but raises questions about how these would be handled.

All who speak accept the need for special treatment for developing countries. A number of developing countries add their own ideas for the development box's contents, including better market access to developed countries' markets and binding commitments on technical assistance. However, views differ on what groups of countries should qualify for what kind of special treatment.

A lot of other developing countries oppose this proposal. They say it would harm trade between developing countries, which should be encouraged instead. They also say some of the ideas are in the opposite direction to the one set in the Doha Ministerial Declaration—the objective of achieving a more market oriented agriculture trading system through reductions in support and protection applies to all WTO members.

Many countries oppose the idea of different sets of rules for developed and developing countries. They caution against adopting policies that increase trade distortion. Some also argue that instead of raising tariffs, developing countries should target low-priced subsidized exports through countervailing duty. Some countries say concerns such as food security and rural development apply to them as well. Many developing countries oppose extending development box provisions, such as those dealing with food security, to developed countries.

Single Commodity Producers Details

The proposal under this heading envisages special treatment for these countries and technical assistance to help them diversify. Among the specific ideas: transparency in the operations of multinational corporations, similar to those applying to state trading enterprises; improved market access (including removal of tariff peaks, tariff escalation and non-tariff barriers); price stabilization schemes; access to technology; diversification and capacity building.

Many developing countries support these points. Others pick points they agree with such as getting rid of tariff peaks and escalation. Some argue that dependency on single commodities can be the result of trade preferences in developed-country markets. Some argue that the question of multinational corporations is a good reason for having negotiations on competition policy. Some also point out that commodity agreements designed to stabilize prices have failed.

Some developing countries say they no longer rely on a small number of commodities because they have successfully diversified into other agricultural products and into other economic sectors such as tourism and manufacturing. They say domestic reform is often needed for any country to make use of new trade opportunities. Some others say diversification is not always possible.

Special and Differential Treatment Details

This debate is similar to the one on the development box, with the added dimension of two papers on programmes to grow crops as substitutes for illicit narcotics. Again, the debate hinges on whether protection and support is needed or whether market orientation (and the reduction of protection and support in developed countries) is the solution; and on whether some proposals might affect trade among developing countries.

Among the specific proposals are better access to export markets; protecting domestic markets for some products by re-evaluating current tariff bindings; and flexibility to support and encourage domestic production. Some developing countries want to be able to use special safeguards in response to import surges. Others advocate using countervailing duty instead—to react to imports of subsidized products.

Many countries note that special and differential treatment has a high priority in the Doha Development Agenda and is an integral part of the negotiations. Some note that the Ministerial Declaration sets special and differential treatment within the overall objective of achieving a fair and market orientated agricultural trading system, meaning that all members would have to participate in reform. Special and differential treatment would be reflected in flexibilities.

Rural Development

Discussion on this topic has been one of the lengthiest in Phase 2. All papers and comments say this is important, particularly in developing countries. But is it also important for developed countries? Broadly, participants give one of three answers: yes, even if details are different; yes, specially for transition economies; no, or yes but there is a significant difference.

Several developing countries advocate various special provisions for dealing with their problems of food security, rural poverty, etc. These include additional transition periods, and a "development box" of measures that would be added to the Green Box.

One proposal is for the development box to incorporate a "positive list" approach, i.e. each member would list the agricultural products it is ready to discipline under the Agriculture Agreement.

Several developed and developing countries emphasize the need for market orientation and the removal of distortions, even if flexibility is allowed to deal with rural poverty. Some warn that each country's measures should not hurt others—they should be targeted, decoupled and transparent, and should move away from border and production measures. Others argue that some price/production intervention is necessary to deal with rural development problems even in developed countries.

TRADE PREFERENCES

Most countries, both developed and developing, say trade preferences are important for poorer countries, and therefore the preferences should not be removed abruptly. But most also acknowledge that preferences will be eroded as tariffs in general are reduced, and so countries enjoying preferential treatment may need help to adjust.

One or two countries argue that they may have to depend on preferences over the longer term because they see little chance of becoming competitive. A few argue that their exports are such a small proportion of world trade that they have little impact on other countries, therefore, others should not be concerned about the preferences remaining in force.

On the other hand, some countries doubt whether preferences are truly beneficial because they encourage small countries to be dependent on a small number of uncompetitive products, discourage diversification and prevent other countries from supplying those products. The countries currently depending on preferences would be better off when major markets liberalize and eliminate subsidies, according to this argument.

A number of developing countries say that the trade preferences cover non-agricultural products as well. Because the subject is now mandated more broadly under the declaration of the Doha Ministerial Conference, these countries say it should be discussed outside the agriculture committee.

Among the details developed in the new proposals and the Phase 2 discussion are:

- Criteria for deciding which countries should be eligible for preferences, e.g. those currently enjoying preferences, with some additions, but perhaps only small players.
- Clearer criteria for "graduation" (determining that a country's products have progressed enough to continue without preferential treatment).
- Ensuring preferences are predictable (including longer or better defined time periods), stable, and have no "reciprocal" conditions attached.

One developed country currently giving trade preferences extensively says that in the long run, free trade agreements would provide more stability, predictability and transparency.

Special products: Under the draft, developing countries would be able to identify some products as "special products" (SP). They would be able to make lower tariff reductions on these products—a simple average reduction of 10%, with a minimum of 5% per product—and tariff quotas on these products would not have to be expanded.

Preferences: This is for "long-standing preferences" that developed countries give to developing countries—and it would apply for products accounting for at least 20% of the developing country's total merchandise exports. In these cases, developed countries would:

- Maintain to the maximum extent technically feasible, nominal margins (i.e. the difference between preferential and normal tariff rates).
- Eliminate of all in-quota duties.
- Apply tariff cuts over 8 years instead of 5 years, with the first installment deferred until the third year.

In addition, countries giving preferences would also provide technical assistance to help the developing country diversify.

Least-developed countries: This group would not have to make reduction commitments, but are encouraged to think about making some commitments "commensurate with their development needs" and in response to requests.

Specific groups of countries: The draft simply says participants would continue to consider proposals on these groups (e.g. small island developing states, vulnerable economies, and transition economies).

'NON-TRADE' CONCERNS: AGRICULTURE CAN SERVE MANY PURPOSES

The Agriculture Agreement provides significant scope for governments to pursue important "non-trade" concerns such as food security, the environment, structural adjustment, rural development, poverty alleviation, and so on. Article 20 says the negotiations have to take non-trade concerns into account. Most countries accept that agriculture is not only about producing food and fibre but also has other functions, including these non-trade objectives. The question debated in the WTO is whether "trade-distorting" subsidies, or subsidies outside the "Green Box", are needed in order to help agriculture perform its many roles.

Some countries say all the objectives can and should be achieved more effectively through "Green Box" subsidies which are targeted directly at these objectives and by definition do not distort trade. Examples include food security stocks, direct payments to producers, structural adjustment assistance, safety-net programmes, environmental programmes, and regional assistance programmes which do not stimulate agricultural production or affect prices. These countries say the onus is on the proponents of non-trade concerns to show that the existing provisions, which were the subject of lengthy negotiations in the Uruguay Round, are inadequate for dealing with these concerns in targeted, non-trade distorting ways.

Other countries say the non-trade concerns are closely linked to production. They believe subsidies based on or related to production are needed for these purposes. For example, rice fields have to be promoted in order to prevent soil erosion, they say.

Countries such as Japan, Rep of Korea and Norway placed a lot of emphasis on the need to tackle agriculture's diversity as part of these non-trade concerns. The EU's proposal says non-trade concerns should be targeted (e.g. environmental protection should be handled through environmental protection programmes), transparent and cause minimal trade distortion.

Many exporting developing countries say proposals to deal with non-trade concerns outside the "Green Box" of non-distorting domestic supports amount to a form of special and differential treatment for rich countries. Several even argue that any economic activity — industry, services and so on — have equal non-trade concerns, and therefore if the WTO is to address this issue, it has to do so in all areas of the negotiations, not only agriculture. Some others say agriculture is special.

Food Security

Is it necessary to protect domestic production in order to ensure food security?

Most countries say this is best handled through a combination of means, but they vary a lot in the emphasis they give to various methods. These include: trade (importing, together with exporting in order to finance imports); stockholding; and domestic production (which can require some support and protection in developing countries).

They differ on whether liberalization and market orientation should be the main route because distortions jeopardize food security (countries advocating substantial liberalization take this view); whether market failures and particular circumstances such as an adverse climate require more emphasis on intervention (importing developing countries, some developed countries favouring continued protection and support); or whether a gradual approach towards liberalization is best (some European countries).

Some developing countries argue that they need to intervene in agricultural trade because they see little prospect of developed countries ceasing to distort markets with subsidies and protection, because at times they lack foreign exchange, and because they need to support small-scale subsistence farming.

Some countries distinguish between short-term and long-term measures and between different problems. One view is that developing countries' short-term problems in obtaining food are best served with well-targeted food aid. In the long-term, the solution is raising incomes, which means liberalization is part of the long-term best solution. However, complete reliance on market forces could lead to specialization in different regions, increasing the risk of acute shortages when weather and other conditions are unfavourable in those regions, and therefore, the best approach is gradual, monitoring the impacts, according to this view.

Some other countries agree that raising incomes is the long-term solution to food security. They further said that for the short-term, the Marrakesh Ministerial Decision on Net Food-Importing Developing Countries and Least Developed Countries, combined with food aid and other emergency measures apply.

International stockholding and a revolving fund: Some countries propose creating an international stockpile. A number of developing countries have proposed a safety-net revolving fund to allow net food-importing developing countries and least developed countries to borrow in order to buy food in times of shortage. Developing countries concerned about food security support the stockpile proposal. Some countries question whether there should be a new fund, preferring existing World Bank and IMF programmes.

6TH MINISTERIAL CONFERENCE AT HONG KONG

The sixth WTO Conference Ministerial was held in **Hong Kong from December 13 - December 18, 2005**. It was considered vital if the **four-year-old Doha Development Agenda** negotiations were to move forward sufficiently to conclude the round in 2006. **In this meeting, countries agreed to phase out all their agricultural export subsidies by the end of 2013,** and terminate any cotton export subsidies by the end of 2006. Further concessions to developing countries included an agreement to introduce duty-free, tariff-free access for goods from the least developed countries, following the everything but arms initiative of the European Union but with up 3% of tariff lines exempted. Other major issues were left for further negotiation to be completed by the end of 2006.

The Ministerial Conference is the highest decision-making body in WTO, meeting at least once every two years and providing political direction for the organization. The Hong Kong Ministerial Conference of the World Trade Organization, which was held from 13 December to 18 December 2005, is the sixth ministerial conference (MC6) of WTO. The 150 WTO member economies aimed to reach a preliminary agreement on liberalization of farm trade by reducing subsidies, and address other issues at the Hong Kong meeting, aiming for a successful conclusion of the Doha Round in 2006.

Doha Development Agenda Carried Forward

The declaration of the "MC4 in Doha", named for the Qatar capital (Doha) has provided the mandate for negotiations on a number of issues on agriculture, concerning the implementation of the agreements which had to be completed in 2000 originally. However, the declaration set 1 January 2005 as the deadline for completing all but two of the agreements.

The Doha round aims to cut trade barriers across a wide range of sectors and is supposed to address the needs of developing countries, for whom agriculture is a particularly sensitive topic. Developing countries say farm trade needs to be tackled first because it is so important to their economies and because it is heavily protected in many rich countries. The 25-nation European Union, in particular, has been under fire for not making further cuts to its farm tariffs and subsidies. A series of meetings between ministers has failed to break the deadlock. The EU says equal attention needs to be paid to manufactured goods, which far outweigh agriculture's importance in global trade.

In the 2003 MC5 in Cancún, Mexico, it was expected all members would reach consensus on how to complete the remaining agreements. However, the meeting got stuck because of discord created by agricultural issues and ended in deadlock on Singapore issues. The original 2005-01-01 deadline was missed. After that, members aimed at finishing the negotiations by the end of 2006.

Therefore, the shelved Doha development agenda will be carried on in the MC6 in Hong Kong. That is why speculation on the chances of success of the MC6 has been rife in recent months.

The November 2001 declaration of the Fourth Ministerial Conference in Doha, Qatar, provides the mandate for negotiations on a range of subjects and other work, including issues concerning the implementation of the present agreements.

The negotiations include those on agriculture and services, which began in early 2000.

The Fifth Ministerial Conference in Cancún, Mexico, in September 2003, was intended as a stock-taking meeting where members would agree on how to complete the rest of the negotiations. But the meeting was soured by discord on agricultural issues, including cotton, and ended in deadlock on the "Singapore issues". Real progress on the Singapore issues and agriculture was not evident until the early hours of 1 August 2004 with a set of decisions in the General Council (sometimes called the July 2004 package).

The Sixth Ministerial Conference in Hong Kong, December 2005, recorded the progress made in the year and a half since then. The final declaration included agreement on a range of questions, which further narrowed down members' differences and edged the talks closer to consensus. A new time table was agreed for 2006 and members resolved to finish the negotiations by the end of the year. By then, the original 1 January 2005 deadline had been missed.

These negotiations will continue, but now with the mandate given by the Doha Declaration, which also includes a series of deadlines. The declaration builds on the work already undertaken, confirms and elaborates the objectives, and sets a time table. Agriculture is now part of the single undertaking in which virtually all the linked negotiations are to end by 1 January 2005.

The declaration reconfirms the long-term objective already agreed in the present WTO Agreement: to establish a fair and market-oriented trading system through a programme of fundamental reform. The programme encompasses strengthened rules, and specific commitments on government support and protection for agriculture. The purpose is to correct and prevent restrictions and distortions in world agricultural markets.

Without prejudging the outcome, member governments commit themselves to comprehensive negotiations aimed at:

Market access: Substantial reductions.

Exports subsidies: Reductions of, with a view to phasing out, all forms of these.

Domestic support: Substantial reductions for supports that distort trade.

The declaration makes special and differential treatment for developing countries integral throughout the negotiations, both in countries' new commitments and in any relevant new or revised rules and disciplines. It says the outcome should be effective in practice and should enable developing countries meet their needs, in particular in food security and rural development.

The ministers also take note of the non-trade concerns (such as environmental protection, food security, rural development, etc.) reflected in the negotiating proposals already submitted. They confirm that the negotiations will take these into account, as provided for in the Agriculture Agreement.

On domestic support, there will be three bands for reductions in Final Bound Total AMS and in the overall cut in trade-distorting domestic support, with higher linear cuts in higher bands. In both cases, the member with the highest level of permitted support will be in the top band, the two members with the second and third highest levels of support will be in the middle band and all other members, including all developing country members, will be in the bottom band. In addition, developed country members in the lower bands with high relative levels of Final Bound Total AMS will make an additional effort in AMS reduction. We also note that there has been some convergence concerning the reductions in Final Bound Total AMS, the overall cut in trade-distorting domestic support and in both product-specific and non-product-specific de minimis limits. Disciplines will be developed to achieve effective cuts in trade-distorting domestic support consistent with the framework. The overall reduction in trade-distorting domestic support will still need to be made even if the sum of the reductions in Final Bound Total AMS, de minimis and Blue Box payments would otherwise be less than that overall reduction. Developing country members with no AMS commitments will be exempt from reductions in de minimis and the overall cut in trade-distorting domestic support. Green Box criteria will be reviewed in line with Paragraph 16 of the framework, inter-alia, to ensure that programmes of developing country members that cause not more than minimal trade-distortion are effectively covered.

We agree to ensure the parallel elimination of all forms of export subsidies and disciplines on all export measures with equivalent effect to be completed by the end of 2013. This will be achieved in a progressive and parallel manner, to be specified in the modalities, so that a substantial part is realized by the end of the first half of the implementation period. We note emerging convergence on some elements of disciplines with respect to export credits, export credit guarantees or insurance programmes with repayment periods of 180 days and below. We agree that such programmes should be self-financing, reflecting market consistency, and that the period should be of a sufficiently short duration so as not to effectively circumvent real commercially-oriented discipline. As a means of ensuring that trade-distorting practices of STEs are eliminated, disciplines relating to exporting STEs will extend to the future use of monopoly powers so that such powers cannot be exercised in any way that would circumvent the direct disciplines on STEs on export subsidies, government financing and the underwriting of losses. On food aid, we reconfirm our commitment to maintain an adequate level and to take into account the interests of food aid recipient countries. To this end, a **safe box** for bona fide food aid will be provided to ensure that there is no unintended impediment to dealing with emergency situations. Beyond that, we will ensure elimination of commercial displacement. To this end, we will agree effective disciplines on in-kind food aid, monetization and re-exports so that there can be no loop-hole for continuing export subsidization. The disciplines on export credits, export credit guarantees or insurance programmes, exporting state trading enterprises and food aid will be completed by 30 April 2006 as part of the modalities, including appropriate provision in favour of least-developed and net food-importing developing countries as provided for in Paragraph 4 of the Marrakesh Decision. The date above for the elimination of all forms of export subsidies, together with the agreed progressivity and parallelism, will be confirmed only upon the completion of the modalities. Developing country members will continue to benefit from the provisions of Article 9.4 of the Agreement on Agriculture for 5 years after the end-date for elimination of all forms of export subsidies.

On market access, we note the progress made on *ad valorem* equivalents. We adopt four bands for structuring tariff cuts, recognizing that we need now to agree on the relevant thresholds — including those applicable for developing country members. We recognize the need to agree on treatment of sensitive products, taking into account all the elements involved. We also note that there have been some recent movements on the designation and treatment of special products and elements of the special safeguard mechanism. Developing country members will have the flexibility to self-designate an appropriate number of tariff lines as special products guided by indicators based on the criteria of food security, livelihood security and rural development. Developing country members will also have the right to have recourse to a special safeguard mechanism based on import quantity and price triggers, with precise arrangements to be further defined. Special products and the special safeguard mechanism shall be an integral part of the modalities and the outcome of negotiations in agriculture.

On other elements of special and differential treatment, we note in particular the consensus that exists in the framework on several issues in all three pillars of domestic support, export competition and market access and that some progress has been made on other special and differential treatment issues.We reaffirm that nothing we have agreed here compromises the agreement already reflected in the framework on other issues including tropical products and products of particular importance to the diversification of production from the growing of illicit narcotic crops, long-standing preferences and preference erosion. However, we recognize that much remains to be done in order to establish modalities and to conclude the negotiations. Therefore, we agree to intensify work on all outstanding issues to fulfil the Doha objectives, in particular, we are resolved to establish modalities no later than 30 April 2006 and to submit comprehensive draft Schedules based on these modalities no later than 31 July 2006.

We recall the mandate given by the members in the decision adopted by the General Council on 1 August 2004 to address cotton ambitiously, expeditiously and specifically, within the agriculture negotiations in relation to all trade-distorting policies affecting the sector in all three pillars of market access, domestic support and export competition, as specified in the Doha text and the July 2004 Framework text. We note the work already undertaken in the Sub-Committee on Cotton and the proposals made with regard to this matter. Without prejudice to members' current WTO rights and obligations, including those flowing from actions taken by the Dispute Settlement Body, we reaffirm our commitment to ensure having an explicit decision on cotton within the agriculture negotiations and through the Sub-Committee on Cotton ambitiously, expeditiously and specifically as follows:

- All forms of export subsidies for cotton will be eliminated by developed countries in 2006.
- On market access, developed countries will give duty and quota free access for cotton exports from least-developed countries (LDCs) from the commencement of the implementation period.
- Members agree that the objective is that, as an outcome for the negotiations, trade distorting domestic subsidies for cotton production be reduced more ambitiously than under whatever general formula is agreed and that it should be implemented over a shorter period of time than generally applicable. We commit ourselves to give priority in the negotiations to reach such an outcome.

In this phase, some countries are proposing the total elimination of all forms of export subsidies, in some cases with deep reductions right at the start of the next period as a "downpayment". Others are prepared to negotiate further progressive reductions without going so far as the subsidies' complete elimination, and without any "downpayment".

Many developing countries argue that their domestic producers are handicapped if they have to face imports whose prices are depressed because of export subsidies, or if they face greater competition in their export markets for the same reason. This group includes countries that are net food importers and also want help to adjust if world prices rise as a result of the negotiations.

In addition, many countries would like to extend and improve the rules for preventing governments getting around ("circumventing") their commitments on export subsidies—including the use of state trading enterprises, food aid and subsidized export credits. **Some countries, such as India, propose additional flexibility for developing countries to allow subsidies on some products to increase when subsidies on other products are reduced.**

Several developing countries complain that the rules are unequal. They object in particular to the fact that developed countries are allowed to continue to spend large amounts on export subsidies while developing countries cannot because they lack the funds, and because only those countries that originally subsidized exports were allowed to continue subsidizing—albeit at reduced levels. One group of developing countries compares the effect of various types of export subsidies with "dumping" that harms their farmers.

As a result of all of these concerns, some proposals envisage sharply different terms for developing countries. ASEAN and India, e.g. propose scrapping all developed countries' export subsidies while allowing developing countries to subsidize for specific purposes such a marketing. Some developing countries say they should be allowed to retain high tariff barriers or to adjust their current tariff limits, in order to protect their farmers—unless export subsidies in rich countries are substantially reduced. Some other developing countries counter that the barriers would also hurt developing countries that want to export to fellow-developing countries.

26

Indian Negotiations on WTO Agreement and Livestock Sector

MC Sharma, Chinmay Joshi, Rupasi Tiwari

Animal husbandry occupies a predominant position in Indian economy with over 75% working population of rural areas dependent on agriculture and animal husbandry. Animal husbandry sector provides large self-employment to millions of households in rural areas both in principal status as well as in subsidiary status.

This includes employment in sale, reprocessing and transport of animal products at secondary market level. Apart from these, large manpower is involved in livestock related activities, viz. manufacture of animal feeds and beverages, manufacture of woolen's fabric, leather from hides and skins. Such approach may be helpful in alleviating poverty and increasing the family income. Livestock rearing is an age-old tradition for millions of rural household. Animal husbandry and livestock sector are among the few growth sectors in rural India and directly linked with the livelihoods of more than 73% of rural households. Livestock wealth of the country is impressive both numerically as well as rich genetic diversity. Of the total buffalo and cattle breeds of the world 76% and 20%, respectively are available in Asia and India alone has 15% and 5% respectively. India accounts for more than 15.7% of the world cattle population while 55% of the world buffaloes population exists in our country. In addition, India has 20 % goats, 4% of sheep and 9% of world camel population. India produces 34 billion eggs (2000-01) and ranks 4th in the world and has produced 47.4 million kg of wool during 2000-01. Cattle population in 1997 was 209.5 million which is on top among countries of the world (FAO, 1999). The estimated growth rate in cattle population from 1992 to 1999 was 2.42%. Buffalo population in 1997 was 91.78 million and estimated growth rate of 10% from 1992-1999 (FAO, 1999). In developing country like India where still almost one-fourth of its gross domestic product (GDP) is obtained from agriculture. Livestock rearing and income obtained from it alone contributes to 9% of the GDP. While the share of the agriculture to the GDP declined from 52% (1950) to 29% (1991), the contribution of livestock sector marginally increased from 8 to 9% to the national GDP. The value of output from animal husbandry and dairying to agriculture over the years has gone up and was 32% in 2000-01. This did not include draught animal power, which is valued between 40-95 billion rupees. The value of output from livestock to agriculture is likely to increase further to higher than 50% by 2020.

Presently India's annual milk production is 85 million tonnes which is number one in the world. Presently annual growth rate of milk production is 4–5% and value of annual milk production alone is estimated to Rs 1,020 billion, which is higher than that of paddy (Rs 811 billion), wheat (Rs 471 billion) and sugarcane (Rs 275 billion). These figures and achievement at world level is credited to White Revolution initiated in 1970 in various phases. Establishment of cooperative dairies and milk collection centres with the help of rural people has done miracles. Despite such impressive figures the average milk production by a cow and buffalo is as low as 2.3 litres and 3.5 litres, respectively. In addition, majority of milk is obtained from buffaloes. Though India stands 1st in milk production but it is attributable to larger number of milch animals rather than production per animal. Per head milk availability is 206 grams which is well below the WHO recommendation of 270 g/day/head. The value of meat (meat, meat products and by-products) estimated at the current prices was Rs 20856 crores during 1999-2000 and export of meat and edible offal touched about Rs 1457 crores during 2000-2001. Leather industry ranks fourth among all export-oriented industries and account for 7–8% of India's total export. Export earnings from livestock and related products rose from about Rs 17 billion in 1994-95 to Rs 35 billion in 2000-01, an increase by 107%. Leather and leather products accounted for around 50%, while meat and meat products accounted for nearly 43% of the total export. The value of output from livestock to agriculture is likely to increase further to more than 50% by 2020. A major proportion of the livestock product in India is consumed internally and export market is negligible (0.35 for eggs, 0.6% of buffalo meat and 0.8% of mutton). Therefore, still the prospects of exploiting animal husbandry and dairying exits and need in this direction require attention.

The major concern of SPS measures for India includes the quality and safety of dairy and meat products. It is imperative that the principle of hazard analysis critical control point (HACCP) systems, code of practices on good animal feed, good hygienic practices (GHP) and good manufacturing practices (GMP) and cold chain system are followed. India should also put in place prevention of infectious and contagious diseases in Animals Act and take effective measures to eradicate "A" category diseases as notified by OIE. For the hygienic practices for milk production, Codex standards are required not only for the livestock products for export conform to stipulated safety and suitability standards but also that the raw milk used in the manufacture of the products is produced using GHP and GMPs. Extensive extension programmes should be implemented to ensure this. The maximum permissible levels of aflatoxins, heavy metals, veterinary drugs, pesticide residues, etc. are increasingly becoming areas of major safety concerns. SPS measures permit members to adopt, if necessary, a higher level of protection based on risk assessment. Better physical infrastructure for reference laboratories for monitoring and surveillance of the contaminants and their levels, strengthening of information systems for risk analysis are needed. The quality of all the livestock products, raw or processed meat for export improvement to meet the international standards. For this, appropriate quality control measures, modern processing and infrastructure facilities should be developed. In order to become significant player in the world market, it is necessary to ensure a sizeable market surplus of exportable farm products.

FOOD SECURITY

It is enshrined in the Preamble to the Agreement on Agriculture (AoA) that commitments under the reform programme for trade in agriculture should be made in an equitable way among all members, having regard to non-trade concerns, including food security. Article 20 of the Agreement, which mandates negotiations for continuation of the reform process, also recognises that non-trade concerns, such as food security should be taken into account in the negotiations. Food security is defined by FAO as the physical and economic access for all people at all times to enough food for an active, healthy life with no risk of losing such access and as such is directly connected with livelihood in the developing countries. The food security concerns can be meaningfully addressed in the current negotiations only by ensuring that disciplines, especially in the area of market access and domestic support, serve the food security interests of developing countries.

Agriculture is a way of life, in most developing agrarian economies. Rapid growth of agriculture is essential for ensuring food security and alleviatior. of poverty. In developing countries, agriculture still contributes significantly to their overall GDP and it employs a large proportion of the work force. The land holdings are, however, very small, unirrigated and dependent on the vagaries of nature. Further, the agricultural practices are labour intensive with relatively low intensity of farm inputs. Consequently, the farm productivity in such countries is low. As most farmers in country like India are engaged in subsistence land farming, their participation in international trade is quite marginal. The food needs and supply gaps in developing countries are developmental problems and thus all their policies for agricultural development aim at harnessing the potential for increasing productivity and production in the agricultural sector. Given these characteristics of agriculture in developing countries with meagre domestic support and the virtual absence of export subsidies, it is obvious that developing countries are not in any way responsible for the current distortions in international trade in agriculture.

The critical importance of the agriculture sector in developing countries as also its distinctive characteristics *vis-à-vis* developed countries can be appreciated from the following factors:

i. Agriculture continues to be the main employer in low-income countries. It employs over 70% of the labour force in low-income countries, 30% in middle-income countries and only 4% in high-income countries.

ii. It is a significant contributor to GDP in developing countries. Between 1990 and 1996, contribution of agriculture as a proportion of GDP was on an average 34% for low income countries as compared to 8% for upper middle income countries, and 1.5% for the high income countries of the OECD.

iii. Agriculture also continues to be an important source of foreign exchange and revenue for developing countries. In 1996 for example, while the 'share of agricultural exports in the total merchandise exports was in excess of

50% for about a quarter of 55 developing countries, this share was in excess of 30% for about half of these countries.

iv. Food consumption accounts for a large share of expenditure out of the total household income in developing countries, while in developed countries, it accounts for a small and decreasing proportion. Therefore, even small changes in agricultural employment opportunities, or prices, can have major socio-economic effects in developing countries. For most developing countries, the need is to raise agricultural productivity and increase production, particularly of basic foodstuffs. In contrast, in developed countries, the primary concern appears to be to maintain some sort of parity of income between the small proportion of the work force in farming and those in industry.

v. The social and economic vulnerability of agriculture in developing countries is generally reflected in parameters such as substantial contribution of agriculture to their GDP, low level of commercialisation of agriculture, low productivity, weak market orientation, preponderance of small and marginal uneconomical operational landholdings, lack of infrastructure, dependence on monsoon, susceptibility to natural calamities, and dependence of a very large percentage of population on agriculture for their livelihood, etc. Such vulnerability fully justifies the extension of special provisions to the developing country members for ensuring their food and livelihood security concerns.

For all the above reasons and also because it would not be possible for developing countries to provide alternative sources of employment for the rural poor, it is critically important that agriculture remains a viable source of livelihood to the large percentage of population dependent on it.

Accordingly, it is felt that food security which is not only of great economic relevance but also a very important socio-political concern in large agrarian economies like India needs to be addressed up-front in the ongoing negotiations on agriculture.

The low-income developing countries would like to be able to produce their food requirements, in the light of constraints that a number of developing countries have faced in the past in procuring their foodgrain requirements from international markets. Moreover, since a majority of the population is dependent on agriculture for their livelihood in these countries, such countries being able to have a certain level of self-sufficiency would also facilitate in taking care of a large number of the work force engaged in agriculture.

The extent to which the food gap of developing countries can be met by imports is also constrained many a times by their meagre foreign exchange resources. The entry of large consuming countries in the world food grain markets can lead to an upswing in the prices, which would in turn compound the problems of these countries. Besides, the world commodity market for basic food grains is significantly more volatile than the domestic food grain market in most of the developing countries. International price fluctuations, if transmitted to the domestic economies of developing countries, can seriously affect the prices of food grains and food entitlement of the poor. The inadequate physical and institutional infrastructure for managing large quantities of import of food grains and their distribution particularly in rural areas further makes it undesirable for the developing countries to depend on imported food for meeting their domestic requirements.

Further, the ability of farmers to respond to market signals through a shift in the cropping pattern or a relocation in order to maintain their income entitlements is hampered on account of low literacy levels, limited infrastructural facilities and dependence of a very large number of farmers and agricultural labourers on this sector.

The income entitlements of majority of people in the developing countries are directly linked to domestic agricultural production. In a liberalized trade policy framework, this entitlement is often threatened due to surge in subsidised imports. Several commodities like wheat, coarse grains, oilseeds, vegetable oils, sugar, dairy products, fruits and vegetables which are of great significance for food security in developing countries have been subjected to high levels of export subsidies by the developed countries. By artificially depressing the international prices, these subsidies in developed countries lower the farm incomes of otherwise efficient producers in importing countries and thus adversely affect their livelihood. It is in this context of high trade distortions being practised in developed countries that the developing country members would require an appropriate level of tariff protection. As such any reduction in tariffs by the developing countries could be considered only after substantial reduction in trade distorting domestic subsidies and elimination of export subsidies. For the same reasons, the developing countries should be allowed to revise the bound levels of their sensitive items, which may have been bound at low levels during the earlier negotiations, to levels at which similar categories of products were bound during the Uruguay Round of negotiations.

FAO in its paper on 'Issues at Stake Relating to Agricultural Development, Trade and Food Security' has concluded: "significant progress in promoting economic growth, reducing poverty and enhancing food security cannot be achieved in most of these countries without developing more fully the potential capacity of the agriculture sector and its contribution to overall economic development". Given the diverse conditions and varying stages of agricultural development in developing countries, the need for making relevant provisions to enable them to pursue policies aimed at increasing agricultural production and productivity is thus necessary. From the present structure of the Green Box, it is observed that most of the provisions are not widely used by the developing world, tailored, as they have been to the conditions prevalent in the developed countries. It is therefore, imperative that the Green Box should have provisions for the general development of agriculture including its diversification in developing countries, which in turn would help them to take care of their rural employment and food security. For instance, input subsidies given by developing countries for crops wherein productivity levels are below the world average should be covered under the Green Box. Sufficient flexibility should, therefore, be allowed to developing countries to administer such policies.

Another possible option for providing the necessary support to the farm sector in developing countries which in turn would lead to increased production helping them to achieve a certain amount of self-sufficiency in food grains could be by way of exempting the product specific support given to low income and resource poor farmers from AMS calculations. This would be in addition to what has already been provided in Article 6.2 of the AoA for exempting non-product specific support provided to low-income resource poor farmers.

Another aspect of AoA to be reviewed is the product coverage as prescribed in Annexure 1 of AoA. It is observed that commodities like rubber, jute, coir and forestry products are excluded from the ambit of the Agreement despite the fact that they are primary agricultural products and are a source of livelihood for a sizeable rural population in developing countries. The justification for inclusion of the above mentioned products is the same if not greater than for products like raw hides and skins, animal hair, furskins, etc. which are already covered under Annexure 1.

Experience in implementation of the Agreement has shown that despite the disciplines mandated under it, the playing field continues to be uneven between the developed and developing countries. The structural imbalances of the Agreement as also the wide divergence in the agricultural policies being practised in various countries appear to be the main contributors to this scenario. The ongoing negotiations, therefore, provide a good opportunity for taking suitable measures for rectification of the anomalies, which have surfaced during the implementation of AoA in the last 6 years. Thus, a number of suitable measures in the areas of market access, domestic support and export subsidies would necessarily have to be addressed in a co-ordinated manner so as to enable the developing countries to take care of their food security and livelihood concerns.

It is by now well established that despite reduction commitments, the level of distortions in agricultural trade continues to be high. The anticipated benefits in terms of an increase in exports for developing countries have consequently not materialized. On the other hand to maintain the income entitlement of people engaged in agriculture, it is imperative that the developing countries are allowed to maintain tariffs commensurate with their development and trade needs while at the same time undertaking relevant measures to enhance productivity and improve the quality of output. In this context, it should also be noted that the "Food Security and Livelihood Concerns" of developing countries are on a totally different plane and should not be confused or equated with the non-trade concerns advocated under "Multi-functionality of Agriculture" by a few developed countries with a view to provide legitimacy to and thereby perpetuate their trade distorting subsidies. A very low percentage of the population in the developed countries is engaged in agriculture and the livelihood of their population is not under any threat as it is in most developing countries. Further, despite having an underdeveloped agricultural sector, developing countries do not wish to practise trade distortions and would instead demand the removal of all trade distorting support from the current Agreement for the entire membership.

PROPOSALS

For large agrarian developing countries like India, food security is an important and integral element of national security. Physical access to food in developing countries can be ensured only through a certain minimum level of self-sufficiency. Further, the subsistence and livelihood of farmers in large agrarian economies can also be seriously jeopardised due to cheap/subsidised imports. Other factors like the limitations of developing country farmers to change to other crops or to shift from agriculture to manufacturing or services, and the inability of developing countries to set apart required foreign exchange resources for making purchases from the volatile global markets, as also the difficulties in ensuring timely distribution of imported food grains in remote and backward areas are also significant issues in safeguarding the food security and livelihood in these countries. Given the fact that more than 50% of the population in most of the developing countries is totally dependant on agriculture for their livelihood, the following measures would constitute a **Food Security Box** for developing countries:

i. All existing provisions of Annexure 2 of AoA except paras. 5, 6 and 7 should be continued, being an integral part of the food security measures required to be taken by developing countries.
ii. All measures taken by the developing countries for poverty alleviation, rural development, rural employment and diversification of agriculture should be exempted from any form of reduction commitments.
iii. Flexibility to be given to developing countries in the manner of providing subsidies to key farm inputs, which nevertheless should continue to be accounted for the non-product specific support AMS calculations.
iv. In addition to the provisions contained in Article 6.2 of AoA, relating to agricultural investment and input subsidies, product specific support given to low income and resource poor farmers should also be excluded for AMS calculations.
v. Negative product specific support to be permitted to be adjusted against positive non-product specific support.
vi. Appropriate level of tariff bindings to be allowed to be maintained by developing countries as a special and differential measure, keeping in mind their developmental needs and high distortions prevalent in the international markets so as to protect the livelihood of their very large percentage of population dependent on agriculture. The appropriate levels of tariff bindings will have to necessarily relate to the trade distortions in the areas of market access, domestic support and export competition being practised by the developed countries.
vii. Low tariff bindings in developing countries, as could not be rationalised in the earlier negotiations, should be allowed to be raised to the ceiling bindings for similar category of products, committed during the Uruguay Round.
viii. A separate safeguard mechanism on the lines of the Special Safeguard provisions (Article 5 of AoA) including a provision for imposition of quantitative restrictions under specified circumstances, should be made available to all developing countries irrespective of tariffication in the event of a surge in the imports or decline in prices and to ensure food and livelihood security of their people.
ix. Developing country members should be exempted from any obligation to provide any minimum market access.

x. The product coverage of the Agreement on Agriculture requires rationalisation by including primary agricultural commodities such as rubber, primary forest produce, jute, coir, abaca and sisal, etc. which are much more agricultural than hides and skins which are already covered under AoA.

PROPOSAL ON MARKET ACCESS

1. One of the important objectives of the world agricultural trade reforms is to expand market access opportunities across products and countries. The process of tariffication and reduction in tariffs was expected to provide market access to products from efficient producers of agricultural commodities. Even after 6 years of implementation of the Agreement on Agriculture (AoA), the access for products from developing countries, however, continues to be impeded in the developed country markets due to their high trade distorting domestic support policies coupled with high tariffs, tariff peaks, tariff escalations and a plethora of non-tariff barriers. A detailed analysis of these factors has already been made in an earlier paper, submitted by a group of developing countries including India.

2. India would further like to highlight the fact that the opening of the markets, in the post-Uruguay Round phase, has taken place mainly in the developing countries. The share of exports from developing countries, which constitute over three-fourths of the WTO membership, continues to remain around 30% of the world trade in agriculture. This is less than what it was 25–30 years ago. The anticipated increase in exports from developing to developed countries, thus, has not materialised. Among the three major developed regions, Western Europe is the most important market for agricultural exports from developing countries, but the share of total agricultural exports from developing countries into Western Europe has declined from 28.5% in 1994 to 28% in 1998. The share of agricultural exports of developing countries into Japan has also fallen from 14.5 to 11.5% during this period.

3. In several country studies done by FAO on implementation of the Agreement on Agriculture in developing countries, it has been observed that there was "asymmetry in the experience between the growth of food imports and the growth of agricultural exports. While trade liberalisation had led to an almost instantaneous surge in food imports, these countries were not able to raise their exports". It has been further observed that the process has marginalised small producers and added to unemployment and poverty. The studies conclude that the challenge for these countries lies in being able to maintain an appropriate mechanism to safeguard the livelihood of the people engaged in agriculture.

4. Given the volatility of agricultural commodity markets and the inability of farmers in developing countries to bear risks arising out of violent fluctuations in international prices, an effective safeguard mechanism for preventing a surge in imports becomes absolutely essential for preserving the livelihood of farmers. The provision of general safeguards available under the Agreement on Safeguards would be extremely difficult to invoke, as farming in developing countries is an unorganised family-based economic

activity involving a majority of the population. Moreover, the time taken to invoke these provisions would render the entire proceedings infructuous, as by the time action is taken, farmers would have already suffered due to the adverse impact of volatile markets. There is thus a requirement for providing an effective safeguard mechanism on the lines of the Special Safeguard provisions (Article 5 of AoA) including provisions to put quantitative restrictions, which could be used by developing countries irrespective of tariffication for all products that they consider sensitive. On the same count, developing country members must be allowed to maintain existing level of tariff bindings keeping in mind their developmental needs and the high distortions prevalent in the international market.

5. It is by now well established that the selective extension of high domestic support and export subsidies to a few commodities in the developed countries has not only eroded the competitiveness of products originating in developing countries but has also introduced an unfair competition for local producers and threatened their livelihood. Therefore, any tariff reduction commitments can be considered by developing countries only after substantial reduction has actually been effected by the developed countries in all the three areas of market access, domestic support and export subsidies.

6. The preamble of the Agreement on Agriculture recognises that the process of reform of trade in agriculture initiated during the Uruguay Round is a continuing process. The mandated negotiations, would only carry forward the commitments made under the reform programme. Thus, it is important that for the country of the negotiations, the reform process should be continued and not come to a standstill. Moreover, experience in the implementation of the agreement is an important component of the ongoing negotiations and it is by now well established that the anticipated benefits of liberalisation of trade in agriculture have not materialised for developing countries. It is, thus, important that the WTO membership particularly the developed countries undertake to carry forward the reform process during the currency of the negotiations at an accelerated pace. As a proof of their commitment to the reform process and also to ensure that the reform process continues even during the negotiations, a down payment by way of bringing down their tariffs by at least 50% from the level existing as on 1.1.2001 during the first year of negotiations itself would go a long way in building confidence among the less developed members of the WTO.

7. It has been observed that many products of export interest to developing countries will continue to face high tariffs as the AoA commitments "required reductions on an unweighted average basis for each country's agricultural products, thereby leading to maintenance of high tariffs on some products like sugar, rice or dairy products by making substantial reductions on less sensitive tariff lines in which there is little trade".

8. The average tariffs in OECD countries in 1995 were 214% for wheat, 197 % for barley, 154% for maize. A joint UNCTAD/WTO Study on the post-Uruguay Round Tariff Environment for exports from developing countries (1997) reports that QUAD countries maintain an extremely large variation of tariff

rates. Their tariff peaks reach 350% and above in extreme cases for some products of interest to developing countries. One-fifth of the peak tariffs of the US, a quarter of those of EU, about 30% of those of Japan and about one-seventh of those of Canada exceed 30%. The study further reports that the most important areas with the highest tariff rates include the major agricultural staple foods, cereals, meat, sugar, milk, butter and cheese as well as tobacco products and cotton. In EU, for instance, the out of quota tariff for bananas is 180%; in Japan these tariffs range between 460 to 600% for dried beans, peas and lentils and in the US, groundnuts in shell attract a tariff of 164%. This study also emphasizes that even after full implementation of the AoA, tariff wedges will continue to be significantly high on account of tariff escalation, which is a major factor preventing developing countries from diversifying and increasing their share of processed agricultural exports. Recently, Japan has levied a tariff of about 1000% on rice.

9. Article 13 of the Agreement on Agriculture is one of the outstanding examples of AoA having actually awarded special and differential treatment in favour of developed countries. During the operation of this clause, developed country support policies have enjoyed exemption from possible countervailing actions in certain situations as specified in the Article. This has further skewed the terms of trade in favour of developed countries. With a view to making the playing field even, it would be appropriate that the peace clause is abolished for developed countries. However, for developing countries, a special and differential treatment should be given for the flexibility of use of peace clause for a period of at least 10 years.

10. The Special Treatment provided under Section A of Annexure 5 of AoA which is presently enjoyed by only 3 or 4 countries for a few agricultural products like rice and cheese, should be done away with and tariff should be the only measure to regulate the imports.

11. The tariff rate quotas (TRQs) established to provide minimum market access opportunities have also perpetrated trade distortions by legitimising quantitative restrictions, generating quota rents and denying market access to new corners. Allocation of quota licences with wide differences between inquota and out of quota tariffs in the OECD food importing countries has a potential to generate excessive quota rents. Non-transparent administration of TRQs and preferential trade arrangements has contributed to low quota fill in several commodities. It is, thus, strongly felt that the TRQ system should not be allowed to be 'embedded' in the trade rules as it could easily become a form of 'managed' trade, which would be a retrograde step in terms of the progressive liberalisation envisaged in the agricultural sector .

PROPOSALS

i. An appropriate formula with a cap on tariff bindings should be evolved to effect substantial reduction in all tariff levels including peak tariffs and tariff escalations in developed countries. The developed countries should make a down payment by way of bringing down the tariff bindings, as on 1.1.2001, by 50% by the end of the year 2001.

ii. As a special and differential measure, the developing country members should be allowed to maintain appropriate levels of tariff bindings keeping in mind their developmental needs and the high distortions prevalent in the international markets. The appropriate levels of tariff bindings will have to necessarily relate to the trade distortions in the areas of market access, domestic support and export competition being practised by the developed countries.

iii. A separate Safeguard mechanism on the lines of the Special Safeguard provisions (Article 5 of AoA) along with a provision for imposition of quantitative restrictions under specified circumstances, should be made available to all developing countries irrespective of tariffication, in the event of a surge in the imports or a decline in prices and to ensure the food and livelihood security of their people.

iv. Even after the abolition of the peace clause (Article 13 of AoA), as a special and differential provision, measures taken by developing countries under Annexure 2 (Green Box) and other domestic support measures conforming to Article 6 of AoA shall be exempted for a period of 10 years from imposition of countervailing duties under the Agreement on Subsidies and Countervailing Measures and Article XVI of GATT 1994 and shall also be exempted from actions based on non-violation nullification or impairment of the benefits of tariff concessions under paragraph 1 (b) of Article XXIII of GATT 1994.

v. Tariff rate quotas (TRQs) should be eventually abolished. In the intervening period, there should, however, be substantial expansion of TRQs administered by developed countries. There should also be greater transparency in administration of TRQs by prescribing guidelines for complete uniformity across countries and products, adopting a common base period for calculating domestic consumption for minimum market access commitment by the developed countries, mandatory filling up of TRQs by developed countries and stricter application of the MFN principle in allocation of TRQs with special preference being given to developing countries having less than $ 1000 per capita annual income. Allocation of TRQs should be for specific products and not for aggregated commodity groups.

vi. Developed country members should not be allowed to use SPS measures for protectionist purposes by prescribing overly stringent trade restrictive SPS measures for denying market access to developing countries.

vii. Developing country members should be exempted from any obligation to provide any minimum market access.

viii. The provision of Special Treatment as provided in Section A of Annexure 5 of AoA, which is enjoyed by a very few countries for a few products, should be removed as it is against the basic principles of GATT.

PROPOSAL ON DOMESTIC SUPPORT

12. The long-term objective of the Agreement on Agriculture (AoA) to "establish a fair and market-oriented agricultural trading system", was sought to be achieved "through the establishment of strengthened and more operationally effective GATT rules and disciplines". One such set of disciplines comprised

the domestic support reduction commitments, which were undertaken under the AoA by member countries with an aim to correct price distortions and allow market forces to determine the level and composition of agricultural production.

13. A significant feature of AoA was the distinction between support measures that were considered trade distorting and therefore, subject to discipline and those with "no or at most minimal trade distorting effects" and which could be allowed to be maintained without any ceiling or reduction commitments. Some countries complied with the reduction commitments regarding aggregate measurement of support (AMS) by restructuring their domestic support policies/programmes. Some of them have also shifted their potentially 'trade distorting' measures from the Blue Box into the Green Box. An analysis based on Secretariat Paper (G/AG/NG/S/12, 15.6.2000) reveals that there is an appreciable increase in expenditure under the Green Box in 1997/98 over the base period in major developed countries. In most cases, it has also resulted in an overall increase in the quantum of support to their agricultural sector. Certain countries have also taken undue advantage by including the quantum of Blue Box support in their initial base period calculations of AMS, as in the subsequent years there were no reduction commitments for this category of Blue Box support. Such countries thus, got the unintended benefit of being able to achieve reduction in their domestic support without actually having to effect any reduction.

14. Among the Green Box measures, the expenditure on 'decoupled income support' and direct income payments has increased substantially during the implementation period. The share of the total direct payments under the Green Box measures is estimated to have increased from 23% in 1995 to 43% in 1998 (G/AG/NG/S/2, 19 April, 2000). The 'decoupled' support and other supports under paras 5, 6 and 7 of Annexure 2 (Green Box) and the production limiting subsidies under Article 6.5 (Blue Box) of AoA are not as minimally trade distorting as is made out on account of the following reasons:

   i. The ability of the farmers to take, risk as well as to make farm investments substantially increases, if support in the form of assured payments including decoupled income support is provided, since such payments entail insurance and wealth effects.

   ii. These direct payments encourage greater use of farm inputs and enhance access to technology leading to over-production, which in turn distorts agricultural markets.

   iii. Decoupled or direct payments can be a powerful incentive to maintain or increase current production in the expectation of receiving higher levels of future support.

   iv. Decoupled or direct payments have been found to increase land values resulting in maintenance of land in farming rather than putting it to some other economically better use.

   v. Decoupled or direct payments heavily subsidise the cost of production, which enables the receivers of such support to capture a substantial share in the export markets at the cost of more efficient producers.

The provisions of Annexure 2 of the AoA particularly paras 5, 6 and 7 have enabled high subsidising countries to enhance their overall level of support to agriculture. This is evident from the producer support estimate (PSE) figures for all OECD countries, which have increased from US$ 246 billion in 1986-88 to US$ 283 billion in 1999. For a few developed countries, the PSE is not only high as compared to the base period but has also risen sharply since 1997. As also borne out by data from OECD, total support estimate (TSE) in OECD countries in 1999 amounted to US$ 361 billion which is much higher than the $308 billion TSE figure during the period 1986-88. This TSE figure of OECD countries is approximately six times of the total value of the current annual agricultural production in India.

Moreover, developing countries suffer from an inherent disadvantage of limited financial resources as compared to resource rich countries, and are, therefore, not in a position to have a high subsidy regime. Article 7.2 (b) of the AoA also institutionalises this disparity by allowing the high subsidising countries to maintain 80% of their base level AMS while prohibiting the low income countries from going beyond the *de minimis level* of 10% of the value of their agricultural production. This makes the AoA provisions inequitous and discriminatory. It is also noted that most of the items in Annexure 2 are not widely used in the developing world, tailored, as they are to the conditions prevalent in the developed countries. Given the diverse conditions and varying stages of agricultural development in developing countries, the need for making some additional provisions to enable them to pursue policies aimed at increasing agricultural production and productivity is thus necessary. For instance, input subsidies given to crops wherein productivity levels are below the world average should be covered under the Green Box. Sufficient flexibility should therefore be allowed to developing countries to administer such policies through the Green Box.

Another possible option for providing the necessary support to the farm sector in developing countries, which in turn would lead to increased production, helping them to achieve a certain amount of self-sufficiency in food grains, could be by way of exempting the product specific support given to low income and resource poor farmers from AMS calculations. This would be in addition to the exemption given to non-product specific support provided to this category of farmers under Article 6.2 of the AoA.

It was expected that with the domestic support reduction commitments under AoA, production of agricultural products (notably cereals) in highly subsidised countries would fall and the output in nonsubsidising and, therefore, low-cost producing countries would expand by 2000. However, as a consequence of the asymmetrical provisions of the AoA and their lackadaisical implementation by the developed countries, the post-AoA experience establishes that the anticipated production changes in terms of levels and locational shifts have not materialised. This is also borne out by the recent FAO production estimates, which indicate that there has been insignificant change in World cereal production between 1995 and 1999.

Moreover, selective extension of high domestic support to a select few commodities in developed countries has effectively neutralised the competitiveness and the potential market access that would have been available to developing countries. For example, commodities of interest to developing countries like dairy, meat, sugar, poultry, cereals and fruits and vegetables, etc. have been extended maximum support/subsidies in developed countries, which has negated the comparative advantage of developing countries in these commodities.

Article 13 of the Agreement on Agriculture is one of the outstanding examples of AoA in fact having accorded a special and differential treatment in favour of developed countries. During the operation of this clause, developed country support policies have enjoyed exemption from countervailing action. This has further skewed the terms of trade in favour of developed countries. With a view to making the playing field even, it would be appropriate if the peace clause were abolished for developed countries. However, developing countries as a special and differential measure should be allowed the use of peace clause for a further period of at least 10 years. It is also felt that a rationalisation of the subsidies/ support exempt under Article 13(a) and (b) is required. While Annexure 2 measures, which are minimally trade distorting, should continue to be exempt under Article 13(a) during its currency for developed countries, the 'trade distorting' measures under Annexure 2 (paras 5, 6 and 7) should actually be clubbed with the measures listed out in Article 13(b) as they are as trade distorting as the Blue Box payments covered under Article 6.5 and thus do not merit separate treatment.

During the course of implementation of AoA, certain operational problems have also been encountered by the developing countries in the calculation of AMS for the purpose of estimating the domestic support. These include effect of inflation and exchange rate fluctuation on the methodology of calculation of AMS. The rate of inflation varies widely between countries. The average prices in developing countries in 1996 were 656% higher than in 1990 compared to only 19% in industrialised countries (International Financial Statistics Yearbook quoted in AIE/33).

The depreciation in currencies has also rendered any comparison between the base year and current year AMS figures quite meaningless. For example, the value of the Indian currency (rupee) in 1999-2000 has depreciated by over 70% of its value in 1986-87 vis-à-vis the US dollar.

In the context of calculation of AMS, it is observed that in calculating the "product specific" or market price support component of AMS, if an applied administered price is lower than the external reference price (ERP), the result will be a negative figure. The non-product specific support, given the nature of methodology of its quantification, will either be zero or a positive figure only. The aggregate measure of support, as the name itself implies, is the sum of all measures comprising domestic support to the agricultural sector. It is only such a summation of negative and positive support, which truly reflects the total domestic support given to the agricultural sector. Thus, negative AMS values, which are indicative of the fact that an administered price is at a lower level than the corresponding external reference price, should be reflected appropriately through negative figures. Members should, accordingly, be able to use negative product specific support to offset positive non-product specific support to arrive at aggregate measure of support under the agreement.

Besides, the provisions for S and D treatment for developing countries also need to be spelt out in terms of concrete obligations taking into account their experience in implementation of the AoA, the differing levels of economic development, the role of agriculture in economics with a large rural population and the need to preserve food and livelihood security taking into account the vulnerability of their agricultural sector.

In view of the uneven playing field due to continued high level of distortions in agricultural trade, it is extremely important that developing countries have the flexibility to use appropriate policies to address the problems facing their agricultural sector. The developing countries do not intend to use these measures for achieving an unjustified share in the world market. The ongoing negotiations are, thus, an appropriate opportunity to take stock of the fact that the trade policies being practiced by developed countries have created serious trade distortions and need to be effectively disciplined. Necessary corrective action will have to be taken to allow the emergence of developing countries as equal trading partners.

The preamble of the Agreement on Agriculture recognises that the process of reform of trade in agriculture initiated during the Uruguay Round is a continuing process. The mandated negotiations would only carry forward the commitments made under the reform programme. Thus, it is important that during the currency of the negotiations the reform process should be continued and not come to a standstill. Moreover, experience in the implementation of the agreement is an important component of the ongoing negotiations and it is by now well established that the anticipated benefits of liberalisation of trade in agriculture have not materialised for developing countries. It is, thus, important that the WTO membership particularly the developed countries undertake to carry forward the reform process during the currency of the negotiations at an accelerated pace. As a proof of their commitment to the reform process and for continuing the reform process, a down payment during the first year of negotiations itself would go a long way in building confidence among the less developed members of the WTO.

PROPOSALS

i. Direct payments along with decoupled income support and governmental financial participation in income insurance and income safety-net programmes (paras 5, 6 and 7 of Annexure 2) as well as direct payments under production limiting programmes (Article 6.5) should be included in the non-product-specific Aggregate Measurement of Support and should be subject to reduction commitment so as not to exceed the *de minimis* level, i.e. 5% (for developed countries) and 10% (for developing countries) of the value of that Member's total agricultural production (Article 6.4).

ii. Product specific support provided to low-income resource poor farmers should be excluded from the AMS calculations, as is the case for the non-product-specific support as per para 6.2 of AoA.

iii. The total domestic support should be brought down below the *de minimis* level within a maximum period of 3 years by developed countries and in 5 years by the developing country members. The developed countries should make a down payment by the end of the year 2001, through a 50% reduction in the domestic support from the level maintained during the year 2000; or by the amount as is higher than the *de minimis*, whichever is lower.

iv. A suitable methodology of notifying the domestic support in a stable currency/basket of currencies should be adopted for taking into account the incidence of inflation and exchange rate variations.

v. Negative product specific support figures should be allowed to be adjusted against the positive non-product-specific AMS support figures.

vi. While product specific support should be calculated at the aggregate level, support to any one particular commodity should not be allowed to exceed the double of the *de minimis* limit of that commodity, as prescribed under Article 6.4.

vii. Support extended under paras. 5,6 and 7 of Annexure 2 should be shifted from Article 13 (a) to 13 (b) of the Peace Clause. However, the Peace Clause must lapse as already provided in AoA.

viii. The provisions of Article 6.4 of AoA should prevail over the stipulation contained in Article 13 (b) (ii) of the Agreement.

ix. After the abolition of the peace clause (Article 13 of AoA), as a special and differential provision, measures under Annexure 2 (Green Box) and other domestic support measures conforming to Article 6 of AoA shall be exempt from imposition of countervailing duties under the Agreement on Subsidies and Countervailing Measures and Article XVI of GATT 1994 and shall also be exempt from actions based on non-violation nullification or impairment of the benefits of tariff concessions under paragraph 1 (b) of Article XXIII of GATT 1994.

x. All measures taken by developing countries for poverty alleviation, rural development, rural employment and diversification of agriculture should be exempted from any reduction commitments.

PROPOSAL ON EXPORT COMPETITION

15. Agriculture is the only sector of the world economy still marked by the existence of export subsidies. The disciplines evolved in the Uruguay Round Agreement on Agriculture have proved to be grossly inadequate to correct these most trade distorting policies maintained by about 25 WTO member countries. The developing country members of WTO have serious concerns in regard to these subsidies as they destabilise and depress the international market prices impacting adversely farm incomes in developing countries.

16. Export subsidies encourage inefficient production of agricultural commodities in developed countries while discouraging domestic production in food importing countries. They also introduce an unfair competition for the local producers and are totally inconsistent with a market-oriented framework for world agricultural trade. The principal commodities, which have high incidence of export subsidies, include wheat, coarse grains, oilseeds, vegetable oil, sugar, dairy products and fruits and vegetables, which also happen to be products of export interest to many developing countries.

17. Under the export subsidy reduction commitments for the developed countries, the value of subsidies is to be reduced by 36% from the base period 1986-90 and the volume of subsidised exports is to be decreased by 21% in 6 years. The measurement of the reductions of the subsidies is to be on the basis of commodity aggregates.

18. The information on the use of subsidies with respect to volume commitments and budgetary outlay commitments indicates that by and large all the countries have complied with their overall reduction commitments at the aggregate level. However, as per the data compiled by WTO Secretariat, the actual use of subsidies in terms both of budgetary outlays and volume has increased for some particular items in major subsidising countries between 1995 and 1998 (G/AG/NG/S/5, 11 May, 2000).

19. The implementation of AoA during the last about 6 years has also revealed that many member countries have shifted export subsidies between products from year to year so as to target a few specific commodities and have also 'rolled over' unused subsidies to the following year resulting in a cumulative depressive effect on prices in that year, eroding the competitive advantage of other exporting countries. There is thus an immediate need to formulate effective measures to prevent the rolling over of unused subsidies to the next year.

20. The export credits, guarantees and insurance programmes have not been included in the export subsidy reduction commitments under AoA. Mainly resource rich countries in order to maintain and enhance their exports operate these schemes, which are actually in the nature of export subsidisation. The absence of clear guidelines governing export subsidisation in the AoA has led to circumvention of export subsidy reduction commitments. The provision of export credit guarantees and price discounts for buyers substantially influences the quantity and direction of exports. The operation of such schemes has also to a great extent neutralised the effects of export subsidy reduction commitments under the Agreement.

21. Article 16 of the Agreement on Agriculture refers to the Ministerial Decision on Measures Concerning Possible Negative Effects of the Reform Programme on Least Developed and Net Food Importing Countries thereby making it an integral part of Agreement. The concept of food aid, a prominent form of external assistance, is by nature and intention specifically designed to enhance food security. It refers to some external resource transfer, normally in kind of food commodities, which provides food directly to beneficiaries in the recipient country or to the government in support of its food security or other developmental objectives. Food aid essentially evolved from surplus disposal programmes of the early 1950s. In recent times, however, it has undergone a lot of changes and has become increasingly complex. Some of the proposals by other member countries have highlighted the fact that the current provisions of Article 10.4 of the Agreement on Agriculture need to be revised and strengthened to prevent the abuse of food aid mechanism. The alarming tendency of donor countries to increase aid with a view to developing their markets negates the very spirit of this mechanism. The

ongoing negotiations should immediately address this issue to bring about greater transparency in the provision of food aid, which should be offered regardless of the world market prices. The recent General Council decision directing the Committee on Agriculture to follow-up on the Ministerial Decision is a first step towards this direction, which, however, needs to be complemented by the entire membership by suggesting suitable guidelines for food aid as distinct from export subsidies.

22. Another significant dimension of the current provisions on disciplining export subsidies under AoA is that countries, which notified the use of export subsidies in their original schedules could continue to use them, albeit in a restrained manner, while the countries which did not notify the use of subsidies in their original schedules are not permitted to introduce them thereafter (Article 3.3). Besides, AoA deprives the developing country members of their right to provide export subsidies, which are otherwise permitted under Article 27, read with Annexure VII of the Agreement on Subsidies and Countervailing Measures (ASCM). There is, thus, every need to restore the rights negotiated by the developing countries under the ASCM.

23. The preamble of AoA recognises that the process of reform of trade in agriculture initiated during Uruguay Round is a continuing one. Thus, it is extremely important that during the currency of the negotiations, the reform process should be continued and not come to a standstill. Moreover, the experience in the implementation of AoA is an important component of the ongoing negotiations and it is by and large well established that the anticipated benefits of liberalisation of trade in agriculture have not materialised for the developing countries. It is therefore important that the WTO membership particularly the developed countries undertake to carry forward the reform process at an accelerated pace even during the negotiations. As a proof of their commitment to the reform process and for carrying it forward, it is proposed that developed countries should make a down payment during the year 2001 by way of effecting a reduction of 50% in the value as well as in the volume of subsidised exports from the level existing on 1.1.2001.

PROPOSALS

i. Export subsidies on all agricultural products should be eliminated in the first 2 years of implementation, both in terms of export subsidy outlays and subsidised volumes. As a down payment, the subsidy outlays and subsidised volumes should be reduced by 50% from the level maintained in the year 2000 by the developed countries by the end of 2001.

ii. During the transition period also, no 'rolling over' of unused export subsidies should be allowed.

iii. All forms of export subsidisation including export credit, guarantees, price discounts and insurance programmes, etc. in developed countries should be added to the export subsidies and should be subjected to the overall disciplines applicable to export subsidies.

iv. Taking into account the needs and special conditions of developing countries:

- The existing special and differential treatment for developing countries under Article 9.4 of the AoA should continue; and
- Special dispensation for developing countries provided under Article 27 read with Annexure VII of the Agreement on Subsidies and Countervailing Measures should prevail over Article 8 of AoA.

v. Article 13 (c), which gives protection to export subsidies that conform to the provisions of part (v) of AoA, should be abolished forthwith.

vi. After the abolition of the peace clause (Article 13 of AoA), the provisions under Article 9.1 (d) and (e) permitted to be used by developing countries without any reduction commitments under Article 9.4 of AoA should be retained as such and should be exempt from countervailing duties and actions based on Article XVI of GATT 1994 and the Agreement on Subsidies and Countervailing Measures.

IMPLICATIONS OF AGREEMENT ON AGRICULTURE FOR INDIA

The Agreement on Agriculture contains provisions in 3 broad areas of trade and agriculture policies: market access, export subsidies and domestic support.

Market Access

For agricultural products is to be governed by a 'tariffs only' regime. That is to say, the agreement states that there can be no restrictions on farm trade except through tariffs. This means that non-tariff barriers such as quantitative restrictions on imports, (i.e. quotas, import restrictions through permits, import licensing, etc.) as were in existence before the Agreement came into being, were to be replaced by tariffs on imports to provide the same level of protection and then were to be followed by progressive reduction of tariff levels. Tariffs resulting from this "tariffication process" as well as other tariffs are to be reduced by a simple average of 36% over 6 years in the case of developed countries and 24% over 10 years in the case of developing countries. **However, developing countries like India who had not converted their quantitative restrictions into tariffs, were allowed to have ceiling bindings which were not subjected to these reduction commitments.**

India had bound its tariffs at 100% for primary products, 150% for processed products and 300% for edible oils, except for certain items (comprising about 119 tariff lines), which were historically bound at a lower level in the earlier negotiations. Out of these low bound tariff lines, bindings on 15 tariff lines which included skimmed milk powder, spelt wheat, corn, paddy, rice, maize, millet, sorghum, rape, colza and mustard oil, fresh grapes, etc. were successfully negotiated under GATT Article XXVIII in December 1999 and the binding levels were suitably revised upward to provide adequate protection to the domestic producers. **India has also not taken any commitment to provide minimum market access opportunities which other countries who had tariffed their QRs had to undertake to the extent of 3% of its domestic consumption going up to 5%, at the end of the implementation period.** Though India is not entitled to use the Special Safeguard Mechanism of the Agreement, which can be used only by countries which had tariffied, yet **it can take safeguard action under the WTO Agreement on Safeguards if there is a surge in imports causing serious injury or if there is a threat of serious injury to the domestic producers.**

Domestic Support

Measures, according to the Agreement, are meant to identify acceptable measures of support to farmers and curtailing unacceptable trade distorting support to farmers. These measures are targetted largely at developed countries where the levels of domestic agricultural support had risen to extremely high levels. Domestic support is divided into two categories viz., (a) support with no, or minimal, distortive effect on trade (often referred to as "Green Box" and "Blue Box" measures) and (b) trade distorting support (often referred to as "Amber Box" measures).

The trade distorting domestic support is measured in terms of what is called the "Total Aggregate Measurement of Support" (Total AMS), which is expressed as a percentage of the total value of agricultural output and includes both product specific and non-product specific support. The Agreement on Agriculture stipulates a reduction commitment of total AMS by 20% for developed countries in 6 years (1995-2000) and by 13-1/3% by developing countries in 10 years (1995-2004), taking 1986-88 as the base period. **However, domestic support given to the agricultural sector up to 10% of the total value of agricultural produce in developing countries and 5% in developed countries is allowed. In other words, AMS within this limit is not subject to any reduction commitment.**

In India, the product-specific support is negative, while the non-product specific support, i.e. subsidies on agricultural inputs, such as, power, irrigation, fertilisers, etc. is well below the permissible level of 10% of the value of agricultural output. **Therefore, India is under no obligation to reduce domestic support currently extended to the agricultural sector.**

Disciplines in the area of **export subsidies** required developed countries to reduce, over a period of 6 years, the base period (1986-90) volume of subsidised exports by 21% and the corresponding budgetary outlays for export subsidies by 36%. For developing countries, these reductions are 14% in volume terms and 24% in budgetary outlays over a period of 10 years.

Export subsidies of the kind listed in the Agreement on Agriculture, which attract reduction commitments, are not extended in India. Also, developing countries are free to provide certain subsidies, such as subsiding of export marketing costs, internal and international transport and freight charges etc. India is making use of these subsidies in certain schemes of Agricultural and Processed Food Products Export Development Authority (APEDA), especially for facilitating export of horticulture products.

CURRENT ASSESSMENT OF IMPLEMENTATION OF AGREEMENT ON AGRICULTURE

It is now an established fact that the Uruguay Round did not bring about trade liberalisation in agriculture to the desired extent. There were no significant reductions in domestic support as well as export subsidies by the developed countries. Although the Agreement on Agriculture achieved a great deal by defining rules for international trade, its achievement in terms of immediate market opening has been limited. **The anticipated gains from agricultural trade liberalisation, therefore, have eluded the developing countries till now.**

During the Uruguay Round, it was expected that following the Agreement, distortions in agricultural trade would be reduced and scope for exports of products from developing countries would increase. The anticipated increase in exports of agricultural products from developing countries has not been realised. It was also expected that the contemplated fair trading regime would help the efficient producers in realising higher prices for their products. On the contrary, prices of most agricultural commodities are declining in the world markets. It was anticipated that due to the reduction in domestic support in developed countries, cereal production would shift from developed to developing countries. Empirical evidence, however, shows that there has not been much change in the pattern of world cereals production and exports.

A number of developed countries have continued to provide high domestic support to their agricultural sectors. At best, the policies in many developed countries have only been cosmetically altered by shifting the support from one "box" to another. **The continuation of the high domestic support to agriculture in many developed countries is a cause of concern as they encourage over-production in these countries leading to low levels of international prices.**

It is obvious, therefore, that benefits to developing countries in terms of increasing their exports will only occur after complete elimination of export subsidies and substantial reduction in domestic support in the developed countries has been effected. In this context, India has demanded a substantial reduction in the trade distorting domestic support and elimination of export subsidies by developed countries.

Market access in the developed countries is also hampered by their maintaining high tariffs on products of interest to developing countries besides a plethora of non-tariff barriers. In a recent study of 14 countries, Food and Agricultural Organisation (FAO) concluded that there was little change in the volume exported or in diversification of products and destination. Tariff peaks continue to block exports from developing countries to the developed world. Tariffs still remain very high in certain sectors, specially, in cereals, sugar and dairy products. Tariff escalation (increase in tariff with successive stages of processing) block exports of value-added products from developing countries to the developed countries. Stringent sanitary and phytosanitary (SPS) measures continue to be a major barrier in diversifying exports in horticulture and meat items. Fresh commitments have, therefore, to be negotiated to substantially improve market access for products of particular interest to developing countries. Since entry of new comers is difficult in the existing tariff quota (TRQ)* regime, India is demanding substantial expansion of TRQs pending their eventual abolition. It

---

* *TRQ is a trading mechanism that provides for the application of a customs duty at a certain lower rate to imports of a particular good up to a specified quantity (in-quota quantity) and at a higher rate on imports of that good when it exceeds the in-quota quantity.*

is (also) essential that administration of tariff quotas should become more transparent and equitable.

To sum up, the expectations about reductions in domestic support or export subsidies prevailing in the developed countries at the time of conclusion of AOA have not materialised. Market access has thus been effectively denied to developing countries.

As far as India is concerned, it has been possible to maintain without any hindrance the domestic policy instruments for promotion of agriculture or for subsidised targeted supply of foodgrains. The domestic policy measures like the operation of the minimum support price (MSP), the public distribution system (PDS) as well as provision of input subsidies to agriculture have not in any way been constrained by the Agreement. In fact, certain provisions contained in Annexure 2 of the Agreement (popularly known as the 'Green Box') give us the flexibility to provide support for, research and extension services, pest and disease control, marketing and promotion services, infrastructure development, payments made for relief from natural disasters, payments under regional assistance programme for disadvantaged regions and payments under environmental programmes.

In the recent budget announcement, a tax holiday for 5 years and 30% deduction of profits from income for the next 5 years to the enterprises engaged in the integrated business of handling, transportation and storage of food grains has been given.

As agriculture constitutes a vital segment of the Indian economy, finding greater market access for India's agricultural products, especially in the developed country markets, would therefore, be one of the important issues during the negotiations. **Food security of our people, protection of the interests of domestic farmers and their livelihood as well as the need for export maximisation will be the guiding principles during the ongoing negotiations.**

MEASURES TO SAFEGUARD INDIAN AGRICULTURE

Some of the measures taken by the government in this regard are:

i. Import duties on a number of agro and other items have been increased. For example, the duty on areca nut has been raised from 35% to 100%, on poultry products from 35% to 100%, on wheat from 0% to 50%, on skimmed milk powder from 0% to 60% for imports beyond the tariff rate quota (TRQ) of 10,000 tonnes; on apple from 35% to 50%, on rice from 0% to 70%, on broken rice and paddy from 0% to 80%, and on sugar from 27.5% to 60%.

ii. In the Budget 2001-2002, customs duty on tea, coffee, copra and coconut as well as desiccated coconut has been increased from the present rate of 35% to 70%. The rate of duty on crude edible oils, except soyabean oil, which ranged from 35% to 55%, has been increased to a uniform rate of 75%. Similarly the duty on refined oils which ranged from 45% to 65% has also been hiked to 85%. Customs duty has also been enhanced on import of crude palm oil by vanaspati manufacturers from 25% to 75%. However, sick vanaspati units would pay @ 55%. It needs to be mentioned in this connection that customs duty on edible oil has to harmonize the interests of both domestic producers and consumers.

The interest of farmers would be adequately safeguarded and the Government would move swiftly whenever there is a perceptible threat on account of imports. It has also been announced in the budget that countervailing duty equivalent to state excise duty would be levied on imported alcoholic beverages.

iii. Import of all packaged commodities has been subjected to compliance of all the conditions of the standards as are applicable on the domestic packaged commodities in accordance with the Weights and Measures (Packaged commodity) Order 1977.

iv. Import of 131 products has been made subject to compliance of the mandatory Indian quality standards as applicable to domestic goods. For compliance of this requirement, all manufacturers/exporters of these products to India are required to register themselves with Bureau of Indian Standards (BIS). The list of 131 products includes various food preservatives and additives, milk powder, infant milk food, etc.

v. An Inter-ministerial Group headed by Commerce Secretary was constituted on 28/7/2000 to assess the likely impact of the removal of QRs on imports and to suggest suitable corrective measures. Departments of Agriculture and Cooperation; Consumer Affairs; Small Scale Industries and Agro and Rural Industries; Chemicals and Petro-chemicals; Fertilisers; Petroleum and Natural Gas; Animal Husbandry and Dairying as well as the Ministries of Heavy Industries and Public Enterprises and Information Technology have been represented in the Group.

Although maintenance of quantitative restrictions (QRs) on imports is not permitted as per Article XI of GATT, the government can, if the situation so warrants, utilise the mechanism of raising the applied tariffs within the bound rates, if such a gap exists and take measures such as anti-dumping action, safeguard actions and imposition of countervailing duties, which are permissible under certain specified circumstances under the WTO Agreements, in order to provide protection to the domestic producers. Imports are being closely monitored and the government is determined to ensure through the appropriate use of the above mechanisms that imports do not cause any serious injury to the domestic producers.

AGRICULTURAL IMPORTS

From the import data for the period April–October 2000, it is seen that the import of wheat, rice, coffee, fresh fruits, millets, sugar cane individually have not been more than Rs 15 crores, which is insignificant compared to the total domestic production of these items.

Increase in imports of certain agricultural commodities like edible oil, areca nut, skimmed milk powder was noticed recently. In case of edible oils (crude and refined), the duties have been regularly revised to check the growth in imports. Similarly import duty on skimmed milk powder and areca nut have also been increased. The increase in duty on skimmed milk powder has been very effective and the imports have come down heavily. The total import of this item, which stood at Rs 101 crores during the year 1999-2000, has come down to less than Rs 3 crores during the first 7 months of the financial year, 2000-2001.

There are apprehensions in certain quarters that the prices of tea, coffee, pepper, natural rubber, raw jute, milk and cream have declined significantly on account of a surge in imports. Whereas prices are mainly a function of demand and supply, the demand for a particular product depends to a great extent on consumer preferences. An analysis of the import data (Table 26.1) reveals that there has been no significant surge in the imports of these items. It will not be correct in general to attribute the present decline in domestic prices of such commodities except edible oils to import surges or to our WTO commitments for the domestic sector.

Table 26.1: Import values of selected agricultural commodities *(Value in Rs. Crore)*

Items	1998-99	1999-2000	1999-2000 (April-November 1999)	2000-2001 (April-November 2000)
Coconut	0	Negligible (0.37)	Negligible (0.01)	0.87
Tea	64.82	25.75	20.23	16.08
Coffee	14.39	6.50	5.31	10.75
Pepper	60.8	47.44	35.00	41.6
Natural rubber	91.17	59.78	45.40	25.5
Raw jute	86.38	143.81	83.78	39.71
Milk and cream	12.31	96.90	91.45	5.66
Edible oil	7588.93	7983.8	6240.61	4472.03

HIGHLIGHTS OF INDIAN PROPOSALS

India has submitted its initial negotiating proposals to the World Trade Organisation (WTO) for the mandated negotiations under the Agreement on Agriculture in the areas of market access, domestic support, export competition and food security with the objective of protecting its food and livelihood security and creating increased market access opportunities with a view to promoting its agricultural exports. These proposals were approved by the Cabinet Committee on WTO matters.

India may consider submitting additional proposals including by way of clarifications or expansion of existing proposals or new issues, depending on the developments in the ongoing negotiations in the WTO Committee on Agriculture.

Indian proposals submitted to WTO can broadly be classified into the following two categories:

i. Increasing the flexibility enjoyed by developing countries by creation of a 'Food Security Box' for providing domestic support to the agriculture sector under the special and differential provisions as also further strengthening of trade defence mechanisms with a view to ensuring the food security and to take care of livelihood concerns.

ii. Demanding of substantial and meaningful reductions in tariffs including elimination of peak tariff and tariff escalation, substantial reductions in domestic support and elimination of export subsidies by the developed countries so as to get meaningful market access opportunities.

The Proposals in the First Category

- Additional flexibility for providing subsidies to key farm inputs for agricultural and rural development.
- Exemption from any reduction commitments of measures taken by developing country members for alleviation of poverty, rural development, rural employment and diversification of agriculture.
- Exclusion from AMS calculations of product specific support given to low income and resource poor farmers.
- Clarifications on certain implementation issues, such as, offsetting of positive non-product specific support with negative product specific support, suitable methodology of notifying domestic support in stable currency to take care of inflation and depreciation.
- Rationalisation of product coverage of AoA by inclusion of certain primary agricultural commodities such as rubber, jute, coir, etc.
- Flexibility enjoyed by developing countries in taking certain measures in accordance with other WTO covered Agreements should not be constrained by the provisions of AoA.
- Maintenance of appropriate level of tariff bindings on agricultural products in developing countries, keeping in mind their developmental needs and high distortions prevalent in the international markets with a view to protect livelihood of their farming population. Also linking the appropriate levels of tariffs in developing countries with trade distortions in the areas of market access, domestic support and export competition.
- Rationalisation of low tariff bindings in developing countries, which could not be rationalised in the earlier negotiations.
- Separate safeguard mechanisms on the lines of SSG including a provision for imposition of QRs in the event of a surge in imports or a decline in international prices, as an S and D measure to protect food security and livelihood concerns.
- No minimum market access commitments for developing countries.

The Proposals in the Second Category

- Blue box and decoupled and direct payments in Green Box to be included in the Amber Box to be subjected to reduction commitments.
- Accelerated reduction in AMS so as to bring it below *de minimis* by the developed countries in 3 years and by the developing countries in 5 years.

- Substantial reduction in tariff bindings including elimination of peak tariffs and tariff escalation in developed countries.
- Expansion and transparent administration of TRQs pending their eventual abolition.
- Elimination through accelerated reduction in export subsidies and disciplining of all forms of export subsidisation, etc.
- Abolition of Peace Clause for developed countries.

QANDA: TRADE IN AGRICULTURE—URUGUAY ROUND AND AFTER: A BRIEF GLIMPSE

Q.1. What was the role of India with regard to agriculture in WTO/GATT?

Ans. India was one of the leading developing nations which initiated from the very beginning of the Uruguay Round of discussions at Punta Del Este in September 1986, that "Agriculture" should be brought within the purview of GATT. The need for liberalisation in the world trade in agriculture was felt due to extensive subsidisation by the developed countries which led to distortion in the prices of agricultural commodities. As a result, the poor and developing countries like India were finding it difficult to have access to the markets of agricultural products in the developed and developing countries.

Q.2. Will the agreement on agriculture jeopardise subsidies to our farm sector?

Ans. There has been a concern that subsidy for Indian farmers will no longer be possible under WTO Agreement on Agriculture.

The concern is misplaced because India is under no obligation under the WTO Agreement on Agriculture to reduce any of the subsidies given to our farmers. This is because the total aggregate value of subsidies given to farmers namely, subsidies on fertilizers, electricity, seeds, pesticides and cost of credit available to all crops as well as agricultural commodities is well below the ceiling prescribed in the Uruguay Round agreement.

An opinion is sometimes expressed that subsidy, both product-specific and non-product-specific, to the farm sector might get jeopardised due to the GATT Accord. Some sort of support, both product-specific and non-product-specific, is needed to achieve the objective of food security and to be self-sufficient in food production. Calculations have been made that in the base years 1986-87, 1987-88 and 1988-89, both product-specific and non-product-specific subsidies provided by the Government of India to the farming sector, without taking into account the concessions provided for in the Agreement, were negative to the extent of Rs 19,000/- crores. This implies that we would have to further subsidize agriculture to the tune of Rs 19,000/- crores to even come in the range of positive subsidies let alone above 10%, which is a near impossibility in the foreseeable future. *Hence the agreement would impose no obligation whatsoever on us to make any reduction in the present levels of agricultural subsidies."*

Moreover, developing countries have been provided three additional exemptions, namely: (1) investment subsidies which are generally available to agriculture; (2) agricultural input subsidies generally available to low-income or resource-poor producers; and (3) domestic support to producers to encourage diversification from growing illicit narcotic crops.

Q.3. Will India's farm sector be affected by imports as a result of the minimum market access provisions?

Ans. The concern about minimum market access in agriculture is also misplaced. India in its schedule filed in the WTO at the time of signing the Uruguay Round had indicated that it was not under any obligation to provide minimum market access, on account of it being under BOP problems. Even in the event of removal of quantitative restrictions (QRs) maintained on balance of payment (BOP) grounds, during the implementation period India would not be obliged to provide any minimum market access. The then Minister for Commerce had stated: "...imports at tariff rate of 100% for primary agricultural products, 150% for processed agricultural products and 300% for edible oils as bound by us, would be prohibitive and make imports an extremely unviable proposition. *Hence the apprehension that the Indian market would be flooded with imported agricultural goods is unfounded".*

Q.4. Supposing import of some articles increases to our detriment, what should we do?

Ans. In case any import surge is noticed or apprehended, Government can suitably calibrate the applied rates of custom duties within the bound rates and can also initiate trade remedial measures including anti-dumping action, imposition of countervailing action or safeguard action under specific circumstances as provided under WTO agreements.

Q.5. Will the WTO agreement affect our public distribution system (PDS)?

Ans. No. It is to be noted that operations of PDS in India are not subsidies to the farmer or the producer, but are consumer subsidies meant for the rural and urban poor to meet their food requirements. Such consumer subsidies are exempt from WTO discipline, and this is clearly written in the Agreement. Further, India has stated in its Schedule of Commitments in WTO that concessional sales of foodgrains through the PDS and other schemes with the objective of meeting the basic food requirements as a social safety net are in conformity with the provisions of the Agreement. The schedule has been verified and accepted by our trading partners. The apprehension is, therefore, baseless.

Q.6. Will the WTO agreement interfere with India's ability to follow its own agricultural policies and programmes?

Ans. No. All our developmental schemes can be continued under the WTO Agreement on Agriculture. These include our subsidies for research, pest and disease control, marketing and promotion services, infrastructural services, including capital expenditure for electricity, roads and other means of transport, marketing and port facilities, irrigation facilities, drainage systems and dams, etc. For developing countries like India, there are some agricultural subsidies which are also permissible and need not be reduced. These are investment subsidies which are generally available to low income and resource poor farmers. The types of subsidies mentioned above account for the bulk of the agricultural subsidies provided in India.

We are carrying on with our policies and programmes. The Government has recently announced the first ever National Policy in Agriculture. Agricultural package for this year, inter-alia, has been designed to stimulate growth through measures to encourage better management of food economy, removal of constraints on the movement of food grains within the country, enhanced credit flow to farm sector through institutional channels (increased to Rs 64,000 crores in 2001-2002, i.e. an increase of 24%), special initiatives like the credit linked subsidy scheme for construction of cold storages and rural godowns, reduction of rate of interest (from 10 to 8.5%) for funding the storage of crops, thus enabling farmers to enhance their holding capacity to sell later at remunerative prices and excise exemptions to food processing, etc. **The Agreement, thus, does not constrain us from following our developmental policy with regard to agriculture.**

Q.7. What is the status of 'food security' in the WTO agreement?

Ans. It is enshrined in the preamble to the Agreement on Agriculture (AoA) that commitments under the reform programme for trade in agriculture should be made in an equitable way among all members, having regard to non-trade concerns, including food security. Article 20 of the Agreement, which mandates negotiations for continuation of the reform process, also recognises that non-trade concerns, such as food security should be taken into account in the negotiations.

Q.8. What is 'food security'?

Ans. Food security as defined by FAO is the physical and economic access for all people at all times to enough food for an active, healthy life with no risk of losing such access and as such is directly connected with livelihood in the developing countries.

The Bali Declaration of the non-aligned movement and other developing countries defined food security as *access to food for a healthy life by all people at all times (NAM, 1994)*. It recognised that, in spite of a substantial increase in the world's food output, the number of people suffering from hunger and malnutrition has increased during the last decade in many developing countries. The Bali Declaration reaffirmed that "food security should be a fundamental goal of development policy as well as a measure of its success".

"A secure food system should be equitable, meaning, as a minimum, dependable access to adequate food for all individuals and groups both now and in the future".

Q.9. What is our position regarding 'food security' in the current negotiations?

Ans. The social and economic vulnerability of agriculture in developing countries is generally reflected in parameters such as substantial contribution of agriculture to their GDP, low level of commercialisation of agriculture, low productivity, weak market orientation, preponderance of small and marginal uneconomical operational landholdings, lack of infrastructure, dependence on monsoon, susceptibility to natural calamities, and dependence of a very large percentage of population on agriculture for their livelihood, etc. Such vulnerability fully justifies the extension of special provisions to the developing country members for ensuring their food and livelihood security concerns.

For all the above reasons and also because it would not be possible for developing countries to provide alternative sources of employment for the rural poor, it is critically important that agriculture remains a viable source of livelihood to the large percentage of population dependent on it.

Accordingly, it is felt that food security which is not only of great economic relevance but also a very important socio-political concern in large agrarian economies like India needs to be addressed upfront in the ongoing negotiations on agriculture.

Q.10. What is the present status of WTO negotiations on agriculture?

Ans. The agreement on agriculture was a part of the Uruguay Round of agreements which were negotiated during the period 1986-1993 and was signed in April 1994 at Marrakesh. It came into force on 1.1.1995. The Final Act of Uruguay Round signed by 120 countries brought in for the first time the liberalisation of world trade in agriculture. It was decided at the time of signing of the agreement in 1994 itself that negotiations for further progressive liberalisation and to take care of problems, issues and concerns arising from the existing agreement on agriculture should start on 1.1. 2000. Accordingly, such mandated negotiations have commenced. Initial proposals for negotiations are being received in the WTO. As agriculture is the bone of contention for developed and developing countries, WTO – watchers feel that the negotiations are likely to continue for a few years as there are serious differences amongst the major players.

Q.11. What are the perceived benefits for developing countries because of the WTO agreement on agriculture?

Ans. The agreement is perceived as likely to create opportunities for our agricultural exports. For that to happen the industrialised countries have to substantially reduce their subsidies and provide increased market access. However, the OECD countries have increased their total support to agriculture from US \$308 bn in 1986-88 to US \$361 bn in 1999. Reduction of their subsidies will naturally raise the prices of agricultural products in the world market and this will make our exports more competitive. Liberalisation measures in agriculture world-wide will create market openings which will be available to us provided we rise up to make use of the opportunities.

India would be a net gainer from trade liberalisation and rural incomes would rise. Countries like India could benefit not only from improved market access opportunities in the developed and developing countries, but also from the reduction of subsidised exports and trade-distorting production incentives prevailing in developing countries".

These are the expectations according to many experts, provided the developed countries agree to substantially reduce their huge subsidies and mega-tariffs according to the letter and spirit of the Accord.

Q.12. How optimistic can we be in thinking that India will succeed in getting the approval of all proposals from all countries at the WTO?

Ans. The extensive use of subsidy and the protectionist measures practised by the developed countries throughout the post World War period led to large scale distortions in the trade in agriculture products, thereby adversely affecting the export potential of the developing countries. Given the intrinsic competitive advantage of the developing countries in agriculture, as well as their dependence on agro-exports for bulk of their export earnings, a restrictive global trade regime in agriculture has been one of the most effective barriers to sustained acceleration of agricultural production and export in the third world countries.

Different countries have different interests in the multilateral regime for agriculture.

As the then Commerce Minister has stated: "When the GATT Accord is analysed, it should be kept in mind that all the provisions of an international Agreement cannot be beneficial to each and every country. Neither the mightiest power like United States of America nor a small tiny island country like Solomon Island can claim that their interests have been fully protected in this multilateral trade agreement. Hence there is one element of trade-off in all such agreements. To achieve something in one sector, it is necessary to make concessions in another." This is the general situation in all multilateral negotiations.

However, we are duty-bound and determined in our efforts to protect our vital interests along with like-minded countries.

Some Data Related to Agriculture Trade in WTO

World trade in agricultural products, 2003

Value $bn	674
Annual change %	
1980-85	–2
1985-90	9
1990-95	7
1995-2000	–1
2001	0
2002	6
2003	15
Share in world merchandise trade %	**9.2**
Share in world exports of primary products %	**41.2**

Source: WTO International Trade Statistics 2004, table IV.3, includes trade between EU members

Top 15 agricultural exporters and importers, 2003

	Value $bn	Share in world%		Value $bn	Share in world %
Exporters			**Importers**		
EU members (15)	284.14	42.2	EU members (15)	308.87	42.8
EU to rest of world	73.38	10.9	EU from rest of world	98.11	13.6
United States	76.24	11.3	United States	77.27	10.7
Canada	33.69	5.0	Japan	58.46	8.1
Brazil	24.21	3.6	China	30.48	4.2
China	22.16	3.3	Canada [c]	18.02	2.5
Australia	16.34	2.4	Korea, Rep. of	15.56	2.2
Thailand [a]	15.08	2.2	Mexico	13.85	1.9
Argentina [b]	12.14	2.1	Russian Fed. [a]	13.73	1.9
Malaysia	11.06	1.6	Hong Kong, China	10.81	-
Mexico	9.98	1.5	retained imports	6.47	0.9
			Taipei, Chinese	7.96	1.1
Indonesia	9.94	1.5	Switzerland	7.12	1.0
New Zealand	9.60	1.4	Saudi Arabia	6.26	0.9
Russian Fed. [a]	9.37	1.4	Thailand [a]	5.72	0.8
Chile	7.47	1.1	Indonesia	5.44	0.8
India [a]	7.03	1.2	Turkey	5.22	0.7
Above 15	**548.44**	**81.8**	**Above 15**	**580.44**	**80.4**

Source: WTO International Trade Statistics 2004, table IV.8. "EU members" includes trade between EU members.

[a] Includes WTO Secretariat estimates.
[b] 2002 instead of 2003
[c] Imports are valued f.o.b.

Agricultural products' share in trade, by region, 2003

	Exports	Imports		Exports	Imports
Share in total merchandise trade %			**Share in primary products trade %**		
World	9.2	9.2	World	41.2	41.2
North America	11.0	6.2	North America	56.6	32.2
Latin America	19.8	9.7	Latin America	47.2	44.0

Agricultural products' share in trade, by region, 2003 (*Contd.*)

Share in total merchandise trade%	Exports	Imports	Share in primary products trade%	Exports	Imports
Western Europe	9.6	10.4	Western Europe	57.6	48.3
C./E. Europe/Baltic States/CIS	8.8	10.1	C./E. Europe/Baltic States/CIS	22.7	47.6
Africa	13.9	15.9	Africa	20.2	59.4
Middle East	3.4	12.4	Middle East	4.4	68.0
Asia	6.3	8.9	Asia	46.3	33.2

Source: WTO International Trade Statistics 2004, table IV.5, includes trade between EU members.

How much do they spend?

Notified domestic support, 1999, and export subsidies, 1998. US$ million.

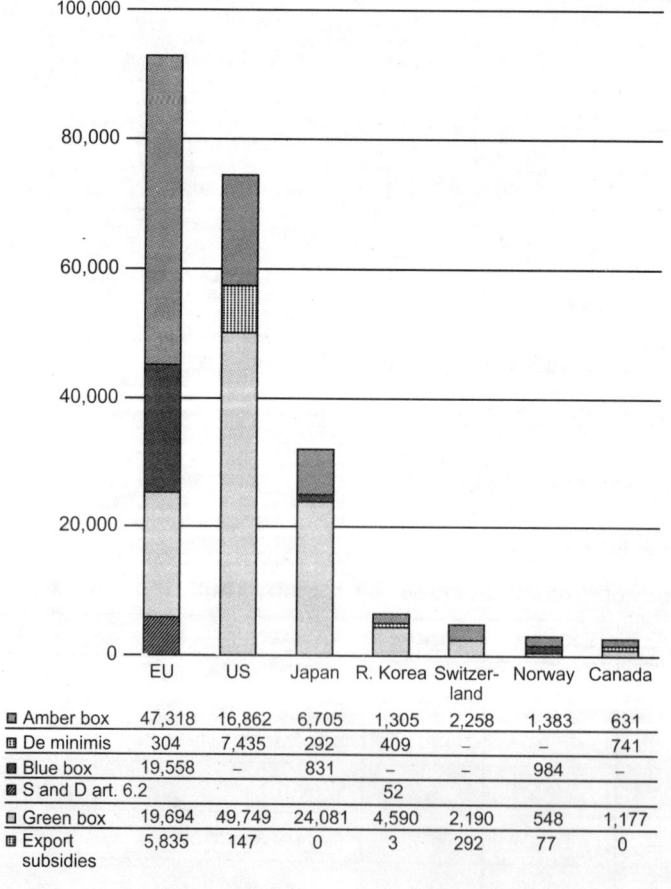

	EU	US	Japan	R. Korea	Switzerland	Norway	Canada
▣ Amber box	47,318	16,862	6,705	1,305	2,258	1,383	631
▣ De minimis	304	7,435	292	409	–	–	741
▣ Blue box	19,558	–	831	–	–	984	–
▨ S and D art. 6.2				52			
▢ Green box	19,694	49,749	24,081	4,590	2,190	548	1,177
▣ Export subsidies	5,835	147	0	3	292	77	0

Source: Member governments' notifications to WTO

PUBLIC DISTRIBUTION SYSTEM

Annexure 2 of the Agreement on Agriculture contains provisions pertaining to public stock holding for food security purposes, permitting governmental stock holding programmes for food security purposes in developing countries whose operation is transparent and conducted in accordance with officially published objective criteria or guidelines shall be considered to be in conformity with the provisions of the Agreement provided that the difference between the acquisition price and the external reference price is accounted for in the AMS.

Thus, there is no constraint on the operation of our public distribution system under the Agreement on Agriculture.

WTO AGREEMENT ON AGRICULTURE (AT A GLANCE)

- **The WTO Agreement on Agriculture was signed as part of the Uruguay Round Agreement in April 1994.** The Uruguay Round of Multilateral Trade Negotiations took place during the period 1986 to1993.
- **The WTO Agreement on Agriculture came into force with effect from 1 January, 1995. It has a 10-year implementation period from 1995 to 2004,** for developing countries.
- The WTO Agreement on Agriculture covers three broad areas of agriculture and trade policy: market access, domestic support and export subsidies.
- **India is under no obligation to reduce domestic support or subsidies** currently extended to agriculture as the support being given is well below the permissible level of 10% of the value of its agricultural output.
- **Under the Agreement, there can be no restrictions on farm trade except through tariffs, i.e. non-tariff barriers such as quantitative restrictions on imports through quotas, import licensing, etc. are to be replaced by tariffs** or duties on imports to provide the same level of protection to domestic agriculture and thereafter, tariff levels are to be progressively reduced. **However, some developing countries like India were permitted to offer ceiling bindings** instead of tariffication on account of the fact that India was maintaining QRs on balance of payment grounds.
- **Reduction commitments on export subsidies do not apply to India** as export subsidies as are subjected to reduction commitments under the Agreement, are not practised in India.
- **The Uruguay Round of Trade Negotiations did not bring about trade liberalisation in agriculture, as expected. There has been no significant reduction in domestic as well as export subsidies given by the developed countries to their agriculture**. The anticipated increase in exports of agricultural products from developing countries, therefore, has not materialised.
- **Continuation of high domestic support to agriculture in many developed countries is a cause for concern as it leads to low international prices for farm produce**.
- **Implementation of the WTO Agreement on Agriculture since 1995 has brought out the inadequacies** inherent in the Agreement. **The ongoing**

negotiations in the WTO on the Agreement on Agriculture present an opportunity for us to rectify these inadequacies and inequalities.

- **Government have taken a series of measures to safeguard our agriculture sector** in the context of phase-out of QRs, i.e. import duties on a large number of agro and other items have been substantially increased and import of 131 products have been made subject to compliance of Indian quality standards as applicable to domestic goods.

- **In the Budget 2001-2002, custom duty on tea, coffee, copra and coconut as well as desiccated coconut has been raised from 35% to 70%. Similarly, duty on refined edible oils except soyabean oil has been raised to a uniform level of 85% and on crude edible oil to 75%.**

- Although maintenance of QRs on imports is not permitted, the **government can, if the situation so warrants, raise the applied tariffs within the bound levels and also take measures such as anti-dumping action, safeguard action, levy of countervailing duties under certain circumstances as permitted under the WTO Agreement**.

- **Government have consulted all stakeholders** in preparing proposals for the WTO negotiations on agriculture. Extensive consultations have been held with the State Governments, farmers' organisations, political parties, NGOs, agricultural universities, experts and academicians and all other stakeholders in formulating the proposals and these consultations will be a continuing process.

27

Creating and Sustaining Organizational Culture: A Dynamic Perspective

Manish Sharma

The idea of viewing organizations as cultures—where there is a system of shared meaning among members—is a relatively recent phenomenon. Until the mid 1980s, organizations were, for most part, simply thought of as rational means by which to coordinate and control a group of people (Robbins, 2003), which have vertical levels, departments, authority relationships, and so forth. But organizations are more than that. They have personalities too, just like individuals which can be rigid or flexible, unfriendly or supportive, innovative or conservative (Weinber, 1998). For example, general electric offices and people are different from the offices and people at general mills. Harvard and MIT are in the same business of education—separated only by the width of the Charles River in Massachusetts, USA, but each has a unique feeling and character beyond its structural characteristics (Case, 1996). Organization theorists now acknowledge this by recognizing the important role that culture plays in the lives of organizational members.

Interestingly, though, the origin of organizational culture as an independent variable affecting an employee's attitude and behaviour can be traced back more than 50 years to the notion of institutionalization. When an organization becomes institutionalized, it takes on a life of its own, apart from its founders and any of its members (Selznick, 1948). For example, Ross Perot created electronic data systems (EDS) in the early 1960s and left in 1987 to establish a new company, Perot Systems. EDS has, however, continued to thrive despite the departure of its founder. Sony, Eastman, Kodak, Gillette, McDonald's, and Disney are a few other examples of organizations that have existed beyond lives of their founders or any one member and have developed their own self-initiated organizational cultures over the period of time (Timmerman, 1996). Additionally, when an organization becomes institutionalized, it becomes valued for itself and not merely for the goods and services it produces. It acquires corporate immortality. If its goods are no longer relevant, it does not go out of business. Rather it redefines itself (Miller, 1994). When the demand for Timex watches declined, the Timex Corporation merely redirected itself into consumer electronics business-making, in addition to watches, clocks, computers, and health care products such as digital thermometers and blood pressure testing devices. Timex Corp took on an existence that went beyond its original mission to manufacture low cost mechanical watches. This sense of redefining itself became a part of Timex's organizational culture (Robbins, 2003).

Hence, institutionalization operates to produce common understandings among members about what is appropriate and, fundamentally, meaningful behaviour (Powell and DiMaggio, 1991). So when an organization takes on institutional permanence, acceptable modes of behaviour, it becomes largely self-evident to its members. This is almost the same thing that organizational culture does. Hence, an understanding of what makes up an organization's culture, and how it is created, sustained, and learned, further enhances the manager's ability to explain and predict the behaviour of people at work. This section leads to an analytical probe into the concept and nature of organizational culture along with a basic reference to its primary characteristics.

ORGANIZATIONAL CULTURE: AN ANALYTICAL OVERVIEW

Armstrong (1999) said that the organizational culture is the pattern of values, norms, beliefs, attitudes and assumptions that may not have been articulated but shape the ways in which people behave and things get done. Values refer to what is believed to be important about how people and the organizations behave. Norms are unwritten rules of behaviour (Armstrong, 1999). This definition emphasizes that organizational culture is concerned with abstractions such as values and norms which pervade the whole or part of an organization. There seems to be wide agreement that organizational culture refers to a system of shared meaning held by members that distinguishes the organization from other organizations (Becker, 1982). This system of shared meaning is a set of key characteristics that the organization values. O'Reilly III, Chatman and Caldwell (1991) suggests that there are seven primary characteristics that, in aggregate, capture the essence of an organization's culture:

- **Innovation and risk-taking:** The degree to which employees are encouraged to be innovative and take risks.
- **Attention to detail:** The degree to which employees are expected to exhibit precision, analysis, and attention to detail.
- **Outcome orientation:** The degree to which management focuses on results or outcomes rather than on the techniques and processes used to achieve those outcomes.
- **People orientation:** The degree to which management decisions take into consideration the effect of outcomes on people within the organization.
- **Team orientation:** The degree to which the work activities are organized around teams rather than individuals.
- **Aggressiveness:** The degree to which people are aggressive and competitive rather than easy-going.
- **Stability:** The degree to which the organizational activities emphasize maintaining the status quo in contrast to growth.

Each of these characteristics consists on a continuum from low to high. Appraising the organization on these seven characteristics, then, gives a composite picture of the organization's culture (Robbins, 2003). This picture becomes the basis for feelings of shared understanding that members have about the organization, how things are done in it, and the way members are supposed to behave. Organizational culture is, therefore concerned with how employees perceive the characteristics of organization's culture, not with whether or not they like them. Organizational culture represents a common perception held by the organization's members. It is widely accepted that individuals with different backgrounds or at different levels in the organization will tend to describe the organization's culture in similar terms (Frost, Moore, Louis, Lundberg and Martin, 1991). It is this 'shared meaning' aspect of organizational culture that makes it such a potent device for guiding and shaping behaviour. That is what determines, e.g. Microsoft's culture which values aggressiveness and risk-taking (Hamm, 1998). This gives the managers the insight and information to better understand the behaviour of Microsoft's executives and employees. It can be concluded that organizational culture provides stability to an organization. Furthermore, every organization has a culture and, depending on its strength, it can have a significant influence on the attitudes and behaviours of organization's members. In order to successfully understand the culture of an organization, it is important first of all to understand how culture begins in an organization.

Beginning of Organizational Culture

An organization's culture does not pop out of thin air. Once established, it rarely fades away. An organization's current customs, traditions, and general ways of doing things are largely due to what it has done before and the degree of success it has had with those endeavours. This leads to the ultimate source of organization's culture: its founders (Schein, 1983). The founders of an organization traditionally have a major impact on that organization's early culture. They have a vision of what organization should be. They are unconstrained by the previous customs and ideologies. The small size that typically characterizes new organizations further facilitates the founder's imposition of their vision on all organizational members.

The process of culture creation occurs in three ways (Schein, 1983): First, founders only hire and keep employees who think and feel the way they do. Second, they indoctrinate and socialize these employees to their way of thinking and feeling. And finally, the founder's own behaviour acts as a role model that encourages employees to identify with them and thereby internalize their beliefs, values and assumptions. When the organization succeeds, the founder's vision is seen as a primary determinant of that success. At this point, the founder's entire personality becomes embedded in the culture of the organization.

To substantiate this, citing the example of **Sony** will be quite appropriate as Sony can truly be viewed as **the Essence of Akio Morita.** Akio Morita, Sony Corporation's co-founder had such a tremendous influence on the company's culture that people often referred to him as Mr.Sony. Morita was described as a passionate lover of music and art, a workaholic, a great socialiser, a brilliant observer of people's behaviour, and a man with an unbounding energy, a relentless drive, and a determined focus. Morita applied these qualities in pursuing his vision of creating a brand name for products that appealed to people worldwide. He chose a short, catchy name for his company so people everywhere could easily pronounce and remember it. Morita began his globalization strategy in the United States, where he moved his family so that he could study American culture and increase Sony's chance of success. Today, Sony is recognized throughout the world as a leading brand name (Adler, 1997).

Citing another recent example, **Southwest Airlines** can be aptly described as **Herbert Kelleher's passion**. The actions of Herbert Kelleher, Southwest Airlines' Chief Executive, had a strong influence on the company's casual, fun-loving culture. He stars in the company's orientation film, where new employees see their leader singing and dancing. Kelleher models the light-hearted behaviour he expects of his employees so they, in turn, know that it is okay as a part of providing exceptional customer service, to have fun with the airline's passengers (Timmerman, 1996).

Similarly, the culture at **Hyundai**, the giant Korean Conglomerate, is largely a reflection of its founder **Chung Ju Yung**. Hyundai's fierce, competitive style and its disciplined, authoritarian nature are the same characteristics used to describe Chung (Gowler, Legge and Clegg, 1993). Other contemporary examples of founders who have had an immeasurable impact on their organization's culture include: Bill Gates at Microsoft, David Packard at Hewlett-Packard, Fred Smith at Federal Express, Mary Kay at Mary Kay Cosmetics, and Richard Branson at the Virgin Group.

Components of Organizational Culture

The culture of an organization represents a complex pattern of shared values, norms and artefacts which are characteristics of the organization (Berman, 1986). Hence, organizational culture can be said to comprise of three different components viz. values, norms and artefacts. These terms are further described below.

Values: Values are the beliefs in what is good for the organization and what should or ought to happen. The 'value set' of an organization may only be recognized at top level, or it may be shared throughout the business, in which case the organization could be described as value-driven. The stronger the values, the more they will influence behaviour. This does not depend upon their having been articulated. Implicit values that are deeply embedded in the culture of the organization and are reinforced by the behaviour of the management can be highly influential, while espoused values that are idealistic and are not expressed in the managerial behaviour may have little or no effect. Some of the most typical areas in which values can be expressed, implicitly, or explicitly are: performance, competence, competitiveness and teamwork (Griffin, 1982).

Norms: Norms are the unwritten rules of behaviour, the 'rules of the game' that provide informal guidelines on how to behave. Norms tell people what they are supposed to be doing, saying, believing and even wearing. They are never expressed in writing—if they were, they would be policies or procedures. They are passed on by the word of mouth or behaviour and can be enforced by the reactions of the people if they are violated. They can exert very powerful influence on the behaviour because of these reactions—people are controlled by the way others react to them. Norms can be very well illustrated by the prevailing work ethics, e.g. 'work hard, play hard', 'come in early, stay late', 'look busy at all times' or 'look relaxed at all times' (Whitsett, 1975).

Artefacts: Artefacts are the visible and tangible aspects of an organization that people hear, say or feel. Artefacts can include such things as the working environment, the tone and language used in letters and memoranda, the manner in which people address each other at meetings or over the telephone, the welcome (or lack of welcome) given to the visitors and the way in which receptionists deal with outside calls. Artefacts can be very revealing (Ford, 1973).

Organizational Culture's Functions

After having described what an organizational culture is, along with its origin and components, it will be appropriate to probe into the wide array of meaningful functions performed by the organizational culture for the organization.

Staw and Cummings (1996) described that organizational culture performs a number of functions within an organization. First, it has a boundary-defining role, i.e. it creates distinctions between one organization and others. Second, it conveys a sense of identity for organizational members. Third, organizational culture facilitates the generation of commitment to something larger than one individual's self-interest. Fourth, it enhances, social system stability. Organizational culture is therefore, the social glue that helps hold the organization together by providing appropriate standards of what employees should say and do. Finally, organizational culture serves as a sense-making and control mechanism that guides and shapes the attitudes and behaviour of the employees. The role of organizational culture in influencing employees' behaviour appears to be increasingly important in today's work-place. As organizations have widened the spans of control, flattened structures, introduced teams, reduced formalization, and empowered employees, the shared meaning provided by a strong culture ensures that everyone is pointed in the same direction (Robbins, 2003). For instance, the employees at Disney theme parks appear to be almost universally attractive, clean and wholesome looking, with bright smiles. That is what the organizational culture at Disney imbibes and conveys. The company selects employees who will maintain that image. And once on the job, a strong organizational culture, supported by the formal rules and regulations, ensures that Disney-theme park employees will act in a relatively uniform and predictable way (Case, 1996). Also, to illustrate the notion of shared meaning, 'Yahoo! Incorporation.' presents a good example. The shared meaning provided by Yahoo! Inc.'s strong organizational culture is stated in the company's motto—'Do what's crazy, but not stupid.' The motto guides employees as they develop entertaining programmes and services that grab the attention of today's internet users. Employee creativity is the key to keeping 'Yahoo!' the leading search engine on the internet. 'Yahoo!' hires young net enthusiastics who thrive in an informal setting where there are few rules and regulations to stifle the creative process (Armstrong, 1999).

Sustaining Organizational Culture

How Employees Adopt Culture

Once an organizational culture is in place, there are practices within the organization that act to maintain it by giving employees a set of similar experiences (Harrison and Carrol, 1991). Culture is transmitted to employees in a number of forms, the most potent being stories, rituals, material symbols and language (Adler, 1997).

Stories: During the days when Henry Ford II was the chairman of the Ford Motor Co., one would have been hard pressed to find a manager who had not heard the story about Mr.Ford reminding his executives, when they got too arrogant, that "its my name that is on the building." The message was clear: Henry Ford II ran the company (Robbins, 2003). Stories such as that circulate through many organizations. They typically contain a narrative of events about the organization's founders, rule-breaking, rags-to-riches successes, reductions in the workforce, relocation of employees, reactions to past mistakes and organizational coping (Deutsch, 1991). For most of the part, these stories develop spontaneously. But some organizations actually try to manage this element of organizational culture's learning. For instance, Krispy Kreme, a large doughnut maker out of North Carolina, USA has a full time 'Minister of Culture' whose primary responsibility is to tape interviews with customers and employees. The stories these people tell are then put into company's video magazine that describes Krispy Kreme's history and values (Case, 1996). These stories anchor the present in the past and provide explanations and legitimacy for current practices.

Rituals: Rituals are repetitive sequences of activities that express and reinforce the key values of the organization; which goals are most important, and which people are important and which are expendable (Kamoche, 1995). One of the best known examples for organizational rituals is Mary Kay Cosmetics' Annual Award Meeting. Looking like a cross between a circus and a Miss America pageant, the meeting takes place over a couple of days in a large auditorium, on a stage in front of a large, cheering audience, with all the participants dressed in glamorous evening clothes. Sales women are rewarded with an array of flashy gifts—gold and diamond pins, fur stoles, pink Cadillacs—based on the success in achieving sales quota. This 'show' acts as a motivator by publicly recognizing outstanding sales performance. In addition, this ritual aspect reinforces Mary Kay's personal determination and optimism, which enabled her to overcome personal hardships, establish her own company, and achieve material success. It conveys to her sales people that reaching their sales quota is important and that through hard work and encouragement they too can achieve success (Beyer and Trice, 1987).

Material symbols: The headquarters of Alcoa, world's leading producer of primary aluminum, fabricated aluminum, and alumina, does not look like a typical head office operation. It has few individual offices. It is essentially made up of cubicles, common areas, and meeting rooms. This informal corporate headquarters convey to the employees that Alcoa values openness, equality, creativity and flexibility (Robbins, 2003). Some corporations provide their top executives with chauffeur-driven limousines and, when they travel by air, unlimited use of the corporate jet. Others may not get to ride in limousines or private jets but they might still get a car and air transportation paid for by the company. Only the car is Chevrolet (with no driver) and the jet seat is in the economy section of a commercial airliner. The layout of the corporate headquarters, the types of automobiles top executives are given, and the presence or absence of corporate aircraft, are a few examples of material symbols. Others include size of offices, the elegance of furnishings, executive perks and dress attires (Rafeli and Pratt, 1993). These material symbols convey to employees who is important, the degree of egalitarianism desired by the top management, and the kinds of behaviour (for example, Risk-taking, conservative, authoritarian, participative, individualistic, social) that are appropriate.

Language: Many organizations and units within the organizations use language as a way to identify its organizational members. By learning this language, members attest to their acceptance of the culture and, in doing so help to preserve it. For example, employees at Tattoo, a marketing services agency in San Francisco, USA use special words to convey the organization's unique culture. They call the Tattoo's three floors of office space the 'hive' because it buzzes with activity as employees move between the floors to work on different client projects. They refer to themselves as 'Tattools', because the company discourages the formal job titles and other symbols of formal authority. Unlike most marketing firms that use market research studies and focus groups for developing brand campaigns, Tattoo uses an intuitive approach it calls 'living the brand'. Employees call client presentations 'collages', a blending of music and visuals intended to show the sensory and emotional aspects of brand (Staw and Cummings, 1996). Hence, organizations, over a period of time, often develop unique terms to describe equipment, offices, key personnel, suppliers, customers, or products that relate to their business. New employees are frequently overwhelmed with acronyms and jargon that, after 6 months on the job, have become fully a part of their language. Once, assimilated, this terminology acts as a common denominator that unites members of a given organizational culture.

Organizational Culture as a Barrier

Every coin has two sides and so has organizational culture. On the one hand, organizational culture plays a very integral part in the organizations' overall conduct (Deal and Kennedy, 1983). Many of its functions are valuable to both the organizations and the employees. Organizational culture enhances organizational commitment and increases the consistency of employee behaviour. These are clearly benefits to organizations (Impoco, 1992). From an employee's standpoint, organizational culture is valuable because it reduces ambiguity. It tells employees how the things are done and what is important (Pascale, 1985). On the other hand, organizational culture can also pose to become a barrier to organizational growth and development. This fact is well-depicted in some potentially dysfunctional aspects of organizational culture and its effects on the organization, especially a strong one, on an organization's effectiveness:

A Barrier to Change

Culture is a liability when shared values are not in agreement with those that will further the organization's effectiveness. This is most likely to occur as an organization's environment is dynamic. When an organization is undergoing rapid change, organization's entrenched culture may no longer be appropriate. So consistency of behaviour is an asset to an organization when it faces a stable environment. It may, however, burden the organization and make it difficult to respond to changes in the environment (Beyer and Trice, 1987). For instance, JC Penney and Sears once ruled the USA's retail department store market. Their executives considered their markets immune to competition. Beginning in the mid 1970s, Wal-Mart did a pretty effective job of humbling Penney's and Sear's managements. General Motors' executives, safe and cloistered in their Detroit headquarters in USA, ignored the aggressive efforts by the Japanese auto firms to penetrate its markets. The result is history. General Motors's market share has been in a free fall for three decades. Toyota, once one of those aggressive Japanese firms that was successfully stealing market share from General Motors, itself became a casualty of its own success. During the first half of 1990s, having been slow to respond to the recreational vehicle market and stuck with a cumbersome vehicle development process, Toyota experienced a serious loss in market share and profit margins (Weinberg, 1996).

A Barrier to Diversity

Hiring new employees who, because of race, gender, disability, or other differences, are not like majority of the organization's members, creates a paradox (Cox, 1993). Management wants new employees to accept the organization's core cultural values. Otherwise, these employees are unlikely to fit in or be accepted. But at the same time, management wants to openly acknowledge and demonstrate support for the differences that these employees bring to the workplace. Strong cultures put considerable pressure on employees to conform. They limit the range of values and styles that are acceptable. In some instances, such as the widely publicized Texaco case (which was settled on behalf of 14000 employees for $ 176 million) in which senior managers made disparaging remarks about minorities; a strong culture that condones prejudice can even undermine formal corporate diversity policies (Labich, 1999). Organizations seek out and hire diverse individuals because of the alternative strengths these people bring to the workplace. Yet, diverse behaviours and strengths are likely to diminish in strong cultures as people attempt to fit in. Strong organizational cultures can, therefore, be liabilities when they effectively eliminate those unique strengths that people of different backgrounds bring to the organization. Moreover, strong organizational cultures can also be liabilities when they support institutional bias or become insensitive to people who are different.

A Barrier to Acquisitions and Mergers

Historically, the key factors that management looked at in making acquisitions or merger decisions were related to financial advantages or product synergy, but, in recent years, organizational cultural compatibility has become the primary concern (Berman, 1986). While a favourable financial statement or product line may be the initial attraction of an acquisition candidate, whether the acquisition actually works seems to have more to do with how well the two organizations' cultures match up. A number of acquisitions consummated in the 1990s already have failed. And primary cause is conflicting organizational cultures. For instance, AT and T's 1991 acquisition of NCR was a disaster. AT and T's unionized employees objected to working in the same building as NCR's non-union staff. Meanwhile, NCR's conservative, centralized culture did not take kindly to AT and T's insistence on calling supervisors 'coaches' and removing executive's office doors. By the time AT and T finally sold NCR, the failure of the deal had cost AT and T more than $ 3 billion. Similarly, Word-Perfect Corp. bought Novell Inc. in 1994 to give it a viable word-processing product to compete against Microsoft. But the employees and the managers from the two organizations could never see eye to eye on important issues. When Word Perfect was sold to Corel Corp. in 1996, Novell got $ 1 billion less than it had paid just two years earlier (Robbins, 2003). Hence, it is clearly evident from the above real-life corporate examples that rigid organizational cultures can pose to be significant barriers to the organization's future growth and development.

Organizational Cultures in the 21st Century

Any group of people who have worked together for some time, any organization of long standing, indeed, any state or national body over a period of time develops a philosophy and a series of traditions. These are unique and they fully define the organization, setting it aside for better or worse from similar organizations (Denison, 1984).

To cite an example from the fast-moving, ever changing information technology world, this paper dwells into Hewlett-Packard which is a leading giant in the computer and information technology business. At Hewlett-Packard, whole of its organizational culture goes under the general heading of the 'H-P Way'. In general terms, 'H-P Way' is the policies and actions that flow from the belief that men and women want to do a good job, a creative job, and that if they are provided with the proper environment, they will do so. But that's only a part of it. Closely coupled with this is the H-P tradition of treating each individual with consideration and respect and recognizing personal achievements. This really catches the essence of the 'H-P Way'. It cannot be described in number and statistics. Basically, it is the spirit, a point of view. It is a feeling that everyone is the part of a team, and that team is Hewlett- Packard. It exists because people have seen that it works, and they believe in it and support it. The belief is that this feeling makes Hewlett-Packard what it is, and that it is worth perpetuating. And this belief forms the crux of Organizational Culture at Hewlett-Packard (Kilmann, 1985).

This example provides some insight into the organizational culture of Hewlett-Packard. In many respects, its culture is unique in itself and is very different from that of IBM or Apple Computers or Texas Instruments. In fact, two organizations might be in essentially the same business, be located in the same geographic area, have similar form of organizational structure, and yet be, somehow, very different as places to work. This difference can be credited, to a large extent, to different organizational cultures unique to an organization itself (Case, 1996). This goes on to substantiate the fact that a strong organizational culture can affect employees' behaviours and commitment to the organization in a significant manner.

Sustaining Basics and Developing Variable Aspects of Organizational Culture: Conclusion

In the end, it would be wise to acknowledge the fact that in order to make organizational cultures work for the organization, we have to sustain some of the basic aspects of the organizational culture as they provide stability to the organization, while developing certain variable aspects of organizational cultures in order to equip the organization to survive in a dynamic environment of today's modern day corporate world. An organization's culture is largely made up of relatively stable characteristics. It develops over many years and is rooted in deeply held values to which employees are strongly committed. In addition, they are a number of forces continually operating to maintain a given culture. These would include written statements about the organization's mission and philosophy, the design of the physical space and buildings, the dominant leadership style, hiring criteria, entrenched rituals, popular stories about key people and events, past promotion practices, the organization's historic performance evaluation criteria, and the organization's formal structure (Beyer and Trice, 1987). Selection and promotion policies are particularly important devices that work for sustaining the basics of organizational culture. Employees choose an organization because they perceive their own values to be a good fit with the organization. They become comfortable with that fit.

Hence, one of the most important managerial implications of organizational culture relates to the selection decisions. Hiring individuals whose values do not align with those of the organization is likely to lead to employees who lack motivation and commitment and who are dissatisfied with their jobs and the organizations. Employees form an overall subjective perception of the organization based on such factors as degree of risk tolerance, team emphasis, and support of people. This overall perception becomes, in effect, the organization's culture or personality (Case, 1996). These favourable or unfavourable perceptions then affect employee performance and satisfaction, with impact being greater for stronger cultures. Just as people's personalities tend to be stable over time, so too strong cultures do. This makes strong cultures difficult for managers to change. When a culture becomes mismatched to its environment, management would want to change it. But changing an organization's culture is a long and difficult process. The result, at least in the short-term, is that managers should treat their organization's culture as relatively fixed. Robbins (2003) says that culture is largely stable in nature but that does not mean it cannot be changed. In the unusual case when an organization confronts a survival-threatening crisis— a crisis that is universally acknowledged as a true life-or-death situation— members of the organization will be responsive to efforts at cultural change. Hence, changing an organization's culture is extremely difficult, but cultures can be changed. Roth (1998) suggests that cultural change is most likely to take place when most or all of the following conditions exists:

First condition is of a **dramatic crisis**. This is the shock that undermines the status quo and calls into question the relevance of the current culture. Examples of this crisis might be a surprising financial setback, the loss of a major client or customer base, or a dramatic technological breakthrough by a competitor.

Second condition is of **turnover in leadership**. This happens basically when the new top leadership, which can provide an alternative set of key values, may be perceived as more capable of responding to the crisis.

Third is the case of **young and small organizations**. The younger the organization the less entrenched its culture will be. Similarly, it is easier for the management to communicate its new values when the organization is small and young.

And finally, there is the case of a **weak culture**. The more widely held the culture and the higher the agreement among members on its values, the more difficult it will be to change. Conversely, weak cultures are more amendable to change than strong ones.

If the preceding conditions exist, the following actions may lead to change: new stories and rituals need to be set in place by top management; employees should be selected and promoted who espouse these new values and the reward system needs to be changed to support the new values. Under the best of conditions, these actions would not result in an immediate or dramatic shift in the prevailing organizational culture. This is because cultural change is a lengthy process—measured in years rather than in months. But cultures can be changed.

28

Micro-credit Facility for Women: The Benign Paradox

Shalini Agarwal, Deepa Vinay, Nirmal Kaur

Woman is often described as the better half of man, but the actual condition of women in the world does not match with this concept. By and large across the world, women have not achieved equality with men.

In India, women constitute about 48% of the population but their participation in economic activity is only 34%. There is a continuing concentration of women in low paid and low status occupations which indicates marginalization of women in the labour force.

There is a common assumption that men are the bread earner and that most of the female work is either done in the leisure time or serves as the procurer of supporting income for the family.

It is believed that economic strength is the basis of social, political and psychological power in the society. Thus, the lower status of women mostly stems from the low economic status and subsequent dependence and lack of decision-making power. A woman will gain visibility and voice, if her economic strength is increased.

With the spread of education and awareness, women have shifted from the limits of kitchen to non-traditional higher levels of activities. In fact women's contribution and participation in economic activity and production of goods and services is much greater than statistics reveal, since much of it takes place in the informal sector and also in the households.

Financial institutions and banks have also set up special cells to assist women entrepreneurs. The result has been the emergence of women entrepreneurs on the economic scene in recent years though the number of enterprises initiated by women is still quite low.

Because for women there are several handicaps to enter into and manage business ownership due to conservative and orthodox Indian society.

Poverty alleviation is about re-distribution, about sacrifices by the rich and about cross-subsidy, i.e. how can the poor be a profitable market, how can their purchase be profitable for them as well as for whoever is selling to them? In most fields, as health, education and basic foodstuff, "doing well doing good" is just not possible; therefore, we need aid from different organizations, taxation and the whole of non-commercial transfer of resources.

Lending money to poor people to enable them to increase their income through micro-enterprise may be one activity where this goal is possible, where every one can benefit, where nobody is the loser and where enlightened self-interest can coincide with the relief of poverty.

While cooperatives, savings and credit groups and micro-credit have been recognized as effective tools for poverty alleviation and economic development in rural areas, community-based saving and credit systems and micro-finance schemes have emerged only quite recently as strategic ways of improving the economic status of the urban poor. This has been partly due to the increasing emphasis on self-employment and the need to find finance and credit mechanism to support small enterprises and self-help activities.

In less than a decade, savings and credit movements and micro-finance schemes have become a vogue within international government and non-government organizations dealing with development issues in slum and squatter communities of Asia.

WHY MICRO-CREDIT?

Micro-credit has everything, i.e. participation, flexibility, community ownership and best of all women's empowerment.

It is a hand-aid solution to poverty and an easy way of side stepping structural issues and making the poor responsible for finding solution to their own problem and if the objective is poverty alleviation rather than its elimination, micro-credit may at best provide better solution.

There are arguments for emphasizing access to micro-credit in poverty alleviation strategies.

- The poor remain enmeshed in poverty because they are unpaid or earn an inadequate return for their time/labour, if they are self-employed.
- Having little or no savings or assets of their own, the poor are cut off from conventional credit sources at market interest rates and forced to borrow from land lords, informal sectors at usurious interest rates.

These two factors, i.e. low income and lack of credit are interdependent. For example, petty traders usually have to borrow to buy the items that they hawk and repay the money back in the evening, which cuts their profit and reduce their income.

Saving and Credit: Benefits

Community-based savings and credit groups have emerged as an effective medium through which credit can reach to the poor. Most of these savings are pioneered by local and international NGOs.

In this scheme, the members of poor community play the central role in accumulating the savings, setting the terms of credit and guaranting that money borrowed are paid back. This helps to strengthen the confidence and commitment of the individual members and helps them to improve their livelihood and lifestyle. It also feeds their capacity for community development.

These groups provide an organizational base in poor communities that can endure. These groups have a continuing relevance to people lives even when their economic situation has significantly improved.

After observing and witnessing the success of different savings and credit schemes, several National government agencies and international and bilateral donors were impressed. Organizations like the Urban Community Development Office in Thailand, established in 1992, promoted the formation of savings and credit groups in urban low income communities and provided them funds in the form of loans for income generating activates and environmental improvement. Supporters of commercially inspired micro-credit like the Consultative Group to Assist the Poorest (CGAP) to the World Bank seems to see micro-lending as an end itself.

Thus, many organizations, provide a base in poor communities that can endure. These groups have a continuing relevance to people lives even when their economic situation has significantly improved.

Saving and Credit: Warrant

Women entrepreneur face problem due to lack of access to funds because women do not possess any tangible security and credit in the market. Since women do not enjoy right over poverty of any forms, they have limited access over external sources of funds.

- There is a tendency among saving and credit institutions to report unrealistic levels of repayment, year in and year out. This creates an unnecessary pressure on their low-income membership and prevents the development of mechanism to deal with default.
- It is seen that these schemes benefit the people on and just below the poverty line than they bring to those who are far below it.
- When these organizations grow big and amounts of money become large, reliable leadership, competent and transparent management is required. There is a chance of corruption or inadequate management system.
- There is concern in some quarters that saving and credit as well as micro-credit organization seek to provide financial services that might be better delivered by other financial institutions.
- Another criticism raised is that micro-finance institutions do not alter the status quo in countries in which they are operating.
- The interest rates from the donor or organizing institution are much higher than the market interest rates.
- Institutional micro-credit, may not be as profitable as appear to have the potential to benefit poor people with little or no subsidy.

The participation of commercial banks in micro-financial is rare. Bank has been reluctant to extend credit to micro-enterprises for a number of reasons, including high risks and transaction costs and the socio-economic and actual barriers between bankers and micro-entrepreneurs. The complex and complicated procedure of bank loans, the delay in obtaining the loans and running around involved, deter many entrepreneurs in establishing enterprise.

VARIOUS SUPPORTIVE AGENCIES INVOLVED IN MICRO-CREDIT

Many NGOs that were formerly confronting the status quo on social and economic issues and decrying the market systems impact on the poor, now devoting the bulk of their efforts to setting up savings and loans group and micro-credit schemes. Whilst international NGOs and bilateral donors are very willing to fund saving and credit movements, multilateral funding agencies are increasingly eager to promote and fund micro-credit or micro-lending schemes.

Witnessing the success of different saving and credit schemes, various national, government agencies, international and bilateral donors become impressed with the impact that even the limited access to credit that community-based schemes provided has on the lives of the poor.

Some of the organizations, which provides micro-credit to the entrepreneurs, are:

- Co-operative, agricultural and rural banks and NABARD, NAFSCOB, state co-operative banks, etc.
- Various nationalized banks like SBI, UCO, Grammin Banks, UBI, OBC, different state banks, etc.
- Various non-government organizations are also working for the same like SEWA.

These banks and organization provides credit through various schemes, like SGSY, Dena Shakti, Mahila Shasktidaran Abhiyan, etc.

There are many organizations which are using saving and credit groups as a vehicle not just for the provision of credit to their membership but also for building members solidarity, self-esteem, political awareness and organizational capacity to address their social political and economical problems. They are focused on empowering their member by promoting saving culture and creating solidarity through group guarantees on individual loans and shared ownership and control to the movement by the membership.

SEWA Bank has been providing banking services to poor, self-employed women in and around the city of Ahmedabad since 1974 this project is assisting the bank to expand its rural operations. SEWA and Coaly International Institute have collaborated to develop training curricle and material to string the ability of community-based groups to manage their own finance and to prude local credit associations, which cut as intermediates between SEWA bank and community groups with bases financial counselling and business planning skills.

Friends of Women's World Banking, India is a non-profit organization and was established as an affiliate at women's worla banking (WWB) in 1982. It was created to extend as well as expand informal created supports and networks within India.

FWWB designed a revolving loan fund while provides collateral-free loans to poor women in rural and urban areas. Loans are given out through women's self-help groups, cooperatives and NGOs. They operate loan facilities that provide for there NGOs, self-help groups and federations. Citibank has pointed hands with FWWB in on-lending funds to women's saving and credit group.

NSIC (National Small Industries Corporation Ltd.) was established in 1955 by the government of India with a view to promote, aid and foster the growth of small industries in the country. It assists the small scale sector in the country. Financial service division of NSIC provides assistance to the small enterprise for production and marketing activities. It also provides working capital finance for meeting emergent needs of small enterprises and export oriented units for export development.

Micro-finance institutions combine the social mission of providing financial services to the lowest income population possible, with the financial objectives of achieving profits with the help of private financial institutions, or self-sufficiency through NGOs.

MICRO-CREDITS TO MICRO-ENTERPRISES: INDIAN CONTENT

Financial assistance to the Swarojgar is provided through loan and subsidy. The latter being minor and enabling component. Major part of investment consists of bank credit. The size of the loan depends on the nature of the project. The loan amount would be equal to the total project cost and the amount of subsidy admissible to the entrepreneurs. These interest rates are as per RBI/NABARD. The banks assess the investment requirement on the basis of unit cost, entrepreneur's needs and the viability of the scheme.

The entrepreneurs are given full amount (loan and subsidy) and they have full freedom to procure the assets themselves. They have to procure the assets within one month. The assets procured should be of standard quality and at economic prices and they should have receipt of the same.

The credit requirements of the entrepreneur are met though multiples doses. They are offered multiple doses of credit over a period of time with a second and subsequent dose enabling them to access higher amount of credit.

Regarding, subsidy, the entrepreneurs under SGSY are entitled for a subsidy of 30% of the project cost. The benefit of subsidy will accrue to the Swarojgari after he/she honors the repayment schedule of the borrowed funds.

Regarding repayment of loans, all SGSY, loans are treated as medium term loans with minimum repayment period of 5 years. Loan installments are fixed as per the unit cost approved by the NABARD. Numbers of installments are fixed as per principal amount.

Entrepreneurs are not entitled for any benefit of subsidy if the loan is fully repaid before a certain fixed period known as the lock-in-period.

In order to promote credit discipline and a sense of accountability of the community, entrepreneur's prompt repayment will entitle to wearies of the 0.5% processing-cum-monitoring fee.

CONCLUSION

There appear to be a number of approaches, where by very small amounts of loan funding can be channeled to poor people and recovered from them in a way that allows them to substantially improve their own livelihoods and also allows the financial institutions to cover the cost.

Financial services can apparently be distributed through numerous alternative channels and each producer has to select the most appropriate "marketing mix" in relations to the particular consumer he wishes to reach and credit is presumably at least as desirable a product as most fast moving consumer goods. Commercial bankers should view micro-credit not as a matter of charity but as a vast and largely untapped market opportunity.

In same circles, the micro-credit approach is being toted as a panacea for a spectrum of problems that ranges from poverty alleviation through small enterprise development to shelter development. The perception is that if you are going to help people to overcome poverty, in addition to helping them increasing their income through better livelihood, you are going to build some carefully targeted tailored credit mechanism including the cost of funds and even to make a modest profit to develop a substantial equity base for future unsubsidized expansion.

Thus, if this change of attitude can be achieved the banks themselves will be able to profitably expand their deposit base and their advances.

29

Quality Control, Grading of Meat and Meat Animals for Entrepreneurship

SK Mendiratta, N Kondaiah

India's economic progress is mainly dependent on agriculture and livestock. The contribution of animal husbandry and dairying to the total gross domestic product (GDP) is around 6%. India has a large livestock population, which accounts for 56% of the world buffalo population (97 million), 15% of world cattle population (185 million) and about 17% of world goat population (125 million). Thus India is world leader in cattle, buffalo and goat population. It holds 5th rank for sheep and poultry population and ranked 17th in pigs.

The assets and market values of outputs from livestock, i.e. cattle, buffalo, sheep, goat, pig and poultry, have been estimated to be around Rs 80,000 crores. Food products like milk, meat and eggs valued at Rs 70,000 crores, work animals contribute Rs 6,000 crores and dung may be worth of Rs 5,000 crores. At present about 14.2 million cattle, 10.3 million buffaloes, 19.2 million sheep, 47 million goats, 16 million pigs and 604 million poultry birds are slaughtered/annum (FAO 2004). Of the total meat production of 5.9 MMT, about 63.4% is coming from cattle and buffaloes, 16% from sheep and goats, 10.5% from poultry and 9.5% from pigs. There are about 3600 licensed slaughterhouses run by local bodies for domestic meat supply and 10 modern abattoirs for export of meat. A number of meat processing units also source carcasses from local slaughterhouses for processing and export of meat.

Meat is becoming an important commodity in the diet of people. The average annual per capita consumption of meat in India is about 5 kg compared to about 80 kg in some developed countries. Need for meat consumption in our country is greater both to utilize as a food resource as well as to meet nutritional requirement. A person's daily protein intake should be 1 g per kilogram of body weight for adequate nutrition and ideally 30 to 50% of the daily protein intake should be animal protein to provide an optimal range of amino acids. Average man needs a minimum 125 g/day meat or meat equivalent food. A 100 g serving of cooked meat from any of the meat animal species provides approximately 10% calories, 50% protein, 35% iron and 25-60% B complex vitamins recommended for an adult. Anaemia caused by lack of iron is one of the major nutritional problems in India and other developing countries particularly in woman and children that can be corrected by meat consumption. In addition, meat production and utilization is an employment and livelihood generating activity for a considerable number of people engaged in the meat and associated sectors.

Large variation is observed in the status of meat sector among the developed and developing countries. In India, meat sector is poorly developed and requires considerable efforts for improving the efficiency and utility of meat animals. Meat animal production is largely an activity of small holders without much emphasis on the efficiency of production. Meat production from cattle and buffaloes is largely a by-product system with use of the animals for meat production after productive or reproductive function is over. Sheep are raised for both meat and wool. Similarly goats are raised for meat and milk. Sheep and goat are largely reared in extensive system with very little practice of supplemental feeding. Pigs are largely reared for meat. However, pig production is largely through scavenging/nomadic system. In contrast to these, poultry production has gained momentum during the last 2-3 decades in our country. Large genetic resources, varying animal production practices and input services contribute for the variability in meat animals and their production potential. The utility of meat animals is further compounded by socio-economic and religious factors with limitations on the rearing, culling, transportation, slaughter and use of meat.

Slaughterhouse facilities in our country are not adequate enough to produce meat under sanitary conditions. Slaughter takes place both in authorized and unauthorized places. There are two distinct levels at which the meat is being produced in India, namely, (a) for international market and (b) for domestic market. The quality and safety of meat for international market is governed by the sanitary and phytosanitary measures given by the Office International des Epizootic (OIE), Paris. These export-oriented integrated abattoir and meat processing facilities produce hygienic meat in good sanitary conditions. For domestic market, the meat is generally produced in municipal slaughterhouses, which are old and sanitary regulations are not very strictly followed. However, the general practice of consuming meat in hot (pre-chilled) condition with adequate cooking ensures safety of the meat from food pathogens and the reported risks are quite a few.

MEAT ANIMAL PRODUCTION

Meat is the common term used to describe the edible portion of animal tissues and any processed or manufactured products prepared from these tissues. Common meat animals are cattle, buffaloes, sheep, goats, pigs and poultry. Red meat refers to the meat obtained from mammals and white meat refers to the meat obtained from poultry. Meats are also identified by the live animal from which they come. Beef refers to the meat from cattle, carabeef (buffalo meat) from buffalo, pork (pig meat) from pigs, chevon (goat meat) from goat, and mutton (sheep meat) from sheep. Poultry meat refers to meat from chickens (chicken meat), ducks (duck meat), turkeys (turkey meat) and quails (quail meat).

Meat production involves complex operations, starting from raising of animal to sale of meat by the retailers or processors. Understanding the factors that affect growth of food animals and carcass yield and quality of meat, is essential to the producer, feeder, buyer and consumers of livestock and meat. Growth and fattening processes are important in meat trade as these aspects affect the efficiency of production and determine profits and losses during production. A number of factors affect the growth of food animals, these include: breed, age, sex, maturity, plane of nutrition, disease and management.

During growth, percent contribution of muscle tissue, bone and fat varies considerably. The optimum weight or age of animal is selected based on relative contribution of muscle tissue, bone and fat to the carcass weight and quality of meat. Muscle tissue is of prime importance because this is the component that ultimately will be consumed as meat. Bone is functionally important during growth of the animal to maximize production efficiency. Optimum quantity of fat is necessary to ensure acceptable eating quality and protect the carcass or cuts during storage and handling.

Major production traits that need to be considered in a meat animal development programme are: reproductive performance, mothering ability, live weight, carcass weight, dressing percentage, fat thickness, marbling, maturity, conformation, growth and feed efficiency, carcass composition, rib eye area (*Longissimus dorsi* muscle cut surface area), kidney, pelvic and heart fat and functional qualities of meat.

SUBJECTIVE EVALUATION OF MEAT ANIMALS

Evaluation of the market value of livestock and livestock products is essential for the economic success of any livestock or meat industry enterprise. When selecting and judging meat animals, the following factors need to be taken into consideration.

General appearance: General appearance of a meat animal refers to quality, type, size and development of animal. Meat animal shall have deep rugged bodied, and masculine in appearance, shall show great power and symmetry of form, clean strong bone, smooth well-balanced finish, graceful, powerful walk, impressive style and carriage. Development of animal should be according to age, preference being given to animals showing superior growth and muscle development.

Conformation: Conformation is the build, outline, or contour of an animal. It is influenced largely by the shape and size of the muscles. Superior conformation contributes to a higher dressing percentage, a higher cutting percentage of meat to bone, and a higher cut-out value in the higher priced cuts.

Muscling: Meat animal should show muscling in the regions of the shoulder, hind quarters, loin, brisket, and neck.

Finish or condition: Finish refers to condition or amount of fat an animal is carrying. It is a major factor affecting dressing percentage, yield of retail cuts and meat quality.

Judging of Live Goat

Different steps are followed for judging different meat animals. In case of goat following steps are followed.

Side View

When viewed from the side, the neck should be short to medium in length, strong, and especially thick at the base, blending smoothly into shoulders and brisket. The rump should be long, broad, and slightly sloping with smooth, even covering of firm flesh. Hips should be wide apart and level with back. Pins wide apart and lower than hips. Tail head slightly above and neatly set between pin bones. The barrel should be uniformly deep and wide. The shoulder should be moderately heavy, strong, and well muscled.

Rear View

From the rear, the hind quarters should be full, wide and deep. Hocks should be wide apart.

Front View

When viewed from the front, the head should be medium in length, strong and masculine in appearance, muzzle broad with large open nostrils, jaw strong and even, eyes full and bright and forehead wide. The forelegs should be medium in length; squarely set, straight; and strong. Bones strong and clean. Large heart girth resulting from long, well-sprung foreribs; wide muscular chest floor between front legs; and fullness at point of elbow. Brisket should be broad, deep, muscular, and firm.

Top View

When viewed from the top, a market goat should be blocky and rectangular in appearance. The back should be broad and strong with even covering of smooth, firm flesh. The loin should be wide, full and deep. Width over the top and behind the shoulder should indicate a good spring of rib.

Almost similar parameters are considered for judging different breeds of sheep for mutton production.

Judging of Live Pig

Skeletal correctness is very important in pigs. Hogs should be free of diseases, injuries and wounds. Weight and age should be according to trade requirements. From side, body should be long and compact. Ham should be well fleshed to hocks. Top should be flat and tail setting should be high. Rump and muscle structure should be correct. Loin should be broad and long. When viewed from front, the hog should be straight legged and have adequate substance of bone. Head should be wide according to breed. When viewed from rear, the hog should stand squarely on its rear legs yet toe out slightly from the pastern down.

Judging of Large Meat Animals

In case of beef, cattle and buffaloes almost similar parameters are considered, however, more emphasis is given on general body conditions like fullness in shoulder, loin and rump regions. Animal should have sloping in shoulder, straight and strong in top. When viewed from front, the feet should point straight forward. From the rear, the animal should show prominent muscling.

TRANSPORTATION OF FOOD ANIMALS

After procurement, meat animals are transported from villages or small towns to bigger markets or slaughter houses. Proper care, management and handling of food animals during transportation is very important for:

- Preventing economic losses incurred on account of injury to animals, death and deterioration of the quality of meat.
- Implementing the existing animal welfare regulations.
- Inadequate ventilation in the transport vehicles causes loss in weight, bruising and suffocation during transport of food animals.
- Seasonal effect is also an important consideration in the transport of animals as extremes of temperatures could result in the death of animals.
- Overcrowding in pens can lead to fighting amongst livestock and the vices such as cannibalism can occur. Similarly, fewer animals than the capacity of the transport vehicle and lack of adequate partitioning in the vehicle may cause the animals to be thrown around and consequently suffer from severe injuries.
- Animals from different sources tend to fight when mixed.
- Stress susceptibility of animals, particularly the pigs and the duration and severity of transport affect the quality of meat markedly. Diseases may also occur as a result of transport stress especially when long distances and periods are involved
- Exhaustion of an animal in the last hours before slaughter may result in dark–firm–dry (DFD) meat that has lower keeping quality. On the other hand, excitation immediately prior to slaughter may result in a very rapid fall of meat pH after slaughter in pale–soft–exudative (PSE) meat, which is objectionable due to decreased yield in curing and cooking.
- When fasted during transit, animals loose weights, however, cattle lose weight less readily than sheep and sheep less readily than pigs. Fasting also results in depletion of glycogen and affects meat quality.

Basic considerations in the shipment and transport of food animals are:

- Selection of best method of transportation.
- Proper feeding prior to loading.
- Animals should be kept quiet—avoiding rough handling and beating.
- Use of partitions when necessary.
- Avoiding shipping during extremes of weather.
- Possession of required certificates, permits and complying with regulations.

Guidelines for Transport of Cattle and Buffaloes by Rail and Road (provided by the Bureau of Indian Standards) (IS: 4157 (Part-II) – 1968)

- Animals should be healthy and in good condition and should be certified by a veterinarian.
- Comfort to animals must be ensured avoiding chances of stampede.
- Proper watering and feeding should be done prior to loading and transport of animals. Optimum ventilation of the transport carriage should be ensured.

- Convenient ramps and platforms should be used for loading and unloading the animals.
- Dung should be removed as frequently as possible to keep the place clean.
- Fire accidents should be avoided by taking proper precautions.
- The average space provided per animal in truck/railway wagon shall not be less than 2 m^2.
- Ordinary goods wagon, when used for transportation, shall carry not more than 10 adult cattle or 15 calves on broad gauge, not more than 6 adult cattle or 9 calves on meter gauge and not more than 4 adult cattle 6 calves on narrow gauge.
- Cattle should be loaded parallel to the rail facing each other.
- Floor padding material shall not be less than 6 cm thick in the wagon.
- As far as possible, animals may be moved only during the nights.
- In case of truck transport vehicle fitted with a special type of tail board and padding around the sides should be used.
- Projecting nails should be removed.
- Animals should preferably face the engine to pervert cattle being frightened. Other merchandise should not be loaded while transporting.
- The speed of the truck shall not exceed 40 km per hour.

The approximate space required per cattle in truck or railway wagon shall be as under (IS14904:2001):

Class and weight of animals (kg)	Space required (sq. m.)	
	Un-horned	Horned
Calves (up to 50 kg)	0.28	0.28
Calves (50–100 kg)	0.62	0.73
Cattle/buffaloes (100–200 kg)	0.62	0.73
Cattle/buffaloes (200–300 kg)	0.86	0.96
Cattle/buffaloes (300–400 kg)	1.06	1.20
Cattle/buffaloes (More than 400 kg)	>1.27 to 1.73	>1.59 to 2.00

These figures may vary depending on animal's weight and size but also on their physical conditions, the meteorological conditions and likely journey time. The space allowance should be increased by at least 10% during hot, humid conditions.

Guidelines for Transport of Sheep and Goats by Rail and Road (IS: 4157 (Part-II)—1983).

- Only healthy animals certified by a veterinarian shall be transported.
- It is desirable not to mix sheep and goats in order to avoid stampede.
- Similarly, male stock shall not be mixed with female stock in the same compartment.

- All objects that can cause injuries shall be removed and vehicle shall be sprayed with suitable disinfectant before loading the animals.
- Floor padding material shall not be less than 5 cm thick.
- Suitable ramps shall be provided for loading and unloading, and extremes of temperatures shall be avoided.

The approximate space required per sheep and goat in truck or railway wagon shall be as under (IS14904:2001):

Class and weight of animals (kg)	Space required (sq. m.)	
	Woolen	Shorn
Lamb (up to 15 kg)	0.15	0.15
Lamb (16–20 kg)	0.18	0.16
Adult sheep/goat (21–25 kg)	0.20	0.18
Adult sheep/goat (26–55 kg)	0.3 to 0.4	0.2 to 0.3
More than 55 kg	>0.40	>0.40

These figures may vary depending on animal's breeds, weight, size and length of fleece, presence or absence of horns as well as their physical conditions, the meteorological conditions and likely journey time. The space allowance should be increased by at least 10% during hot, humid conditions.

Guidelines for Transport of Poultry (IS: 5238 (Part-II)—1982)

- Poultry shall be healthy and in good condition and certified by veterinarian.
- Poultry transported in the same container shall be of the same species and of the same age group.
- During hot weather, watering should he ensured every 6 hours.
- Overcrowding shall be avoided.
- Poultry should not be exposed to rain or extreme temperatures.
- Containers used to transport poultry shall be of such material that will not collapse or crumble and shall be ventilated.

Floor space and dimensions of containers for transportation of poultry are as under:

Kind of poultry	Minimum floor space cm²	Dimension			Maximum number in a container
		Length cm	Width cm	Height cm	
Month old chicken	75	60	30	18	24
Three-month old chicken	230	55	50	35	12
Adult chicken stock	480	115	50	45	12

Contd.

Kind of poultry	Minimum floor space cm²	Dimension			Maximum number in a container
		Length cm	Width cm	Height cm	
Geese and Turkey-Young	900	120	75	75	10
Geese and Turkey-Growing	1300	75	35	75	2
Geese and Turkey-Grown up	1900	55	35	75	1

MEAT INSPECTION

Animals are thoroughly inspected before and after slaughter. Although inspection procedures vary from country to country, they are centred around the same basic principles and may be performed by government officials, veterinarians, or plant personnel. In general, these programmes include antemortem inspection, postmortem inspection, sanitation facilities and equipment, labels and standards, compliance, residue monitoring and evaluation. Different countries have set different guidelines for meat inspection procedures. Considering these, FAO has also prepared concise guidelines on the meat inspection, which has been adopted by many countries. In general, the objectives of meat inspection programme are:

- To ensure that only apparently healthy, physiologically normal animals are slaughtered for human consumption and that abnormal animals are separated and dealt with accordingly.
- To ensure that meat from animals is free from disease, wholesome and of no risk to human health.

ANTEMORTEM INSPECTION

Antemortem inspection identifies animals not fit for human consumption. Here animals that are down, disabled, diseased, or dead (known as 4D animals) are removed from the food chain and labelled "condemned." Other animals showing signs of being sick are labelled "suspect" and are segregated from healthy animals for more thorough inspection during processing procedures. Antemortem examination helps in diagnosing certain diseases that cannot be easily diagnosed during postmortem. Diseases that can be detected at antemortem are: tuberculosis, actinobacillosis, FMD, anthrax, rabies, tetanus, black quarter, mastitis, etc.

Major objectives of antemortem inspection are to:

- Screen all animals destined to slaughter.
- Ensure that animals are properly rested and that proper clinical information, which will assist in the disease diagnosis and judgement, is obtained.
- Reduce contamination on the killing floor by separating the dirty animals and condemning the diseased animals if required by regulation.

- Ensure that injured animals or those with pain and suffering receive emergency slaughter and that animals are treated humanely.
- Identify reportable animal diseases to prevent killing floor contamination.
- Identify sick animals and those treated with antibiotics, chemotherapeutic agents, insecticides and pesticides.
- Require and ensure the cleaning and disinfection of trucks used to transport livestock.

Postmortem Inspection

Postmortem inspection is extremely important phase of meat inspection. Routine postmortem examination of a carcass should be carried out as soon as possible after the completion of dressing in order to detect any abnormalities so that products only conditionally fit for human consumption are not passed as food. All organs and carcass portions should be kept together and correlated for inspection before they are removed from the slaughter floor. Postmortem inspection of the head, viscera, and carcasses helps to identify whole carcasses, individual parts, or organs that are not wholesome or safe for human consumption. In general, postmortem inspection involves:

- Viewing, incision, palpation and olfaction techniques.
- Classifying the lesions into one of two major categories—acute or chronic.
- Establishing whether the condition is localized or generalized, and the extent of systemic changes in other organs or tissues.
- Determining the significance of primary and systemic pathological lesions and their relevance to major organs and systems, particularly the liver, kidneys, heart, spleen and lymphatic system.
- Coordinating all the components of antemortem and postmortem findings to make a final diagnosis.
- Submitting the samples to the laboratory for diagnostic support, if abattoir has holding and refrigeration facilities for carcasses under detention.
- Trimming or condemnation of any portion of a carcass or whole carcass that is abnormal or diseased.

MEAT GRADING

Meat grading segregates meat into different classes based on expected eating quality (e.g. appearance, tenderness, juiciness, and flavour) and expected yield of saleable meat from a carcass. Grading of carcass is based on standards, and standards are based on measurable attributes that describe the value and utility of the product. In contrast to meat-inspection procedures, meat-grading systems vary significantly throughout the world. Different countries have different meat quality standards. For example, in the United States, cattle are raised primarily for the production of steaks and are fattened with high-quality grain feed in order to achieve a high amount of marbling throughout the muscles of the animal. Therefore, greater marbling levels improve the USDA quality grade. However, in Australia cattle are raised primarily for the production of ground beef products, and the highest quality grades are given to the leanest cuts of meat.

Some of the characteristics of meat used to assess quality and assign grades include: conformation of the carcass; thickness of external fat; colour, texture, and firmness of the lean meat; colour and shape of the bones; level of marbling; flank streaking; and degree of leanness. These factors are good indicators of different characteristics important to consumers.

Importance of Grading in Meat Trade

Grading is considered essential and beneficial to producer, processor and purchaser of meat.

Grading is important to the *producer* at the farm because:

i. He gets a higher income for his produce by way of sorting and fixing a differential rating for the various groups.
ii. It enables him to adopt modern animal production programmes consistent with the market demands.
iii. It ensures a healthy competition amongst producer to produce better quality of livestock.

Grading is important to the *processor* at the packing plant because:

i. He gets a higher income by way of sorting and differential pricing of the carcasses and cuts.
ii. It enables him to satisfy a wide variety of consumers and thereby his business turnover is increased.
iii. He could conserve his valuable time by placing orders through telephones, etc. since he is assured of the quality being ordered by him.

Grading is important to the *purchaser* at the retail counter because:

i. He is assured of the quality of the product being purchased.
ii. He is free to choose, depending upon his purse and taste.
iii. He is fully satisfied with the expenditure.
iv. The grade of the product forms a good guide to his cooking procedures.

Different Meat Grades

Two major purposes underlying grading are:

i. To find out the expected palatability characteristics of meat and this consideration is termed as "quality grade."
ii. To find out the expected yield to trimmed, boneless, retail cuts from a carcass and this consideration is termed as "yield grade".

Because of the large biological variation in the characteristics of meat animals and their carcasses, the task of grading is complex and difficult.

a. In the case of beef, lamb and mutton, separate standards have been developed for quality grades and yield grades. These carcasses can be graded for quality only, yield only or both.
b. The standards for grades of veal and calf are primarily quality grades.
c. The standards for grades of pork are essentially yield grades but limited consideration is also given to differences in quality.

Meat grading in USA is considered as the best in the world for obvious reasons of higher per capita income and better standards of living. Grades for different type of meat adopted by USDA are summarized in Table 29.1.

Table 29.1: Grades for meat (United States Department of Agriculture)

Kind	Class	Grade names
Beef quality grades	Steer, heifer, cow	Prime, choice, select, standard, commercial, utility, cutter, canner
	Bullock	Prime, choice, select, standard, utility
Beef yield grades	All classes	1, 2, 3, 4, 5
Calf and veal quality grades	All classes	Prime, choice, good, standard, utility, cull
Lamb and mutton quality grades	Lamb, yearling mutton	Prime, choice, good, utility
	Mutton	Choice, good, utility, cull
Lamb yield grades	All classes	1, 2, 3, 4, 5
Pork carcasses	Barrow, gilt	US no. 1, US no. 2, US no. 3, US no. 4, U.S. no. 5, utility
	Sows	US no. 1, US no. 2, US no. 3, US no. 4, US no. 5, utility, cull
Chicken	All classes	A, B, C

Retail Meat Cutting

Whole carcasses are usually fabricated into more manageable primal (major) or subprimal (minor) cuts. In developed countries, different primal and subprimal cuts are usually packaged separately and sold to retailers that further fabricate them into variety of products.

Pork Fabrication

Pork carcasses are usually divided into two sides, and each side is divided into four lean cuts plus other wholesale cuts. The four lean cuts are the ham, loin, Boston butt (Boston shoulder), and picnic shoulder.

Beef Fabrication

Beef carcasses are split into two sides, each side is divided into quarters, the forequarter and hindquarter, between the 12th and 13th ribs. The major wholesale cuts fabricated from the forequarter are the chuck, brisket, foreshank, rib, and shortplate. The hindquarter produces the short loin, sirloin, rump, round, and flank.

Lamb Fabrication

Lamb carcasses are divided into two halves, the foresaddle and hindsaddle. The foresaddle produces the major wholesale cuts of the neck, shoulder, rib, breast, and foreshank. The hindsaddle produces the major wholesale cuts of the loin, sirloin, leg, and hindshank.

Qualities of Meat

Meat quality is defined by the yield, compositional, technological, wholesomeness and palatability characteristics such as appearance, juiciness, tenderness and flavour. The relative importance of these quality characteristics differs for different type of consumers.

Yield and Gross Composition

This comprises of the quantity of salable meat obtained from meat animal, ratio of fat to lean, and muscle size and shape. Minimum level of fat is desirable as majority of consumers prefer higher ratio of muscle to fat. In another words, the amounts of lean that can be recovered from carcass indicate the quality of meat. This is also important from economic point of view.

Appearance and Technological Characteristics

The visual identification of quality meat is based on color, marbling and water holding capacity. The meat should have a normal colour that is uniform throughout the entire cut. In general, colour of meat should be bright red or pink. Brown, purple or grey colour of meat is not desirable. Muscle tissue should also have marbling, i.e. small streaks of fat within the muscle. The marbling will increase the juiciness, tenderness and flavour the product.

pH and water holding capacity are two important technological characteristics of meat. These ultimately influence the cooking yield, juiciness and tenderness of meat. Water holding capacity can be witnessed by carefully observing the meat surface or bottom of the retail package. There should not be any excess water oozing out of meat surface. Higher water holding indicate more yield and higher juiciness of cooked product. Type and level of fat and chemical composition of lean also greatly influence the technological characteristics of meat.

Wholesomeness

Besides, good technological properties, meat should be safe to eat, free from parasites, microbial pathogens and hazardous chemicals. There is growing concern among the consumers that meat should come from animal that are reared and slaughtered as per approved norms and laws.

Palatability Characteristics

It encompasses juiciness, tenderness and flavour. Juiciness depends on the amount of fat and water retained in a cooked meat product. Juiciness increases flavour and tenderness of meat. Time and method of cooking also greatly affect juiciness.

Tenderness can be attributed to a person's perception of meat, such as: softness to tongue, resistance to tooth pressure, ease of fragmentation, mealiness, adhesion and residue after chewing. Tenderness is influenced by several factors, such as the animal's age, sex or the muscle location.

Meat flavour is believed to be due to the breakdown products of ATP or energy, sulfur and nitrogen compounds and water soluble components of the muscle. Each species have a slightly different flavor due to difference in composition of fat within the muscle. Animals with different uses and different diets will deposit fat that contains different products. The fat melts during cooking and gives each species its own distinctive flavour.

Factors affecting Quality of Fresh Meat

Quality characteristics of meat refer to different attributes that determine its degree of acceptance by the consumer. These depend on different independent but interacting production and processing factors. They are broadly classified into pre-slaughter and post-slaughter factors.

Important factors affecting the basic composition and quality are given below:

Species

Meat of different species differ in composition, postmortem glycolysis, tenderness, colour, flavour and functional characteristics. The colour intensity differences between species are primarily caused by differing concentrations of myoglobin. The beef has the highest concentration of myoglobin. Lamb is intermediate in colour and pork is lightest in colour.

Heredity

Different breeds differ in growth potential and quality characteristics. Many physical properties of meat are greatly influenced by genetic factors. For example, colour and firmness of pork and beef are estimated to be approximately 30% inheritable. Marbling in pork is approximately 25% inheritable. Tenderness in beef may be up to 60% inheritable while tenderness in pork is only 30% inheritable. Improvements to the end quality of meat can be made by careful selection of livestock breeds and strains.

Sex

Different levels of sex hormones generally cause variations in meat quality. Female animals have tendency to deposit more fat than males. Degree of tenderness also differs in male and females. Male animal usually produces darker meat than females. The meat of boars often has an unpleasant odour. This odour is most often noted during cooking and may go unnoticed after cooking.

Age

Irrespective of species, breed or sex, the composition of muscles varies with increasing animal age. The degree of intra- and inter-molecular cross-linking between the polypeptide in collagen increases with increasing animal age. Thus, young animals produce more tender meat than old. Fattening is also closely related to age of animals/birds. Meat flavour also intensifies with age. The flavour of meat of older animals, especially sheep, may be so intense that some find it to be objectionable. Animal age also causes darkening of meat due to increased levels of myoglobin.

Muscle Location and Activity

Some muscles yield more tender meat than others. Muscles that are free to shorten during rigor mortis are generally less tender. Another factor affecting meat tenderness is the strength and usage of the muscle. With increase in muscular activity, connective tissue increases, which causes toughness. Muscular activity also affects composition of muscle tissue.

Nutritional Factors

Quality and quantity of nutrients in feed and plane of nutrition also affect quality of meat. Certain feeding regimes and particular substances in the diet of livestock can affect the quality of meat. Starchy foods and sugars fed before slaughter can help restore depleted muscle glycogen levels to allow development of a normal postmortem pH. Abnormal flavours in sheep meat have been reported from lambs grazing on certain strains of clover and other legumes. An undesirable "grassy" flavour may result from compounds found in forage.

Managemental Factors

Managemental factors like temperature and humidity also affect quality of meat. *Uses of chemicals, growth promoters, antibiotics, harmones, etc.* have influence on quality of meat in one way or other.

Pre-slaughter Fasting

Longer or shorter fasting period than the recommended, adversely affect quality of meat.

Method of Stunning and Killing

Different slaughtering methods (Jhatka, Halal, Kosher, etc.) have different impact on quality of meat, e.g. Jhatka meat has good colour but shorter shelf life in comparison to Halal meat.

Chilling and Ageing

Time and temperature of chilling effect rigor mortis development and quality of meat.

Major Changes in Muscle Postmortem

After slaughter of animal, the life-sustaining processes slowly cease, causing significant changes in the postmortem (after death) muscle. These changes represent the conversion of muscle to meat.

pH Changes

After exsanguination, oxygen is no longer available to the muscle cells, and anaerobic glycolysis becomes the only means of energy production available. As a result, glycogen stores are completely converted to lactic acid, resulting the pH to drop. Generally, the pH declines from approximately 7.0 to 7.2 in living muscle to a postmortem ultimate pH of approximately 5.4 to 5.5 in meat.

Protein Changes

When the energy reserves are depleted, the myofibrillar proteins, actin and myosin lose their extensibility and the muscles become stiff. This condition is commonly referred to as rigor mortis. The time an animal requires to enter rigor mortis is dependent on the species, the chilling rate of the carcass and the amount of stress the animal experiences before slaughter.

In resolution of rigor mortis, the stiffness in the muscle tissues begins to decrease due to the enzymatic breakdown of structural proteins. This phenomenon can continue for weeks after slaughter in a process referred to as aging of meat. This aging effect produces meats that are more tender and palatable.

Postmortem Quality Problems

Meat quality may be affected by both the preslaughter handling of the live animals and the post slaughter handling of the carcasses. Some of the common problems associated with improper handling of meat animals or meat are:

DFD Meat

Dark, firm and dry (DFD) meat is the result of an ultimate pH that is higher than normal. DFD meat is often the result of animals experiencing extreme stress or exercise of the muscles before slaughter. Stress and exercise use up the animal's glycogen reserves, and, therefore, postmortem lactic acid production through anaerobic glycolysis is diminished. The resulting postmortem pH of DFD meat is 6.2 to 6.5, compared with an ultimate pH value of 5.4 or 5.5 for normal meat. The dry appearance of this meat is thought to be a result of an unusually high water-holding capacity, causing the muscle fibres to swell with tightly held water. Because of its water content, this meat is actually juicier when cooked and eaten. However, its dark colour and dry appearance result in a lack of consumer appeal.

PSE Meat

Pale, soft and exudative (PSE) meat is the result of a rapid postmortem pH decline while the muscle temperature is too high. This combination of low pH and high temperature adversely affects muscle proteins, reducing their ability to hold water and causing them to reflect light from the surface of the meat so the meat appears pale. PSE meat is especially problematic in the pork industry. It is known to be stress-related and inheritable.

Cold Shortening

Cold shortening is the result of the rapid chilling of carcasses immediately after slaughter, before the glycogen in the muscle has been converted to lactic acid. With glycogen still present as an energy source, the cold temperature induces an irreversible contraction of the muscle (i.e. the actin and myosin filaments shorten). Cold shortening causes meat to be as much as five times tougher than normal. This condition generally occurs in lean beef and lamb carcasses that have higher proportions of red muscle fibres and very little exterior fat covering.

Electrical stimulation (the application of high-voltage electrical current to carcasses immediately postmortem) reduces or eliminates this condition by forcing muscle contractions and using up muscle glycogen. *Thaw rigor* is a similar condition that results when meat is frozen before it enters rigor mortis. When this meat is thawed, the leftover glycogen allows for muscle contraction and the meat becomes extremely tough.

REGULATIONS IN MEAT SECTOR

India has comprehensive legislation as well as a good administrative system to ensure the food safety and quality of the meat production for domestic consumption and export. Meat Food Products Order regulates processed meat products in the country. Meat processors have to obtain license under the order for manufacture and sale of meat products.

Slaughter of meat animals is a state subject regulated under State Animal Preservation Acts and Rules made there under. For establishment of slaughterhouses, clearances from local body, city development authority, state pollution control board, airports development authority, state industries department and Ministry of Defence are required. Meat inspection is carried out by veterinarian appointed by local body. Meat hygiene is regulated as per bye-laws of the local body. Meat hygiene is also covered under The Prevention of Food Adulteration Act, 1954.

Water (prevention and control of pollution) Act, 1974; Air (Prevention and control of pollution) Act, 1981 and Environment (protection) Act, 1986 stipulate requirements for abattoirs. Motor vehicles transport Act and the prevention of cruelty to animals Act, 1960 are also relevant in meat sector. Meat Food Products Order, 1973 regulates meat food products in the country.

Meat export is regulated as per Export (quality control and inspection) Act, 1963 and the Export (quality control and inspection) Rules, 1964. Export of fresh and frozen meat is regulated as per Raw Meat (chilled/frozen) (quality control and inspection) Rules 1992 and meat products under Processed Meat (quality control and inspection) Rules, 1995. Export of animal casings is regulated as per Plant Registration and Animal Casings Rules, 1995.

Animal products export is also subjected to World Trade Organization (WTO) agreements particularly Agreement on the application of Sanitary and Phytosanitary Measures (SPS Agreement) and Agreement on Technical Barriers to Trade (TBT Agreement). SPS Agreement recognizes standards developed by OIE (Office International Epizootics), which has developed International Animal Health Code. The aim of this code is to facilitate international trade in animals and animal products through the definition of health condition governing such trade so as to avoid the risk of spreading animal diseases. Bilateral agreements are also important in the trade of animal products.

Some of the important laws/acts and government bodies connected with meat are given below.

Meat Food Products Order (1973) including amendments up to 2005: The order is implemented by Directorate of Marking and Inspection. It controls production, quality and distribution of raw and processed products.

Export Quality Control and Inspection Act (1963): This act was promulgated to promote export trade by ensuring exports of international quality products. The Export Inspection Council has been established to ensure compulsory quality control and inspection of various commodities.

APEDA: Agricultural and Processed Food Products Export Development Authority (APEDA), Ministry of Commerce, Government of India encourages export of agro and processed food products including meat and meat products and approves Meat plants for export of meat through the activity of Meat Plant registration.

Prevention of Food Adulteration Act (PFA Act, 1954): This is the basic food act which empowers the central Government to make rules and amend the existing ones. Central Committee Food Standards (CCFA) has been constituted at the centre to advise the Central and State Governments on matters of administration of the act.

Bureau of Indian Standards (BIS): BIS (Certification marks) Act 1952 provides third party assurance/guarantee for the consumers. Under this system, BIS issues license to a food manufacturing unit which complies with the specifications laid down in the relevant Indian Standards.

Codex Alimentarius: Codex Alimentarius has now been established as the benchmark for ensuring food safety and consumer protection. Codex develops commodity standards which are product specific and general standards (standards on guidelines, code of practices, reduction of contaminants, sampling procedures, etc.) which have across the board application to all foods and are not product specific. FAO's manual of food quality control and food for export has become standard reference in the improvement of quality of food for national and international trade. Continuous surveillance of product by way of sampling and laboratory analysis is essential to ensure that contaminant levels comply with those prescribed by importing countries.

The important laws that are related to slaughter dictate that:

- Every meat animal must be certified healthy and free from disease by a municipal veterinarian before it can be slaughtered for meat.
- Animals must be rested for 24 hours, given abundant water and rendered unconscious before slaughtering.
- No pregnant animal may be slaughtered.
- Only permitted animals as per law to be slaughtered.
- No animal may be slaughtered except at a municipal or registered slaughterhouse.
- No animal shall be slaughtered in view of another animal.
- Vide a notification dated 31st August 1978 by the Ministry of Civil Aviation, it is illegal to slaughter or flay animals or deposit slaughterhouse waste within a radius of 10 km from airports.
- Under the Water Pollution Act, it is illegal for slaughterhouse waste to be deposited into any water resource.

- No person can in any public place or public street, carry meat exposed to public view (State Municipal Acts, e.g. Section 397 of Delhi Municipal Act).
- No person can sell meat, fish or chicken or use any premises for this purpose unless he has permission from the Municipal Commissioner.
- If it is suspected that any animal for human consumption is being sold or kept for sale in an unregistered place, the Commissioner or anyone authorised by him may at any time by day or night without any notice, enter and inspect such place.
- Anybody who kills or sells any animal without such a licence can have the animal summarily removed and the shop shut down.
- All licensed butcher shops are required to follow the ISI code of health and hygiene standards.
- The butcher shop must have a glass front to keep off flies.
- It must have sufficient running water.
- It must have a proper waste disposal facility. Blood and faeces cannot be sent down public drains.
- If animals are being kept on the premises, they must be provided proper food, water and shelter which means shade from the heat and protection from the cold (PCA Section 11).
- Keeping chickens stuffed into cages is illegal as it denies them opportunity to exercise and causes unnecessary suffering (PCA Section 11).
- Keeping animals constantly tethered or on short ropes/chains is illegal (PCA Section 11).
- Every slaughterhouse has a maximum number of animals that are permitted to be slaughtered.

30

Expectations from Veterinary Professional

MC Sharma, Gunjan Das

The animal husbandry sector is harboring a wonderful livestock wealth having very significant role in providing subsidiary to major sources of income to the large numbers of cultivators, small farmers, marginal farmers and agricultural labourers. Milk enterprise generates income on regular basis as against the crop enterprise. The provision of assured market for the milk leads to their increased participation and the availability of cash income encourages them to take up to social development programmes. The continuing economic and public sector reforms have necessitated the process of decentralization of governmental responsibilities in many sectors and there is no difference as far as animal husbandry is concerned in general which prompted the role of veterinarian for the upliftment of this profession cannot be overlooked. The veterinary profession as we know it today is *The Gentle Doctor,* who takes care of ailment of all companions, domestic and wild animals. Veterinary medicine's principle is focused on diseases and disease prevention in large animal species but it also recognized a more humane and compassionate role for veterinarians in their care for companion and other animals. The development of exclusively small animal practices in the mid-twentieth century has driven the expectations of the society and needs for veterinarians and they require our immediate attention. Veterinarians are very much needed in biomedical research and the full array of careers in public practice. Expectations for food supply veterinarians are rapidly changing with new roles being defined and some traditional roles being unfilled.

This profession works for improved quality livestock and livestock products contributing fully to food security and poverty eradication through increased quality livestock and livestock products in an environment friendly manner and also committed to protect the environment, upholding animal welfare, avoidance of conflict of interest, equality and social justice, commitment to excellence and capacity development, networking and collaboration. Increasing population, urbanization and income in developing countries are catalyzing a massive global increase in demand for food of animal origin. Such a demand-driven growth, which is taking place mostly in developing countries, will call for greater emphasis on harvesting, storing and processing facilities of food of animal origin and veterinary professionals shall play the pivotal role in satisfying consumer demand for foods of animal origin, improve nutrition, income and employment opportunities. Veterinarians have no option but to improve productivity of our livestock through scientific breeding, feeding, healthcare and management. Use of technological and marketing interventions in production, processing and distribution of livestock products should be central theme of any future programme for livestock development.

HISTORICAL PERSPECTIVE OF VETERINARY SCIENCE

From time immemorial human had interactions with many of the wild animals in their environment. They have always found animals interesting and companions. Animal-based products are used as food, useful implements, clothing, writing media, etc. apart from these; humans have regularly been able to utilize some species of animals for transport of people, goods, and equipment, for peaceful purposes and military campaigns, etc. Human relationships with animals have been and still are difficult. Human being tried to understand their illness and often recognized that many of these same illnesses seemed to attack their animals as well.

Hippocrates, the father of Medicine has evolved the theory of disease due to imbalance of body humours (fluids). The Chinese used herbal medicine and other treatments to attempt to cure themselves and their favourite/most valuable animals. Historical information in China depicts that there are records dating to 4000-3000 BC that record the use of herbs for curative purposes for humans and animals. Egyptian hieroglyphics from around 3500 BC prove the presence of numerous types of domesticated animals. The first individual to be considered a veterinarian is Urlagaldinna. The Greek Scientist, Alcmaeon (c. 500 BC) was the first person known to have dissected animals for scientific purposes. In India there are records that animal hospitals were established in India during the Brahaman era and the reign of King Ashoka (273-232 BC). During the period of Greco-Roman, there were a number of individuals who recorded the current knowledge regarding animal care and disease. Aristotle (384-322 BC) recorded much of the knowledge regarding animals. He predicted that animals were different and yet some showed similar characteristics to humans. Columella, a Roman scholar was a very prolific writer on the topic of animal care and breeding. He used the term "veterinarius" for individual who is a caretaker of pigs, sheep and cattle. During the end of 16th century, there are many indications to animal plagues and their devastating effects on farmers' productivity. A plague in European cattle in 1711, namely Rinderpest as a contagious viral cattle disease. After this outbreak of plague it was in 1762 that Claude Bourgelat in Lyons, France established the first veterinary school in the world. In about AD 500 Roman wrote a book on what is the task of veterinarians followed by a book called Anatomy of the Horse and was written by an Italian, Carlo Ruini, in 1598. The first school that taught people about scientific veterinary was in Europe in the mid-eighteenth century less than three hundred years ago. In ancient India, treatment of animals was generally confined to Ayurveda medicine. Salihotra was denoted as horse doctor, apart from that Vaisampayana, Nakula and Palkapya contributed highly in animal prctices through sanskrit treaties on animals.

DEVELOPMENT AND MODERNIZATION OF VETERINARY SCIENCE

The veterinary science started developing on the line of scientific trends after the invention of microscope by Antony Van Lewenhoek. In the twentieth century, progress in veterinary science continued to advance gradually through educational institutions and associations were founded and evolved to communicate the advances to the veterinary community. Their major responsibility were to control and eradication of major epidemic farm animal diseases, the control of imported and exported animals and animal products, the operation of animal health laboratories and treatment of the animals within them, and other animal welfare matters. "Operation Flood", the largest dairy development programme in the world has modernized Indian dairy industry and linked producer and consumers through establishing a national milk grid. The organization of cooperatives of milk producers was a major part of the program, which gave opportunities to the farmers for production, and marketing of their produce.

Technological progress in the production, processing, and distribution of livestock products will be the focus now. Rapid advances in feed improvement; genetic and reproductive technologies and health coverage offer scope for overcoming many of the technical problems posed by increased livestock production. Future growth prospects in developing livestock for food security and the livelihoods of the rural poor and for environmental sustainability are crucial. Biotechnological tools offer an opportunity for an rapid expansion and better management of livestock production and health management through novel, cost-effective and dependable means of vaccine production and diagnostics, development of genetic resistant animal varieties to diseases and increasing the fertility potential of the pedigreed dairy animals. The molecular biological technique such as PCR, RAPD-PCR, gene probes, REA, cloning are very useful for the rapid and sensitive diagnosis of animal diseases. "Therapeutic and preventive approaches to deal with diseases of farm and companion Animals" is in concurrence with the revolutionary phase through which livestock sector is passing in India.

VETERINARY SCIENCE

Veterinary science graduates will find many exciting opportunities to work with animals and the general public in a variety of ways. If you are a caring person and compassionate to animals, you may want to explore the educational and career options within the field of veterinary science. Veterinary science plays a vital role in the maintenance and healthcare of pets, zoo animals, and livestock. Apart from these also meet the healthcare and maintenance needs of animals; some individuals working in veterinary science use their skills to work on zoonotic diseases affecting both animals and humans, viz. anthrax, leptospirosis, brucellosis, rabies, etc. Veterinarian research has always played a vital role in understanding human heart disease, organ transplant procedures, and a variety of drug therapies. Despite the fact that, the field of veterinary science is exciting and rewarding, working with animals requires patience, care and flexibility. Veterinary science is a field with many aspects and individuals working in the field of veterinary science are veterinarians, animal care and service workers, and veterinary technologists or technical personnel.

Role of Veterinary Professionals

Apart from being caring about animals, a good veterinarian must have good dexterity, human communication skills, and management skills. Veterinarians generally diagnose animal health issues, vaccinate animals against diseases, and medicate animals experiencing illness or infection and if necessary they also perform surgery. Small animal veterinarians are vital educators, enabling pet owners to optimally nourish, breed, maintain, and care for their pets. Veterinarians who work with large animals primarily focus on animals associated with farms, ranches, or zoos. These veterinarians usually drive to the animals' living quarters and examine and treat them on site. Large animal veterinarians are key to a large animal's long-term health care plan by offering preventative care. They not only test for and vaccinate against certain diseases, but they also consult with farmers. This network of information restricts the spread of diseases and illness in regional populations and ensures health for the whole community. Veterinarians are committed and often work out doors, in all kinds of weather, and with animals in a variety of states for overall well-being of animals.

Veterinarians not only work as animal caretakers and animal trainers but are also responsible for the cleanliness, maintenance, Grooming and repair of animal habitats, such as cages or staged natural environments and thus ensuring health of the animals. In zoos, veterinarians closely observe animals for signs of illness or injury, monitor eating patterns for other signs of imbalance and treat the ailing animals. Veterinarians conduct clinical trial, perform various medical tests, often perform blood or urine tests, prepare tissue samples.

Desirable Characteristics of a Veterinary Professional

1. In-depth/advanced knowledge base of veterinary medical science and comparative biomedicine as described in the curriculum requirements.
2. Essentials of scientific and professional behaviour to include thoroughness, reliability, efficiency, and critical analysis.
3. Possess problem solving and critical thinking skills.
4. Experience in scientific investigation and scientific processes.
5. Skill in oral and written communication.
6. Integrated general understanding of the world, its cultures and people.
7. In-depth/advanced understanding of the concepts and principles of the biological sciences.
8. Skills in finding and using information and the management of information.
9. Skills and desire for sustained scholarship and lifelong commitment to learning and professional development.
10. Commitment to betterment of humanity and improvement of one's community, society, and the profession.
11. Business and management skills including management of one's personal affairs.

12. Compassion for people, animals, and a reverence for life.
13. Personal integrity and high ethical standards.
14. Dedication and sincerity towards veterinary profession
15. Vets should have knowledge of veterinary jurisprudence and ethics for animal welfare.
16. Moreover, veterinarian should be a good and positive human being who can understand the problem of other people.

Definition of Client's Expectations

People's expectations include what is assumed, desired, wished and hoped for. In the word 'expected', one can perceive the necessity and potential for dissatisfaction if this expectation is not, or no longer fulfilled. In other words, clients may be initially impressed because a service was beyond their expectation. However, it then may become a need and is requested. This is the continuing challenge of trying to achieve excellence in client service by exceeding client expectations. A few years ago, when you called a veterinary clinic, or any consumer service oriented business, you received the typical welcome such as "Hello". Today, a correct welcome would be along the lines of, "Welcome to the Samaritan Animal Hospital, Gail speaking, how can I help you?", to the point that when we do not receive such a type of personal greeting, one wonders if he or she did not dial the wrong number? There are several kinds of expectations. Those that are expressed by clients, so-called 'explicit' expectations, and those that are not expressed, so-called 'implicit' expectations. It is quite important to know what our client's implicit expectations are since, by definition, these will not be mentioned by people. A perfect example is the fact that people expect the personnel and staff in a veterinary clinic to have a 'professional, medical look' (white or medical types of clothes). Intact dress code for a professional is highly essential, which provides the feeling and belongingness for the profession and also render awareness of his duty. There should be different dress code for a veterinary professional and his subordinate or assisting staffs, which will help the owner to recognize the vets. If it is not the case, people may be surprised or even upset but they will not mention it—it is implicit for them. Veterinarians specifically need to have a good understanding of this category of expectations.

Expectation from Veterinary Professional

To talk about the expectations from a veterinary professional include many but to mention few are health protection of the national herd by ensuring effective control of disease, including common, zoonotic, and exotic disease, satisfactory animal welfare and environmentally sound production and processing systems, assuring high quality and safe food, efficient and effective private and public veterinary services, economic competitiveness of livestock and livestock product at home or abroad. Expectations relating to veterinary in the public interest are health protection of the national herd and effective control of disease, protection of the national herd and effective control of animal and zoonotic disease. The main veterinary related threats are from, the introduction of seriously damaging disease, e.g. foot and mouth disease, classical swine fever, rabies, avian influenza, equine infectious anaemia, mastitis, haemorhagic septicaemia, anthrax and BQ, the loss of export status especially to elite markets, customer and consumer resistance to real or perceived "substandard" quality livestock and product.

The community expects that all animals, will be protected through effective clinical practice, surveillance and control of disease, especially zoonotic and exotic disease, up-to-date and effective production, hygienic husbandry and welfare practices. As far as satisfactory animal welfare and environmentally sound production, processing, and animal waste disposal systems are concerned the society expects that all animal husbandry practices should be welfare friendly, environmentally sound, and sustainable, there should be compliance with animal welfare and environment directives and regulations, such as, caging, tethering, transportation, further to mad cow disease, any worthwhile system for the destructive disposal of fallen animals and hazardous animal waste is a better option that recycling into the food chain, the veterinary professional should come forward for a significant input as well as a leader role in many of these developments. Further, expectations in relation to assured quality and safety of food are controlling specific diseases, animal remedies, residue levels, exclusion of certain animal products from the food chain, all participants in the food chain from production to consumption will operate and comply with proper practice. Nevertheless, expected private and public veterinary services are effective animal heath, welfare and disease control programmes both at farm and national level, application of effective clinical practice using modern technology in diagnosis, disease control. The expectation from a professional for sustained production of animal and animal products are satisfactory production systems, high standard veterinary public and private services, safety and quality validation, with product appropriately labeled and correct professional and commercial certification.

A study in Turkey was conducted to determine peoples' expectations from veterinarians and how satisfied they were with the care they received. It was shown that most of the clients expected a high level of interest from veterinarians prior to consultation. They were also more concerned about their emotions than the health of their pets. The clients were highly satisfied by their veterinarians, where cat owners were more satisfied than dog owners. These results show that client expectation is not only limited to pet health, and that client satisfaction is related to counseling services as much as veterinary medical services.

The expectations from the zoo veterinarians in respect to practical basics of parasitology, haematology, postmortem examination, minor and major surgical interventions and follow-up cases of wild animals help the zoo animals to be in sound health. A zoo veterinarian should not be arrogant towards keepers, as they know much more about zoo-animals than some times the veterinary professionals. Hygiene and sanitation are very essential. Veterinary professionals in the zoo should be practical, polite, punctual and should try to understand animal behaviour.

The Indian Veterinary Association was established in the year 1922 and was registered as an Association under the Registration of Societies Act, as Reg.S.No. 96 of 1967. The expectations from the professionals of this association are to promote the advancement of veterinary science in all its aspects; to uphold the dignity and honour of the profession and to safeguard its rights and interests; to initiate, encourage and support veterinary research; education, employment and improving working conditions; to help organize and affiliate branches in different states and territories of the Indian Union, etc. Veterinary extension activities must be of high standard so that what so ever newer technological know-how has developed by the veterinary profession, it can reach to ultimate users, i.e. livestock owner and/or clients. Till today linkage of veterinary and animal husbandry is not so strong as in case of other profession like agriculture and medical profession. Central government or state govt. have to organize regular extension activities so that health and production of livestock sector may improve in this country as our economy and livelihood security is based on animal husbandry.

Other Potentials of Veterinary Profession to Meet Expectations of the Country

Today's veterinarians are in the distinctive position of being the only doctors skilled to protect the health of both animals and people. They are not only educated to meet the health needs of every species of animal but they play an important role in environmental protection, food safety, and public health. Veterinarians consistently rank among the most respected professionals in the country. Veterinarians serve the public by preventing animal disease and promoting food safety. They ensure that food products are safe and wholesome through carefully monitored inspection programmes. They help preventing the introduction of foreign diseases into the country, supervise interstate shipments of animals, test for diseases, and manage, prevent and eradicate diseases such as tuberculosis, brucellosis, and rabies that pose threats to animal and human health. Employment opportunities for veterinarians are almost endless and include private or corporate clinical practice, teaching and research, regulatory medicine, public health, and military service.

Veterinarians use their education to teach veterinary students, other medical professionals, and scientists about the deadly nature of the zoonotic diseases. Faculty members conduct research, teach, and develop continuing education programmes to help practising veterinarians acquire new knowledge and skills. Veterinarians employed in research at universities, colleges, governmental agencies, or in industry are dedicated to find new ways to prevent and treat animal and human health disorders. The society should credit veterinarians for many important contributions to human health. Veterinarians working in pharmaceutical firms develop, test, and supervise the production of drugs and biological products, such as antibiotics and vaccines, for human and animal use. These veterinarians usually have specialized education in fields such as pharmacology, virology, bacteriology, laboratory animal medicine, or pathology. Veterinarians are also employed in management, technical sales and services, and other positions in agribusinesses, pet food companies, and pharmaceutical companies. They serve as epidemiologists, working in environmental pollution studies. Apart from these, veterinarians in the country are serving in remount veterinary corps (RVC) in protecting the country against bioterrorism, veterinary care of government-owned animals, and professional in DRDO (Defense Research

Development Organization) work on the line of development of biomedical research. Veterinary officers with special training in laboratory animal medicine, pathology, microbiology, or related disciplines, conduct research in military and other governmental agencies. In fact, RVC is highly essential and a dedicated corps in Indian army, reason being all the supplies in border areas of our country are maintained by the animals like donkey, mules, horses and camels.

CONCLUSION

Contemporary veterinarians are exceptionally dedicated and willing to work long, difficult hours to save the life of an animal or help solve a public health crisis. Individuals who are interested in veterinary profession should have an inquiring mind and keen powers of observation. Veterinarians must maintain a lifelong interest in scientific learning, and must genuinely like and understand animals. Veterinarians should be able to meet, talk, and work well with a variety of people. Compassion is an essential attribute for success, especially for veterinarians working with pet owners who form strong bonds with their pets. Veterinarians manage private or corporate clinical practice, governmental agencies, and public health programmes. In the face of exceptional competition, the veterinarian must provide their patients and clients with the best scope of medical and surgical care and also a variety of services and products related to their animal's wellness. Most owners look forward to these services and products to be provided by the veterinarian. Owners seek necessary advice at the veterinary practice, but also about products and animal health services. It is therefore compulsory that veterinarians know and try to come as close as possible to the expectations of their clients.

The Indian Society for Veterinary Medicine (ISVM) established in 1981 is a professional organization of veterinary physicians of India. The primary objective of the society is to bring the different members working all over the country together and provide a common platform to project the scientific, technical and clinical information pertaining to livestock health.

31

Eco-jobs and Sustainable Development through Livestock

MC Sharma, Gunjan Das, Rupasi Tiwari

The Republic of India, is a sovereign country in South Asia. It is the seventh largest country by geographical area, the second most populous country and the most populous liberal democracy in the world. The geography of India is having a diverse landscape ranging from snow-clad mountain ranges, deserts to plains, hills and plateaus. India has a long coastline of over seven thousand kilometers most of which lies on a peninsula, which protrudes into the Indian Ocean. Western India is bound by the Arabian Sea and eastern India, the Bay of Bengal. India covers an amazing 3,214 km from north to south, and 2,933 km from east to west. The coastline adds up to over 6,000 km. China situated beyond the northeastern border of India with the Himalayas towering between the two countries. To the west of India is Pakistan, an independent nation. There are five main geographical regions in India, i.e. Himalayan range, Indo-Gangetic plains, Thar desert, Deccan plateau, Western and Eastern Ghats, Coastal plains. The climate of India varies from tropical in the south to more temperate and alpine in the Himalayan north, where elevated regions receive sustained winter snowfall. India's climate is strongly influenced by the Himalayas and the Thar desert.

Post-independence, India has gradually opened up its markets through economic reforms and reduced government controls on foreign trade and investment. With a GDP growth rate of 9.4% in 2006-07, the Indian economy is among the fastest growing in the world. The Indian economy has grown steadily over the last two decades; however, its growth has been uneven when compared to different social groups, economic groups, geographic regions, and rural and urban areas.

Livestock is an important component of our country playing an important role for socioeconomic development of India. Seventy per cent of the rural households generate their livelihood from livestock and agriculture. Over the past 9 five-year plans, the allocation of funds to animal husbandry has come down from about 1.2% to about 0.2% in the 9th plan. The allocation has come down in case of the dairy sector too. In the 8th five-year plan dairying was allocated close to 91% of total plan investment on animal husbandry, but it has come down to 14% in 10th plan outlay.

BRIEF HISTORY OF LIVESTOCK PRODUCTION SYSTEMS OF INDIA

Consistent development of agriculture and livestock sector is embedded in the green and white revolutions that resulted in high-producing, resource-intensive breeds. The mainland of our country consists of four broad geographical areas viz. the Northern Mountains, the Indo-Gangetic plains, the Southern Peninsula bounded by the Western and Eastern Ghats, and lastly the coastal plains and islands. Likewise, livestock production systems, in the country can broadly be described under four categories, i.e. pastoral, forest-based, mixed crop-livestock and commercial production systems. As the former three have subsisted and developed in the country since time immemorial and the latter is a relatively recent occurrence, which is in vogue only in developed countries.

Integrated crop and livestock farming and pasture/grazing management are the two widespread production systems found across our country. In integrated crop and livestock farming system, farmers obtain their livelihood somewhat equally from agriculture and livestock but in the second system farmer's livelihoods depend primarily upon their livestock, which are entirely maintained on grazing. In harsh climatic conditions, there is reduced livestock productivity, which has historically played an important role in people's livelihoods.

Livestocks are efficient utilisers of the available biomass thus, contributing to the grasslands by diffusing valuable grass seeds, checking unnecessary weeds and by fertilizing the soil with their dung and urine. Nevertheless, they consume grass that is unsuitable for human consumption and convert it to a range of valuable animal products like milk, meat, wool, manure, and draught power. Farmers have developed their own mechanisms to cope with the reality of scarce water, biodiversity, dryland cropping practices and the careful selection and breeding of a range of livestock species and breeds in drought prone areas.

LIVESTOCK SECTOR AND RURAL ECONOMY

Our country has observed an exceptional growth in the dairy and livestock industry for the last few decades. Animal husbandry sector provides large self-employment to millions of households in rural areas, which has helped in achieving a remarkable improvement in respect to milk production. Apart from achieving a sustainable goal for milk production and disease prevention, stress should also be given to develop database to take up future strategies for overall well-being of animal husbandry sector including dairying and creating environment friendly jobs for the rural households. The livestock sector facilitates poor and landless farmers to earn by using common-land resources and crop byproducts that would otherwise become waste maintaining ecological balance.

Sustainable Development of Livestock Sector

Animal husbandry and dairying is high priority area as for as sustainable development is concerned. The need of the day is a sustainable and economically feasible livestock farming including poultry farming for generation of employment through entrepreneurship. The overall growth rate for India is fixed around 6%. The rural women play a major role in maintaining animal husbandry by directly involving into breeding, feeding, management and care of animals and thus being a part of sustainable animal husbandry development. Development of this sector can result in a more reasonable improvement of the rural economy and contribute to reduction of poverty. For an economically viable livestock development, technological support is crucial not only for productivity but also to decrease the unit cost of production.

Livestock sector plays a crucial role in sustaining rural economy and livelihood through generation of eco-jobs for rural people. Livestock rearing in India is mainly practiced as a backyard production system wherein the farmers rear a few livestock specially for meeting the household requirements. Thus, by being as an important means of income and employment for these house holds livestock helps alleviate poverty and help income generation. The livestock sector contribution to the agricultural gross domestic product has risen from about 17% in 1980-81 to 26% now. Further it has been found that most of the livestock population is owned by the small and marginal farmers, who possess 71% of cattle, 63% of buffaloes, 66% of small ruminants, 70% of pigs and 74% of poultry. This implies that marginal and small holders derive a considerable proportion of their income from livestock. Livestock sector not only provides food and nutritional security but also acts as a subsidiary source of income for the farmers, in the mixed crop-livestock systems. Further the livestock provide draught power and act as a source of organic manure to crop sector. It also produces hides, skins, bones, blood and fiber for different industries helping the growth of the animal husbandry sector simultaneously with generating eco-jobs for rural households.

Eco-jobs and Livestock Sector Development for Sustainable Livelihood
Eco-jobs

Eco-jobs are knowledge intensive commenced by the digital, space and biotechnological revolutions, provides infrequent opportunities for realizing the goal of jobs for all.

Sustainable livelihood opportunities hold the key to both peace and progress through generation of eco-jobs in the rural areas. In the era of globalization the livestock sector is facing severe problems in respect to production, marketing and export of livestock product, which earn livelihood for rural people. This can be overcome if we make sustainable livelihoods opportunities for marginal landless farmers by providing them the facility and education of eco-jobs. Strategy building in this direction will help through location-specific jobs, livestock resources of the area, development of technology-driven projects, women's participation in rural economy building, infrastructure development for small-scale livestock production system and utilization of livestock waste. Development of eco-enterprises for livestock, poultry, and dairy sectors will assist the country to progress rapidly in the technological transformation in animal husbandry of small rural and urban enterprises.

India is largely rural with more than 60% of our population dependent on agriculture and allied activities. Ecologically sound agriculture is knowledge intensive. Farm women and men need dynamic information relating to meteorological, management and marketing factors as these are related to animal husbandry. The new approach to productivity improvement and employment generation is also information and knowledge intensive. There is presently a disconnection between what farm families need by way of dynamic information and what the conventional extension agencies are able to provide. It is also important to address the need for demand driven and value added information, which is time and location specific. Apart from information related to farming of animals, the rural people urgently need access to healthcare information. Increased health expenditure is an important cause of farmers' indebtedness, leading occasionally to suicides. Information on the health status of livestock and poultry for livelihoods of poor and the marginal farmers in rural India need attention. There is also need for promoting functional literacy among the adult illiterate and making learning joyful for the young through interactive methodologies.

Rural Knowledge Centres (RKC)

These were founded by Dr Swaminathan for overall development of rural people and make them self-sufficient in terms of livelihood.

RKCs provide several micro-enterprises training programmes such as production of *Trichogramma chilonis*, *Trichoderma viridae*, vermicompost, manufacturing products from agricultural and livestock waste, backyard ornamental fish breeding, sea farming, cage fishing, sea weed farming, aquaculture estates, pens culture in estuaries, edible oyster production, ornamental fish growing, training and creating eco-jobs like organic animal production, climate change analysts, energy specialists, aqua-cultural veterinarians, etc. generating awareness on the value of natural resources like mangroves, coral reefs, etc. These centres also offer computer aided learning for the rural children, distribution of quality literacy on phytosanitary measures.

It arranges interdisciplinary research and education for sustainable use of natural resources leading to the strengthening of the ecological basis. It also ensures sustainable income and generation of eco-jobs for the poor rural population. Organizing workshops and seminars for policy makers for widespread adoption of ecotechnologies in agriculture including animal husbandry sector, while encouraging the efficient use of energy and natural resources.

Eco-jobs and Field Schemes

It helps in the creation of eco-jobs and the development of bio-villages imparting knowledge of ecotechnic for the well-being of livestock sector in rural areas. These also identify useful models of traditional ecological knowledge and management useful for ecotechnic applications by using natural resources and bye products of animal's origin for sustainable economy of the rural households.

Example: Animal husbandry focusing in indigenous practices to enhance the capacity of the farmers in animal health care aspects. Soil testing and the establishment of low cost soil testing facilities at the village level and area-specific mineral supplementation for achieving maximum production of livestock with minimum possible expenditure. Mineral mixture prepared for Uttaranchal and Uttar Pradesh helping the rural people in respect to more productivity by their livestock. Eco-jobs facilitate women farmers to develop eco-friendly prawn farming models.

Eco-jobs and Sustainable Livestock Sector

It can be defined in terms of social sustainability. The concept of sustainable agriculture in prosperous nations is different from the concept in a poor nation. In developed countries, the problem is to preserve the high standard of living they have already achieved. In the poor countries, the problem is to get some standard of living for most of the people. They look at sustainability from a more environmental perspective, while for us sustainability is environmental, social and related to gender equality. That's what we do on our research programme. We put a matrix of questions: is it socially sustainable? Is it pro-women? Is it ecologically sustainable? And of course, is it economically viable?

According to Lester Brown, the writer of Eco-Economy, How do we achieve sustainable economic transformation, when all decision-makers—whether political leaders, corporate planners, investment bankers or individual consumers—are guided by market signals, not the principles of ecological sustainability?' The answer to this challenge lies in achieving a paradigm shift to an eco-economy. The prospects now available for implementing environment-friendly technologies in the area of agriculture and many of the eco-friendly technologies have good merits in animal husbandry like, taking the Indian Dairy Industry as an example. India is now the world leader in milk production. However, India's dairy industry is largely based on the use of agricultural residues as feed and not grains, which is due to the capability of ruminating animals to digest cellulose. This is an example of the technology of production by masses, in contrast to the mass production technologies adopted in industrialized countries. The book indicates the uncommon opportunities now available for eco-jobs and eco-entrepreneurship. Hereafter, good ecology will be good business and it is hence in the long-term interests of industry that they adopt environmentally benign technologies. Agriculture, comprising crop and animal husbandry, fisheries, forestry and agro-processing, is the backbone of the livelihood security system of rural areas, where more than 70% of India's population live. A considerable proportion of this population has no assets like land, livestock, fishpond or any commercially viable enterprise. The poor are also often illiterate. Therefore, the Virtual Academy will give particular emphasis to fostering sustainable livelihood options both in the farm and non-farm sectors.

32

Role of Animal Husbandry for Livelihood Security to Indian Farming Community

MC Sharma, Rupasi Tiwari, Gunjan Das

Livestock is an important source of income generation and employment in rural sector. They contribute to household income besides assisting in crop production through draught power, fuel gas and manure. Livestock represents the only way in which man can use natural vegetation. Because of the high quality protein they contain, livestock products play an important role in export earnings. They also provide rich edible food by converting waste and byproducts of crop production. Livestock sector makes multifarious contributions to the rural development in the country. Animal husbandry plays a vital role in the development of livestock for increasing the production potential of milk, meat and egg which are required for better nutrition for the human beings apart from providing subsidiary income, particularly to the rural poor. It has grown into an industry with the application of advanced scientific methods.

Not only does it provide food and nutritional security but also acts as a subsidiary source of income for the farmers, in the mixed crop-livestock systems. Further the livestock in such systems supplies draught power and organic manure to crop sector and hides, skins, bones, blood and fibre to the industries.

CONTRIBUTIONS OF LIVESTOCK SECTOR

Livestock rearing in India is mainly practiced as a backyard production system wherein the farmers rear a few livestock specially for meeting the household requirements and the excess milk is sold in such units. Thus, by being an important means of income and employment for these house holds livestock helps alleviate poverty and smoothen income distribution. In addition, livestock asset can be easily converted into cash, and thus acts as cushion against shocks of crop failure particularly in the less favoured environments. Further it has been found that most of the livestock population is owned by the small and marginal farmers, who possess 71% of cattle, 63% of buffaloes, 66% of small ruminants, 70% of pigs and 74% of poultry. This implies that marginal and small holders derive a considerable proportion of their income from livestock. Evidences indicate that increase in income from livestock in rural areas reduce income inequality.

India has witnessed a phenomenal growth in the dairy and livestock development for the last three decades. In our country, animal husbandry sector provides large self-employment to millions of households in rural. Indian dairy sector has achieved a remarkable boost in respect of milk production by providing nutritional security and livelihood to the farmers all over the country and been instrumental in bringing up socio-economic changes. As we know, agriculture and livestock productivity go hand in hand, combating and knowledge of some impotent diseases, which cause great economic loss to the nation, should be taken care of. Besides achieving a sustainable goal for milk production and disease prevention emphasis should also be given to develop database to take up future strategies for overall well-being of animal husbandry sector including dairying. The livestock sector is an important segment of agricultural sector in India. Presently, the contribution of this sector to the agricultural gross domestic product has risen from about 17% in 1980-81 to 26% now. The value of output from meat at current prices was Rs 29,319 crores during 2003-2004 and export of meat and meat products was Rs 1720 crores during 2004-2005. Total export earning from livestock, poultry and related products was 5120 crores in 2004-05 out of the total exports. Leathers sector accounted for 2660 crores in value terms. The value of output from livestock to agriculture is likely to increase further to higher than 50% by 2020.

India has largest livestock population in the world as well as larger number of breeds of cattle (30), buffalo (10), goat (20) and sheep (42) indicating pool of richest germplasm of livestock in world. Of the total buffalo and cattle breeds of the world; around 76% and 20% respectively are available in Asia and 15% and 5% in India. According to the livestock census (2003), there are 185.18 million cattle, 97.79 million buffaloes, 61.47 million sheep, 124.39 million goats, 13.52 million pigs and 489 million poultry. The dairy farmers have done a great job of making India the highest producer of milk in the world with 97 million tones in 2005-06, which was 22.5 million tones during 1970-71. Per head milk availability is 254 grams estimated during 2005-06, which has increased from the 127 grams during 1979-80. Though India stands 1st in milk production and there is substantial improvement with respect to per capita milk consumption, it is imperative to state that the per capita milk consumption is still below the WHO recommendation of 278 grams per head per day. Our country has achieved annual growth rates of 4–5% for milk, meat and egg production during the last decade. The value of output from animal husbandry and dairying to agriculture over the years has increased and is about 34.59% of the gross domestic product. At present, agriculture is contributing approximately 24% GDP, out of it livestock sector contribute 25%. Animal husbandry sector contribute 6 to 8% growth rate as compare to the 2% crop production per year, which will help the agricultural sector to achieve a target of 4% increase in growth as a whole. The value of milk (Rs 1,020 billion) was higher than that of paddy (Rs 811 billion), wheat (Rs 471 billion) and sugarcane (Rs 275 billion). The value of meat groups (meat, meat products and by products) estimated at the current prices was Rs 20856 crores during 1999-2000 and export of meat and edible offal touched about Rs 1457 crores during 2000-2001.

ANIMAL PRODUCTION

Livestock sector plays a critical role in the welfare of India's rural population. It contributes 9% to gross domestic product (GDP) and employs 8% of the labour force. This sector is emerging as an important growth leverage of the Indian economy. As a component of agricultural sector, its share in gross domestic product has been rising gradually, while that of crop sector has been on the decline. In recent years, livestock output has grown at a rate of about 5% a year, higher than the growth in agricultural sector. This enterprise provides a flow of essential food products, draught power, manure, employment, income, and export earnings. Distribution of livestock wealth is more unrestricted, compared to land. Therefore, from the equity and livelihood perspective it is considered an important component in poverty alleviation programmes. Population of some of the purebred small ruminants, equines, pigs and pack animals has come down considerably and such breeds have come to the category of threatened breeds in the country. The farms or the farmers unit in their respective breeding tract are to be established with cent per cent central assistance for breeds of these animals wherein their population is less than 10,000 with active participation of state governments and NGOs, etc.

A new centrally sponsored scheme for conservation of threatened breeds has been started during 10th five-year plan with a budget outlay of Rs 1500 lakh. During 2005-06, an amount of Rs 406.92 lakh has been released for conservation of several indigenous breeds of animal, which really need to be conserved.

Cattle and Buffalo Production

Since mid-sixties a broad framework of the cattle and buffalo breeding policy is being followed which, envisaged selective breeding of indigenous breeds in their breeding tracts and use of such improved breeds for upgrading of the non-descript stock. Production of quality indigenous bulls has been a long-neglected area and would require a major thrust in order to harvest the best male germplasm available in the country. The present production capacity of frozen semen doses is about 30 million against the estimated requirement of 65 million doses annually. Except for a few pockets in important breeding tracts and in sperm stations, indigenous bulls of unknown pedigree and with poor quality semen are generally used. Crossbreeding, which was to be taken up in a restricted manner and in areas of low producing cattle, has now spread indiscriminately all over the country. Continuous emphasis on cross-breeding with exotic breeds even in the tracts of indigenous breeds led to the near extinction of some of the known breeds. Further, the indiscriminate use of contaminated semen or infected bulls results in the spread of sexually transmitted diseases like infectious bovine rhinotracheitis (IBR), brucellosis, tuberculosis, vibriosis, trichomoniasis, etc. at an alarming rate.

Of total buffalo population of 152 million, India possesses 92.2 million buffaloes (53%) while China and Pakistan have 22.8 and 20.2 million buffaloes, respectively. The excellent dairy type buffalo breeds such present in India and are known for high fat content in their milk. In comparison to cattle, buffaloes are more versatile in terms of adverse climatic condition. Population of Indian buffaloes mostly consists of riverine buffaloes. There are 18 River buffalo breeds in South Asia, the best known breeds used for both milch and draught purposes are Murrah, Nili/Ravi, Jafarabadi, Surti, Mehsana and Nagpuri. Of all the domestic animals, the Asian water buffalo holds the greatest promise and potential for production. Most of the buffaloes of the Indian subcontinent belong to a non-descript group known as the Desi buffalo. The production of buffalo milk in the Asian-Pacific region exceeds 45 million tonnes annually of which over 30 million tonnes are produced in India alone. The individual 3,000 litre-per-lactation female, considered a record 30 years ago, is now common. There are many which yield 4,000 litres in a lactation of 300 days. Out of total buffalo milk production of 54.9 million tons of world, India produces 34.8 million tons while share of China and Pakistan is 2.2 and 14.8 million tons, respectively. India, being the world largest buffalo milk producer recorded 20.0 and 29.3 million tons in 1982 and 1992, respectively, with a growth rate of 3.3% per year.

Twenty-seven acknowledged indigenous breeds of cattle and seven breeds of buffaloes are there in India. Several govt. sponsored schemes are being implemented for genetic improvement of cattle and buffalo with a view to enhance the per capita availability of consumption of milk through increased milk production. The National Project for Cattle and Buffalo Breeding envisages 100% grant-in-aid to implementing agencies. The project will also promote about 14,000 private artificial insemination (AI) practitioners and buildup an annual frozen semen production capacity of 66 million doses. Since inception, 26 states have been assisted with Rs 202.52 crore up to 31 March 2005 for participating in the project. A Central Herd Registration Scheme for identification and location of superior germplasm of cattle and buffaloes, propagation of superior germ stock, regulating the sale and purchase, help in formation of breeders' society and to meet requirement of superior bulls in different parts of the country is also being implemented. The Government has established Central Herd Registration Unit in four breeding tracts, viz. Rohtak, Ahmedabad, Ongole, Ajmer. The seven Central Cattle Breeding Farms at Suratgarh (Rajasthan), Chiplima and Sunabeda (Orissa), Dhamrod (Gujarat), Hessarghatta (Karnataka), Alamadi (Tamil Nadu) and Andeshnagar (Uttar Pradesh) are involved in scientific breeding programmes of cattle and buffaloes. The Central Frozen Semen Production and Training Institute, Hessarghatta (Karnataka) produced 13.43 lakh doses and supplied 14.74 lakh doses of frozen semen of high pedigreed Sahiwal, Red Sindhi, Holstein Friesian, Jersey, crossbred and Murrah buffalo to different States for their AI Programmes.

The performance of cross-breds was much higher than indigenous breeds. The Friesian crosses had higher milk yield, longer productive life and completed more number of lactations than other breed crosses. Variability in performance of cross-breds under field conditions could be ascribed to different availability of inputs, agro-ecological conditions, type of farmer and the indigenous and exotic breeds used in crossbreeding. Cross-bred cattle have higher milk productivity and reproductive efficiency, hence is more profitable than buffaloes and local cattle.

Central Cattle Development Organizations (CCDO)

Central cattle development organizations include the 7 central cattle breeding farms, the Central Frozen Semen Production and Training Institute, Hessarghatta and the 4 central herd registration units, which have been established by the department in different regions of the country for production of genetically superior breed of bull calves, good quality frozen semen and identification of location of superior germplasms of cattle and buffaloes, to meet the requirement of bulls and frozen semen doses in different parts of the country.

Central Cattle Breeding Farms (CCBF)

The Central Cattle Breeding Farms located at Suratgarh (Rajasthan), Chiplima and Sunabeda (Orissa), Dhamrod (Gujarat), Hessarghatta (Karnataka), Alamadhi (Tamil Nadu) and Andeshnagar (UP). These are maintaining bull mothers of important cattle and buffalo breeds which include Tharparkar, Red Sindhi, Jersey, Holstein Friesian, Crossbred (HF × Tharparkar, Jersey × Red Sindhi), Surti and Murrah. The farms produce bull calves from these bull mothers and supply high pedigree bull calves and bulls to the State Governments and other breeding organisations for production of frozen semen. The farms provide breeding facilities to the cows and buffaloes of the nearby villages free of cost and also conduct training of farmers in dairy farming under Animal Husbandry Extension Programme.

Central Frozen Semen Production and Training Institute, Hessarghatta

A premier institute producing frozen semen doses of indigenous exotic and cross-breed cattle bulls and Murrah buffalo bulls for use in artificial insemination. The institute also provides training in frozen semen technology to technical officers of the State Governments.

National Project for Cattle and Buffalo Breeding (NPCBB)

Government of India has initiated a major programme from October 2000, "National Project for Cattle and Buffalo Breeding"(NPCBB) over a period of 10 years for genetic improvement of cattle and buffaloes. National Project for Cattle and Buffalo Breeding envisages genetic upgradation and development of indigenous breeds on priority basis.

Buffalo Production

India is a country of rich resources and agriculture is a livelihood of about 70% people and livestock is part and parcel of it. India is richest in bovine population, highest in milk production, and buffalo is major milch animal of the country. To further advance, the animal agriculture in general and buffalo production in particular through balanced feeding, appropriate breeding, management and health care, a regional focus becomes inevitable. The water buffalo species are divided into two types, the swamp buffalo and the riverine buffalo. Swamp buffaloes are lighter in weight (males approximately 650-700 kg and females 500 kg mature weight) and have a lower milk production capacity, i.e. 430 to 620 kg of milk per lactation. These buffaloes are used mainly for draught power in rice cultivation in the paddy fields of Southeast Asia. The riverine buffalo, on the other hand, is heavier (males approximately 900-1000 kg and females 550 kg mature weight). Their milk production capacity is far higher than that of swamp buffaloes, ranging from 1 000 to 2 000 kg per lactation and varying among countries and strains. These domesticated buffalo has been little exposed to human interference such as artificial breeding because of its already perfect adaptation to the harsh environment in the swampy rice fields of Asia. Water buffalo is potentially a most important tropical bovine species, especially in very hot areas where rivers and swamps abound.

Challenges and Opportunities for Indian Meat Industry

   i. Setting up of the state-of-the-art abattoir-cum-meat processing plants.
   ii. Packaging of technologies to raise male buffalo calves for meat production
  iii. Buffalo rearing under contractual farming as backward integration to the modern abattoirs for meat production
  iv. Establishing disease-free zones for rearing animals

If the green revolution had led to self-sufficiency in food grains, the white revolution saw India occupy the number one position in milk production in the world, and the blue revolution brought about increase in fish production, India is now on the edge to attain the pink revolution through buffalo meat production and achieving the number one position in meat production which could be achieved by reducing the mortality rate in male buffalo calves (80%), and rearing the animals scientifically for quality meat production.

The production of buffalo milk in the Asian-Pacific region exceeds 45 million tonnes annually, of which over 30 million tonnes are produced in India alone. With selective breeding, improved management and the establishment of more dairy herds, milk yields are increasing worldwide. Buffaloes are the most multipurpose of all work animals in the assortment of tasks, which they can be taught to undertake. Presently, the output of thousands of buffaloes is in the form of work energy rather than the direct provision of food as milk or meat. Buffalo is remarkable for its feed conversion ability, but we do not yet understand how, or why, or whether that capacity can be further improved. The young buffalo calf achieves a daily weight gain of 800 grams without any supplement feed. Similarly, the power of the full-grown work-buffalo does not come from high-level nutrients.

Milk Production

Milk is an important and a cheap source of nutrition in rural areas of India. Small scale producer only produce about 9 liters per day while large-scale farms produce at least 55 liters per day. Average milk production per household has a direct association with farm size, and so is the percent share of milk sold. The average per capita consumption of milk per day is higher for large-scale producers compared to smallholders. In the western part of India, some of the farmers sell a large proportion of their milk to dairy cooperatives and in turn, purchase ghee from them for home consumption. The average price an Indian dairy farm family gets for buffalo milk was about 11.6 rupees per liter in both regions, while the price received for cow milk was higher in the northern region compared to the western region.

Sheep and Goat Production

Sheep and goats are important species of livestock for India. They contribute greatly to the agrarian economy, especially in areas where crop and dairy farming are not economical, and play an important role in the livelihood of a large proportion of small and marginal farmers and landless labourers. Small ruminants especially goats contribute to the livelihoods of millions of rural poor in most of the developing countries of the Asia and Africa, where 95% of the world's goat population is concentrated and also the majority of world's poor live. Goat production has witnessed excellent growth over the years despite a negative campaign against it for its perceived adverse impact on vegetation, forest and grazing lands. Small ruminants are well integrated in the farming systems of the small and marginal farmers of India who find in goats a vast potential for their socio-economic upliftment. Women were found to be particularly more inclined towards goats while men were more focused on large animals. Goats offer a strong opportunity to development agencies for suitable interventions including micro-credit, extension, technical and marketing support especially to women, landless and small farmers. Small farmers and landless agricultural labourers are increasingly relying on goats for meeting their cash requirements. Livestock Census (2003), showed there are about 561.47 million sheep and 124.36 million goats in the country. About five million farming family in the country are engaged in the rearing of small ruminants. Main reasons for low productivity by small ruminants are poor exploitation of genetic potential of indigenous animals, low absorption of available technology, inadequate resource of feed and fodder, insufficient health cover, inadequate marketing and credit support, etc. The estimated wool production was about 485 lakh kg during 2003-2004. The production of wool was 44.50 million kg during 2004-05. The expected wool production during 2005-06 stands at 50.0 million kg. The Central Sheep Breeding Farm, Hissar is trying to produce superior quality breeds of sheep, which would be disease resistance, having good feed conversion ratio and superior cross-bred.

Goats contribute 35% of the total meat and 3% of the total milk produced in the country (NCA, 1976). India exported wool and woolens worth $143.7 miilion (Rs 1 150 million) in 1978–79. Export earnings from finished leather and leather goods, including raw and processed sheep- and goat-skins, reached $326.1 million (Rs 2 609 million) during 1978–79 (EPCFL and IM, 1980). In 1978, there were 40.43 million sheep and 70.20 million goats in India, producing 118 million kg of mutton and 276 million kg of chevon, 717 million kg of milk, 33.3 million kg of wool and 26 117 and 71 148 million tonnes of fresh sheep and goat-skins, respectively (FAO, 1979).

The output of Indian sheep and goats is low, yet considering the nutritional and physical environmental conditions under which they are reared, it cannot be considered inefficient which can be attributed to inadequate grazing resources, disease problems and serious lack of organized efforts for genetic improvement.

Indian sheep and goats breed throughout the year with no control on the breeding season. Sheep and goat mortality is quite high due to several dreaded diseases, i.e. sheep pox, enterotoxaemia and anthrax in sheep, and pneumonia, PPR clostridial diseases and lumbar paralysis in goats are common and result in high mortality. Apart form these, some internal parasites also cause large morbidity and economic loss.

Goat population and productivity per animal in India has increased at the fastest rate among all major livestock species during last two decades. Organised marketing and prevention of emerging diseases will help in more milk and meat production from goat population of India. The goat improvement programme is to be given a push through extending credit to the poor landless farmers. There has been negligible increase in the sheep population in the last decade. Production of wool has increased from 43.3 million kg in 1996-97 to 49.0 million kg in 2001-02. The 9th 5-year plan target of wood production (54.0 million kg) was not achieved. To enhance the quality and quantity of carpet wool, shepherds need incentives like credit, health coverage, breed improvement programmes and timely disposal of wool and surplus animals at a reasonable price in the sheep rearing states of India.

Poultry Production

Poultry industry has done a tremendous improvement from a backyard activity to an organised, scientific and vibrant industry. It is estimated that the egg production in the country is about 33.6 billion numbers (2001-02) against the 9th 5-year plan target of 35 billion numbers. The most overwhelming growth among the livestock products has been recorded in eggs and poultry meat. This achievement in poultry development attributed to the private sector for commercial pure-line breeding. However, despite the huge investment made, mostly by the private sector, the poultry-processing sector is incurring losses. Poultry farming should be declared as an agricultural activity. The poultry production model in vogue (high input-high output using commercially developed strain of birds) has been primarily responsible for the rapid growth in production of eggs and broiler meat in the country, but it is successful mainly in large scale units (more than 1,000 units of birds). Due to high feed cost, non-availability of credit and marketing support, most of the small farmers have become contract farmers and are exploited by middlemen. Interventions by government organizations are required for the promotion of poultry in rural areas. Indigenous poultry breeds, including the improved strains that can survive with low quality raw feed and better resistance against diseases, can be reared under free range conditions by rural unemployed youth and women for some additional income and employment.

Poultry industry in India has made remarkable progress during the last three decades evolving from backyard ventures to a full-fledged commercial agro-industrial business mainly due to widespread research and development initiated by the government and subsequently taken up by the organized private sector. Presently, India ranks among the top 5 egg producing nations in the world with the total annual egg production of about 40.4 billion in 2003-04. Very recently, the private organizations are very well placed to meet the requirement of high producing birds suited only for the intensive organized poultry sector, but the unorganized sector, which contributes a substantial proportion of egg production, is still neglected. Poultry is the fastest growing sector of Indian agriculture. Broiler production was started as a novelty in early 1970s and has turned out to be popular with its rearing of 750 million in year 2000. The steep growth in broiler production is also reflected in the increased number of broiler hatcheries from 77 in 1980 to over 750 in the year 2000. Broiler production in 1993 was estimated to be 300 million broilers and with spurt in Broiler production in 90's the expected production in 1998 is approximately 800 million broilers and with poultry industries annual growth around 15 to 20% per annum, the sky is the limit for Poultry in India.

The value of productivity from poultry sector is nearly 20000 crores and it provides direct or indirect employment to over 2 million people. About 25% of the total egg production in the country comes from Desi poultry, which is unorganized rural backyard system. A target for achieving production of over 52 billion eggs by 2011-12, at a growth rate of 4.3% has been visualized by the Government of India. Poultry sector, besides employment generation and subsidiary income increase, provides nutritional security especially to the rural poor. Further, landless labourers derive more than 50% of their income from livestock especially poultry.

Central Poultry Development Organizations

During the 10th five-year-plan, it was decided to combine all the existing 13 Central Poultry Development Organizations region-wise into 4 centres so as to convert the poultry developmental activities in a single window system encouraging backyard/rural poultry production. Diversification of poultry production by taking up production of Duck, Turkey, Japanese quail and Guinea fowl, etc.

India has almost all major commercial breeds of chicks from America, England and Europe. India is self-reliant in feed ingrediant production and local feed plants produce, quality feed for poultry sector. Before taking up a new poultry project, the basic consideration is about its financial viability and technical feasibility. For this, a farmer/extension worker needs to know about the size of capital investment, down-to-earth guidelines to evaluate the economics of the project, comparative data on a layer/broiler farm unit. After that, a project has to be prepared. These and other aspects will be presented here. Hatchery management has undergone remarkable changes in recent years. Its role in disease control, in incubating eggs and hatching chicks is very important in achieving optimum success in the number of first-quality chicks. Pellet feed has a positive effect on broiler growth and feed conversion owing to increased feed consumption, less feed wastage, reduced bulkiness of feed and more homogenous feed. Besides, each pellet is complete feed and toxic pathogens and anti-nutritional factors are destroyed during pellet production.

Swine Production

Swine production is of significant importance, particularly in the northeastern region of the country. Livestock in this region comprises cattle, buffalo, sheep, goat and pig. Many tribal populations have no habit of rearing cattle for milk production due to shortage of feed and fodder and absence of commercialized dairy and piggery and therefore, animals are reared largely for meat. Pig husbandry has flourished much in the animal husbandry sector in the northeastern region inhabited by tribal people. The region also has a substantial pig population, which constitutes around 30% of the country's pig population. The bulk of the population is, however, of the indigenous type whose growth and productivity is very low. The major difficulty in pig development is the acute shortage of breeding males. Cross-breeding policy can bring improvement with subsidies provided to the small and marginal pig rearers.

A profitable sector of north-east region without much investment in housing and feeding practice. Pork can replace animal protein and this is cheap and easily available, moreover swine also have better immunity so, cost due to treatment is largely neglected. Among farm animals, pigs have special importance, as it is one of the most profitable animals farming particularly the northeastern region. As per the latest livestock census, the pig population of the country increased from 13.29 million in 1997 to 14.14 million in 2003, with an annual growth rate of 1.25% (Livestock Census, 2003). In the north-east region, the highest population is in Assam (12.62 lac) followed by Nagaland (6.44 lac), Meghalaya (2.94 lac), Mizoram 180 thousands, Manipur 400 thousands, Arunachal Pradesh 250 thousands, Tripura 235 thousands and Sikkim 30 thousands (1997). Pig husbandry is the most important activity in the animal husbandry sector in the northeastern region inhabited by tribal people. The pig sheds are made up of locally available bamboo, wooden planks which is cost effective and feeder and waters are also made up of wooden planks. Feed provided to pigs are locally available grasses, i.e. tapioca, sweet potato leaves and tubers along with small concentrate and 1.53 kg kithcen waste/pig/day. Generally, 10 quintal leftover feed (Kitchen, hotel waste) can increase 20-45 kg in weight of pigs provided the waste should be free from any toxic particle ensured by proper boiling a common practice. The pork can be sold very easily in local market and other factory can also buy swine for making pork product. Swine production can be a source of employment for landless tribes and unemployed persons to increase their development and food which is not edible for human being can be used in swine feeding.

The pig is one of the most efficient food converting animals among domesticated livestock, and can play an important role in improving the socio-economic status of the weaker sections of the society.

Exotic breeds of pigs like Large white Yorkshire, Hampshire, Berkshire, Saddleback are maintained in the 200 pig breeding farms of state governments, agricultural universities and Krishi Vigyan Kendra. The department was implementing a centrally sponsored scheme "Assistance to States for Intregrated Piggery Development" since 1991-92. Though it was discontinued after the 9th 5-year plan, it is being revived 2005-06 onwards as a component of the new macro-scheme "National Project for Improvement of Poultry and Small Animals". A major constraint in piggery development is lack of adequate high quality breeding stock. To overcome this problem, exotic breeds of 280 pigs of Large

White Yorkshire, Landrace and Hampshire were imported by this department for state government pig farms, from USA during 1999-2000. These pigs have now started producing piglets. There are more than 128 lakh pigs in the country of which approximately 14.5% are graded and exotic variety. There are about 158 pig breeding farms in the country run by the state governments/union territories. Exotic breeds like Large White Yorkshire, Hampshire and Landrace are maintained at these farms. A new scheme on piggery development, viz. 'Integrated Piggery Development' has been initiated, on the basis of evaluation of the earlier scheme by NABARD, during 2006-07. Integrated piggery development scheme will be part of a new restructured centrally sponsored macro-management scheme, viz. National Project for Improvement of Poultry and Small Animals.

EXISTING PROBLEMS LIMITING ANIMAL HUSBANDRY AND DAIRYING

Opportunities for small to medium-scale commercial animal production reflect global patterns of urbanization, economic development and globalization. These changes provide chances for farmers to move from subsistence production to market oriented production. In the mature, developed economies, food costs are a relatively small percentage of disposable income as food security has been essentially achieved, and per capita consumption of animal product is stable or declining. In these economies, issues of food quality, food safety and respect for animal welfare and the environment are gaining importance. Farmers in developing nations must also address these issues if they aspire to market products in the developed nations.

Twenty-three per cent of the world's population living in developed countries presently consumes three to four times meat and fish and five to six times milk per capita than those in developing countries. A change has, however, occurred in the last few decades leading to increase in consumption of animal products in developing countries. From the early 1970s to the mid 1990s, consumption in developed countries has grown by 70 million metric tons. In value and caloric terms, meat consumption in developing countries increased by more than three times the increase in developed countries. Milk consumption in the developing world increased by more than twice as much as milk consumption in the developed world in terms of quantity, money value and calories. The consumption of food of animal origin, however, is still small. Income increase would make people more conscious for consuming more of these items resulting in improved overall nutrition.

WTO IN RELATION TO LIVESTOCK SECTOR

The livestock sector as an industry was recognized after several rounds of negotiations in the Uruguay Round (1986-1994) of General Agreement on trade and Tariffs (GATT). At present, WTO has about 6 agreements directly related to agriculture. These include Trade-related Aspects of Intellectual Property Rights (TRIPs), Agreement on Agriculture (AOA), Application of Sanitary and Phytosanitary Measures (SPS), Technical Barriers to Trade, Anti-dumping, Subsidies and Countervailing Measures and Safeguards.

The basis and objective of the WTO is to establish a level and market oriented trading system through progressive reduction in agricultural support. The major components of the market access under WTO directly related to livestock sector is reduction in tariff and synchronization of the non-tariff barriers, reduction of government subsidies and opening and access to the market.

With the constitution of WTO the whole world is going to be single market with all type of products across the border. To minimize the probability of disguised restrictions on international trade, two agreements are in WTO regime. The Sanitary and Phytosanitary Measures (SPS) and Technical Barriers to Trade (TBT).

The ministerial conference of WTO at Doha from 9-14 November 2001 highlighted the continued recognition of special and differential treatment for the developing countries and of food security and rural development of domestic support. From Indian perspective, it was felt that the progressive reforms in agriculture would require elimination of large-scale domestic support and other trade distorting subsidies. It would also require the removal of all unfair barriers facing farm exports of the developing countries. The large rural populations in developing countries are critically dependent on agriculture there is a need to adequately provide for their food and livelihood security. It is particularly important that negotiations should be held for extending geographical indications to products. Also there should not be any misappropriation of the biological and genetic resources and traditional knowledge of the developing countries. This could have far reaching implications on the availability of affordable plant-based medicines.

The major SPS concern for India includes the quality and safety of dairy and meat products. It is imperative that the principle of hazard analysis critical control point (HACCP) systems, Code of practices on good animal feed, good hygienic practices (GHP) and good manufacturing practices (GMP) and cold chain system are followed. India should also put in place prevention of infectious and contagious diseases in Animals Act and take effective measures to eradicate "A" category disease as notified by OIE. For the hygienic practices for milk production, Codex standards are required not only for the livestock product for export conform to stipulated safety and suitability standards but also that the raw milk used in the manufacture of the products is produced using GHP and GMPs. Extensive extension programmes should be implemented to ensure this. The maximum permissible levels of aflatoxins, heavy metals, veterinary drugs, pesticide residues, etc. are increasingly becoming areas of major safety concerns. SPS measures permit members to adopt, if necessary, a higher level of protection based on risk assessment. Better physical infrastructure for reference laboratories for monitoring and surveillance of the contaminants and their levels, strengthening of information systems for risk analysis are needed. The quality of all the livestock products, raw or processed meat for export has to improve to meet the international standards. For this, appropriate quality control measures, modern processing and infrastructure facilities should be developed. In order to become significant player in the world market, it is necessary to ensure a sizeable market surplus of exportable farm products.

MEASURES TO SUSTAIN ECONOMY FROM ANIMAL HUSBANDRY AND DAIRYING

Animal husbandry and dairying needs organisation in more efficient way so as to obtains maximum production. Governments, NGOs and SHGs should take initiative in this direction and promote establishment of cooperative dairy farms, piggery, poultry farms, goat farms and sheep farms. In addition, non-convention animal rearing such as rabbit, ducks, turkey, etc. should also be promoted. Special attention should be paid for the development of micro-enterprises for value addition of these livestock products that will not only fetch more profit but also help increase our export share of livestock products in the world. Government has taken initiation in this direction by giving loans and subsidies for such establishments. However, much remains undone. The quality of all livestock products, raw or processed meat for export has to be improved to meet the international standards. For this, appropriate quality control measures, modern processing and infrastructure facilities should be developed. In order to become a significant player in the world market, it is necessary to ensure a sizeable market surplus of the exportable farm products. The productivity growth should also be higher in order to offset the effect of cost reducing technological innovation expected to be adopted by the developed nations. It will also help in reducing the problem of inflation on cost production. In addition, the information system needs to be strengthened. The various government agencies involved in export and import should be under one umbrella.

ANIMAL HEALTH TECHNOLOGIES DEVELOPED AT IVRI, IZATNAGAR, INDIA

Indian Veterinary Research Institute is a premier veterinary research organization of South East Asia founded in 1889. The Indian Veterinary Research Institute (IVRI) is perhaps the only organization in South-East Asia, where integrated training and research facilities in livestock health, production, technology and extension are existing simultaneously under one umbrella. The remarkable contributions of this institute has helped the country to make significant progress in the field of animal health and production. The major landmark achievement of the institute was the development of Rinderpest vaccine, through which this deadly disease of livestock was eradicated from the country. This institute is further well known all over the world for its impressive contribution in the various aspects of livestock and poultry health and production technology. This institute is mainly aimed at conducting research, providing postgraduate education and transfer of technology in all areas of animal sciences. Further it is also acting as a national referral centre for veterinary type cultures, disease diagnosis, biological and immuno-diagnostics, etc.

A major focus of research at this institute has been the development of sensitive and specific diagnostics and immunoprophylactics. Till now the institute has developed 44 immunobiologicals against many bacterial, viral and parasitic diseases of economic importance such as HS, FMD, swine fever, PPR, enterotoxaemia, sheep pox, goat pox, buffalo pox, anthrax, black quarter, etc. Institute has patented/registered for patent 40 technologies and commercialized 5 technologies to commercial houses, i.e. OI in all, crstoscope, area specific mineral mixture; FMD and PPR vaccine. Through a number of national and international research projects, the institute is constantly generating newer technologies in the field of animal health and production. The technology developed by the institute and its researchers have been given recognitions and awards at various national and international level. The institute has generated a large number of vaccines, diagnostics, immunobiologicals and other animal production technologies, which are being used by the livestock owners and field veterinary practitioners. These technologies have improved livestock health and production potential to a large extent and the livestock mortality has drastically reduced. A large number of the technologies have been developed by IVRI, which have already been transferred to the farmers and end users in the past years.

CONSTRAINTS OF LIVESTOCK SECTOR

Unorganized Production

Although the milk industry under organized sector has fast growth in the last three decades, it handles only about 30–35% of the milk marketed whereas 65–70% of the market share is still in the hands of unorganized sector. Innumerable vendors, small processors, merchants, manufacturers and retailers of indigenous milk products characterise the unorganized sector. Time has come to bring about structural changes in the unorganized sector.

Inadequacy of Fodder Availability

The inadequacy in fodder availability, both dry and green, has been one of the major problems in development of animal husbandry and dairying sector. It is estimated that during years 2000, the availability of fodder remained in short supply by about 47%. The shortage remained deficit that of dry fodder by 22%. Due to the extensive use of combine harvesters, especially in states like Punjab and Haryana, a large portion of the paddy and wheat straw is either left and burnt or becomes unfit for fodder purpose. In the coming years, the use of machinery is projected to increase which will further affect the availability of crop residues. Quality fodder seeds are a major constraint for fodder production.

Inadequate Market Facility

India has over 2000 markets where livestock are traded which are not developed on scientific lines. Market facilities are generally inadequate and if available are poorly maintained. Wholesale marketing margins amount to about 30% of the consumer price. Singh et al. (2004) in his study on livestock economy in UP was found that market for livestock products was major constraints of milk producers.

Inadequate Disease Prevention Measures

In 1977, FAO/IAEA recommended accreditation of veterinary laboratories for disease diagnosis and for surveillance data to control disease. In spite of the fact, India controlled African horse sickness, Equine influenza and Equine infectious anaemia and recently Rinderpest, but international authorities have not yet accepted our assessment that India is free from disease. In order to bring transparency, OIE certification is becoming mandatory with authenticated data to support our claim for the freedom from the diseases. Use of quality assured diagnostic system, surveillance and monitoring would assist regional or national control and eradication programme of diseases.

Presently, India is producing 21 viral, 13 bacterial and 1 protozoal vaccine and 11 diagnostic reagents. These immunobiologicals are being produced in bout 27 biological production units. Most of the biologicals produced in the state unit lack consistency for quality products and suffer from appropriate technical inputs and inspection system.

Inadequate Credit Facilities and Financial Supports

Public sector lending in livestock sector is abysmally low and such inadequate credit support leads to poor capital formation. The livestock farmers are mainly dependent on the financial intermediaries and bearing a higher interest rate. The share of animal husbandry and dairying sector was received only 5.7% of total ground level credit offered through NABARD for agricultural and allied sectors during 1999-2000, and this support is given in the form of only term loan to the tune of Rs 2366 crore. No production credit or short-term credit was given to this sector. The concept of working capital loan as has been in operation for small-scale sector is not offered the livestock sector.

Poor Livestock Health Services

In most of states, livestock health services are facing problems due to negligence of state government. Due to inadequate finance support, most of veterinary hospitals and dispensaries have very poor infrastructure and human resources. Though the Veterinary Council of India (VCI) recommended one veterinarian per 5000 animal populations, but it was not at all implemented in most of states. Even in the states like Maharashtra where milk industry has developed well, the ratio of veterinarian to animal population is nearly 1:10000–15000, which is far wide than the recommended level.

Lack of Product Processing Facilities

Though in milk sector, India have made some progress in processing the milk into milk products, but it still not up to the mark and most of milk is sold as raw milk in open market without any processing and poor hygienic conditions. Regarding the meat at present in India has only 3600 slaughterhouses out of these only 2700 registered. The concept of frozen meat transport is not all developed in India.

Heavy Subsidies in the Developed Countries

Since January 1995, the agreement of WTO, quantitative restrictions have been removed on the export and import of live animals and animal products including milk. Import tariff by and large for the range animal products is bound at 100%. The problem Indian farmers facing with respect to livestock products are not as much the low tariff rates but the heavy subsidies given to farmers in the develop countries especially the EEC countries who have huge surpluses to dispose off, which create unhealthy competition in the world market. India does not provide any product specific subsidy to any livestock product.

Technical Barriers

Raising the level of quality standards to internationally competitive levels in one of the major challenges. There are technical barriers, however, as the phytosanitary measures, which need to be overcome by maintaining hygienic conditions and preventing the incidence of animal diseases. Failure to enforce strict implementation of sanitary and hygienic measures and to adopt improvements in the slaughter and processing of animal has stood in the way of harnessing the export potential of livestock product sector particularly the quality conscious.

FOCUS AND STRATEGY IN TENTH PLAN

Animal husbandry and dairying will receive high priority in the efforts for generating wealth and employment, increasing the availability of animal protein in the food basket and for generating exportable surpluses. The overall focus will be on four broad pillars, viz.

  i. Removing policy distortions that is hindering the natural growth of livestock production;
 ii. Building participatory institutions of collective action for small-scale farmers that allow them to get vertically integrated with livestock processors and input suppliers;
iii. Creating an environment in which farmers will increase investment in ways that will improve productivity in the livestock sector; and
 iv. Promoting effective regulatory institutions to deal with the threat of environmental and health crises stemming from livestock. The 10th 5-year plan target for milk production is set at 108.4 mt envisaging an annual growth rate of 6%. Egg and wool production targets are set at 43.4 billion numbers and 63.7 million kg, respectively. The allocation for animal husbandry, dairying and fishery is Rs 2500 crore during the 10th plan.

FUTURE STRATEGIES

Organization of Production System

There is an urgent need to give a fillip for the organized production of various livestock products. Government shall endeavour to provide fiscal and policy support to help development of small scale sector dairies so that more unorganized sector is brought under the ambit of cooperative/private organized sector and quality assurance programmes. Further use of information technology in village dairy cooperative societies would enable the farmers to capitalize on opportunities and protect them from exploitation.

Region Specific Approach

Within the country, there are wide variations in productivity levels. Punjab, Haryana, Andhra Pradesh may have attained productivity levels of the world standard. But other regions are way behind. Similarly, pig husbandry is the most important activity in the North Eastern region inhabited by strong consumer base of tribal people. Though, this region has a substantial pig population, which constitutes around 25% of the country's pig population, but bulk of the population, however, is indigenous type whose growth and productivity is very low. Therefore, region-specific strategies should be adopted to realize the full potential of yield in every region taking into account the agronomic, climatic and environmental conditions. Ducks are very popular around coastal areas. The focus shall be to replace local ducks with improved egg and meat type breeds. Programmes on other avian species like quails, guinea fowl and turkey shall be strengthened.

Fodder Availability

In area of fodder production, some strategies like establishment of fodder banks, fodder treatment, enrichment of straw with urea and molasses, use of chaff cutters, hay/silage demonstrations, production of fodder seed and emphasis on fodder production are needed to obtain optimum production in livestock sector. Preparation of database on various feeds and fodder resources, feeding practices and consumption patterns in various agro-climatic zones is necessary. Practical use of biotechnological techniques such as recombinant microbes to digest straws, neutralize lignin and its by-products. Efforts should be made to increase area under fodder crops and agro-forestry by using uncultivated, barren and fallow lends. Feeds quality standards for compound feed shall be continuously adopted to help protect interest of livestock owners.

Reduction of Surplus Cattle

The issue of reduction of surplus cattle was dealt in the Second Five Year Plan but so far it not addressed adequately. It is noticed that the fodder and other resources of the country were grossly inadequate even for maintaining the existing cattle population. Therefore, government should recognize that culling and utilization of surplus animals is an established norm for animal production and improvement. States should take a realistic view of the fodder resources available in defining the scope of bans on the slaughter of cattle. Government should support to voluntary organizations to take responsibility of unserviceable and unproductive cattle, where such animal can be maintained with minimum cost.

Cost-effective Ways of Rearing the Calves

The premature death of buffalo and cross-bred males is a loss of great potential for meat production. The mortality rate in urban buffalo calves is reported to be 60–90% for various reasons and there are about 5.74 million buffalo calves that need to be saved from early death. If their survival is ensured and fattened it could be an assured source of raw material for high quality meat production. There is need to evolve and adopt cost-effective way of rearing of such calf.

Rural-based Abattoirs with Processing Facilities

Establishment or rural abattoir linked with consumption centres at cities and town could be an alternative with many added advantages. Establishing rural-based abattoirs (RBA) with processing facilities in animal tracts would drastically reduce the need for transportation of live animals to urban areas for slaughter.

There should be at least one carcass utilization plant in each district so that dead and fall animals are processed and farmers are paid for hide and bone.

Intellectual Property Rights

Urgent steps are needed to protect the intellectual property rights of region specific livestock's, which proved their production potential such as Vechchoor. Kasaragod cattle, Malabari goat, Black Beatle goat of Kerala.

Adoption of Appropriate Technology

Technology supported and demand driven livestock growth will be the future engine for growth. New commercially viable technologies of production should be adopted for the efficient use of the existing resources and to fulfill the local demands as well as for tapping the external markets of livestock products. There is need for transition from subsistent livestock farming to sustainable and financially viable livestock farming, which will generate wealth and self-employment through entrepreneurship.

Adequate and Timely Financial Support

Financing should be done against model projects that have demonstrated their economic viability. The venture capital fund should be created in the Department of Animal Husbandry and Dairying (in collaboration with NABARD) for establishment of infrastructure by private entrepreneurs like veterinary hospitals, vaccine production units, feed plants, fodder seed production facilities, processing plants for western and indigenous dairy, meat and egg products, semen production units including bull mother farms and network for delivery of semen to the farmers. Such provision will help the entrepreneur to avoid rushing to the bank for further financial help and make a long wait by which time the activity might suffer irreparable loss. Introduction of Dairy and Poultry Farmers Credit Card (Like Kisan Credit Card) would solve the problem of working capital.

Remunerative Prices

Problems of livestock sector are compounded by non-remunerative prices of livestock products, an issue which has not received the attention of the government. Development of marketing network and remunerative prices support to the producers will be a great incentive for higher animal productivity both in quality and quantity. Creation of a permanent institution in the line of commission on agricultural costs and prices (CACP) should be formed which will estimate the cost of production of various livestock products and suggest remunerative price so that farmers are not exploited.

Livestock Extension Services

Presently livestock extension is attached with agriculture extension. Livestock extension is primarily based on delivery of services and inputs. It needs to be treated differently from crop related extension activities because livestock are kept with multiple objectives ranging from income generation, food, fuel and fertilizer production to socio-cultural linkage, which makes change process much more difficult. Panchayats, Cooperatives and NGOs should play a leading role in generating dedicated band of service providers at the farmer's doorstep in their respective areas. There is a need for establishment of a fully operational Directorate of Extension in the Departmental and a National Institute of Livestock Extension (NILE) in the country.

Gender Issue

Involvement of women is more in livestock keeping, compared to crop production. Most training and TOT programmes are men oriented, so is the extension material and these do not suit women in view of different perceptions, priorities, other duties and higher illiteracy amongst them. For livestock extension to be effective, we need more sustained effort, greater interaction with farmers with participatory and systems approach and due consideration of socio-cultural aspects. Gender issue acquires much more importance in livestock development processes and inclusion of women in the extension team is necessary for faster impact.

Effective Coverage of Livestock Insurance Scheme

Issue of financial loss during natural calamities and disaster will require attention and suitable programme need to be developed since such asset loss can drive the poor into destitution. Remunerative livestock production system will call for protection against the risks due to natural calamities, diseases, outbreaks, extreme market fluctuations, etc. The insurance coverage for such exigencies will be encouraged particularly for owners below the poverty line.

Effective Monitoring of Management of Dairy Co-operative

Though, the co-operative approach of dairy development has been successful in India, but due to incompetent management of dairy co-operatives facing various problems. Out of 168 milk unions, 105 milk unions were running in loss as on 2000. These loss making unions handled about 35% of the milk of the cooperative sector. Investment in the dairy sector has been reduced drastically in the 9th 5-year plan. Therefore, this issue should be addressed by effective monitoring and regulations.

Specialized Veterinary Services

In areas having highly productive and valuable animals, there is need for making available specialized veterinary services. As presently, the animal health care service is almost free, it is becoming increasingly difficult for the state to strengthen such services. There is a class of livestock owners who can afford to pay for the services, such owners shall be charged for the services provided. This will not only help the state to improve animal health services but also attract private investment. A research study conducted by Ahuja Vinod et al (2003) in state of Gujarat, Rajasthan and Kerala shows farmers are ready to day for such services.

Import Duty

Import duty on equipment, medicines, feed additives, etc. should be rationalized for promoting animal rearing by farmers.

Information System

Database for livestock sector are not only poor but lack authenticity. There are large data gaps. These gaps would be identified and steps taken to generate and disseminate. The required information for proper planning and programme implementation.

Effective Breeding Strategy

The current yield levels for crossbred, indigenous cows and buffaloes of 1800, 900 and 1200 kg per year respectively could safely be increased to the targeted levels through of selection and progeny testing of bulls for milk and providing breeding and other input services at the farmers, door. The newer breeding and reproductive technologies like open nucleus breeding system (ONBS) and embryo transfer (ET) shall be an integrated part of breed improvement. Efforts are required to increase artificial insemination (AI) rate in certain state.

QUALITY STANDARD OF LIVESTOCK PRODUCTS

With a view to compete in international market in respect of quality standards, methods of collection, storage, transport and processing of milk have to be modernized to ensure quality and hygiene synchronizing with international standards. Suitable legislation/administrative mechanism would be brought in place to ensure that milk is handled in most scientific conditions and reaches the customer without any contamination or any other health hazard agent.

Registration of the all slaughterhouses in the city/town is must for clean meat production it should be located keeping in view environmental angle and logistic support. Machinery is required to be put in place to provide support for creation of necessary infrastructure for rural slaughter houses, transport arrangements, cold storage and marking. Large modern abattoirs shall be encouraged for production of quality meat. Regulatory supervision of export oriented slaughter is necessary in order to synchronize with global health standards to augment export. Quality processing, attractive packaging, cold chain and suitable marketing network should be made an integral part of the production and processing.

Disease-free Zone

In view of the large size of the country, it may not be possible to control and eradicate livestock diseases from the entire country at one point of time and creation of disease free zone with respect to a specific disease is a recognized method of solving this problem in a phased manner. To start with, foot and mouth disease-free zones are sought to be created in areas with export potential. The zone concept should be focused to the areas where there is export potential for meat, milk, skin/hide and other livestock products or the area from where the disease could be easily controlled and animals and animal products could be exported.

Health Aspect

There is need for a position of controller veterinary vaccines, biological and drugs, who would be responsible for the harmonization of veterinary vaccines, drugs and diagnostic reagents. Introducing quality management system shall strengthen facilities for specific and general disease diagnosis. An inventory of traditional Indian medicinal practice for animal health shall be prepared and used. Other alternate systems of medicine adopted in the country shall be used for ailments against which they are effective. Special emphasis will be laid for control of zoonotic to safeguard human health and food safety.

Effective Quarantine Mechanism

Creation of animal quarantine certification and enforcement authority, Quarantine facilities shall be further strengthened and strict zoo sanitary and quarantine procedures followed to prevent ingress of exotic diseases. The system of export health certification shall be synchronized with global standards to promote export. With a view to control inter-state transmission of diseases, the movement of livestock from one state to another shall be regulated through central legislative backup. Mechanism for emergency preparedness against emerging and exotic diseases shall be put in place. A system of reliable and prompt disease reporting, forecasting and creation of database for all important diseases will be put in place.

Veterinary Educational System and Human Resources

Since 1994, Veterinary Council of India came into force for regulation of veterinary education in India. But so far only five states have taken initiatives for establishment of separate animal science and veterinary universities. Still in most of the states, veterinary education system is under the state agriculture universities and has very poor infrastructures facilities and faculties due to negligence of agriculture universities.

Therefore, other states should be take responsibility to separate out veterinary education as a separate entity with strong financial support for creation of qualitative and quantitative human resources.

NEGOTIATIONS IN INTERNATIONAL MARKET

A major difficulty faced by India in the international market is the high level of domestic support and export subsidies given by developed countries for agri-exports. Hence it is imperative to evolve concrete strategies to make Indian agriculture competition and enhance its efficiency.

The present scenario has resulted into new priorities and calls for meaningful role of extension education to exploit the opportunities for desired gains.

The present paper tried to analyze the strengths, constraints, opportunities and future strategies of livestock sector in India. The present scenario has resulted into new priorities and calls for the meaningful role of veterinary extension to exploit the opportunities for desired gains. The strong animal/veterinary research and extension base coupled with the hard work of the livestock owners and appropriate policy efforts will definitely play a vital role for ushering white revolution and achieving the red revolution in India.

Recommendations on Animal Husbandry and Dairy Sectors (state ministers' conference on animal husbandry dairying and fisheries on 3rd February 2003 in Vigyan Bhavan, New Delhi)

1. Improvement of the livestock breeding is important but also increased remuneration to the farmers.
2. Charges for the services like artificial insemination can also be levied for other services so that the quality of services can be improved and the fund so received can again be ploughed back for the development of animal husbandry.
3. Disease control is of immense importance from the farmers' point of view. Therefore, a massive programme is required to eradicate some of the diseases like foot and moth disease.
4. There is need to form a separate body for carrying out research in the field of animal husbandry. This body may be called the Indian Council of Veterinary Research so that better synergies can be developed between the farmers and various research institutions.
5. Promotion of milk and milk products through the mid-day meal programme.
6. The Government of India may take up with the state governments the issue of fodder development on wastelands and degraded lands so as to over come the deficit in fodder supply.
7. Development of poultry and small ruminants like sheep, goats are very important from the point of view of small and marginal farmers and specially in the hilly and backward areas of the country.
8. Livestock policies must reflect the regional cattle wealth of the country and ensure preservation of the indigenous breeds of livestock.

For Indian livestock sector to emerge successful in the fast changing global scenario and an unqualified need to produce more food in term of quality, quantity and availability for the booming domestic population, there is a need to introspect and project itself with renewed vigour at every possible opportunity that globalization shall provide. For this, areas should be identified for immediate attention. These includes biotechnology, conservation, effective management, use of bioresources, management of IPR related tasks, post-harvest management of the product, safe delivery in the consumer market, more investment in the indigenous product, etc. In addition, thrust in the direction of building infrastructure for promoting livestock health and production is needed in the form of development of veterinary hospitals in every village, polyclinic with facility of modern laboratories at least at district level and appointment of subject specialist at these laboratories and polyclinics. Funds provided by Indian Government is very less compared to the share of agriculture in the GDP compared to other developed countries. If conclusive results with respect to sustaining our country economics by development of animal husbandry and dairying are to be achieved, it is possible only by problem oriented research and release of funds for such practical based research.

In order to forage balance in trade, WTO agreements in relevant cases are expected to create/enhance opportunities for agribusiness, particularly in improved packages/methods of farming that require regulated use of chemicals inputs, post-harvest processing and value addition and packaging. Overall, the impact of further challenges and opportunities with increased scope of converting challenges into opportunities. Capital flow is essential prerequisite for sustained/

enhanced entrepreneurship, partnerships and synergies wherein the former is bound to increase with the application of legislative and regulatory provisions as per the various WTO agreements. The globalization process has thrown open opportunities for active contribution of scientist. The globalization process will induce the private sector to go in for research on its own. In future, public-private partnership for carrying out research in the areas of mutual continence is, therefore, relevant and important. The linkage between the public research and the private industrial sectors may help in strengthening production/export of the export-oriented products. Research can be positively reorganized based on the feedback of the exporters. Also requisite and logical decision has to be taken for any offer of investment in public sector particularly the multinationals while taking due note of emerging bio-concerns of the developing countries, such as bio-survey, bio-piracy, bio-partnership, bio-safety, etc.

33

Project Planning

Deepa Vinay

Entrepreneur, entrepreneurship and enterprise go hand in hand. It has to be stressed that people are the most valuable resource within any country. There exist a strong linkage between the training, attitudes and goals of people and the level of economic growth within a country. An essential ingredient for the earner growth of any country is the key individuals who promote change and development. These persons may be called entrepreneur. These entrepreneurs take numerous decisions to convert their business idea into a running concern. In setting up of an enterprise, decision-making process start with project selection. Infect project selection is the first corner stone to be laid down in setting up an enterprise.

Any proposed activity whose cost and benefit to some extent can be isolated, where cost must be incurred before benefits are known, is known as project. Project can be major or minor. Thus any single proposed activity which involves expenditure and returns, and about which any decision must be made is known as project. Project can have urgent priority or may be of simple in nature but understanding the goal of a project is must. The goal of the project may be:

- To make profit irrespective of benefit to many or most of the community.
- To employ many of the people of community on the project irrespective of profits.
- To make some profit while bringing benefit to many or most of the community.

Any scheme, design, or proposal of some thing intended or devised to achieve is called project. There are three basic attributes of project.

a. A course of action.
b. Specific objectives.
c. Definite time perspective.

Every project has a starting point and an end point with specific objectives.

CLASSIFICATION OF PROJECT

The project can be classified on the basis of its nature.

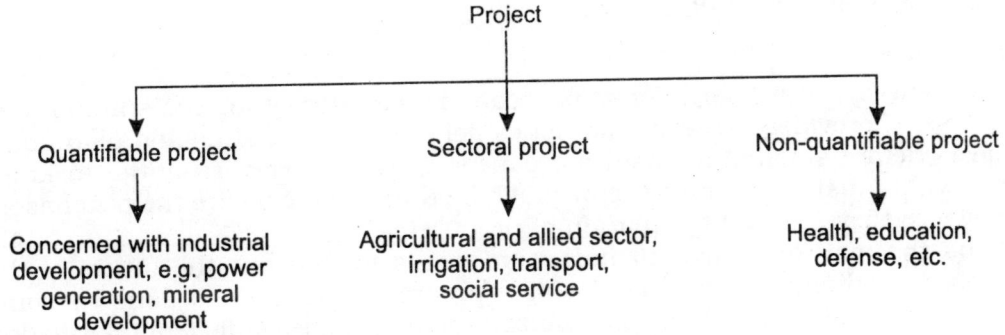

PROJECT IDENTIFICATION

The selection of a right project goes to validate "the trite proposition well begun is half done". Any project idea which have a good market, can be identified as best project.

Project selection process starts with idea generation. Ideas can be discovered from various internal and external sources. These may include:

i. Knowledge of potential customer needs.
ii. Watching emerging trends in demands for certain products.
iii. Scope for producing substitute product.
iv. Professional magazines.
v. Success stories of known entrepreneur.

Planning a project is a very important task and should be taken up with great care, as the efficiency of the whole project largely depends upon its planning (Fig. 33.1). While planning a project, each and every detail should be worked out in anticipation considering all the relevant provision in advance.

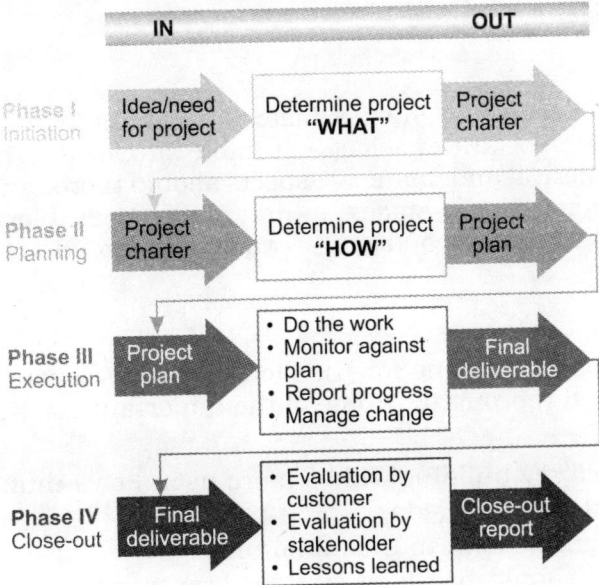

Fig. 33.1: Project management frameworks

FUNCTIONS IN PROJECT PLANNING

Market Survey

Market survey, in a board sense is a commercial survey for the suitability of business. It provides necessary statistics helpful for forecasting and planning a project. Before starting a business, market survey is very essential to know about what must be produced, how much be produced, who are the purchasers and where they are located, margin of profit, etc.

Thus the main objective of market survey is to find out the future of the proposed products. In the initial stage, preliminary survey is done by some experienced analyst and if this preliminary survey supplies sufficient information that there is no profitable market for the product to be manufactured then further detailed survey is not required. If preliminary survey provides some hope then only detailed survey is done.

Project Capacity

After conducting the market survey, capacity of the project must be decided considering the amount of money which can be invested for the particular type of product and how the money can be arranged, i.e. by partnership, through banks, financing corporations or shares. While deciding the capacity of the project, following are the factors which should also be considered.

1. Demand of the product in the market.
2. Whether the demand is regular or fluctuating
3. Quantity of power, water, land and raw material available.
4. Type of business organization.
5. Nature of the product.
6. Investment capacity.

Selection of Site

When it has been decided to start a factory for manufacturing a particular product, it is most important to select a suitable site for it. While selecting the site technical, commercial and financial aspects should thoroughly be considered. Site should be selected in two stages, in first stage general location for factory should be decided and in second stage exact site should be selected in this location.

Plant Layout

For the construction of building for the factory and its layout, several factors should be considered thoroughly. Some of the important considerations in this respect are:

1. Whether single storey building will be more useful or a multistory building.
2. Provisions for future expansion.
3. Material movement be kept to the minimum.
4. Flow of material should be along straight line to minimise the production delays.

5. Flexibility for future changes.
6. Easy to supervise.
7. Proper lighting and ventilation.

Design and Drawing

Having been decided about the product to be manufactured, it must be designed. The work of design should be done very carefully by the experienced designer considering all the relevant factors. After designing the product, its detailed drawings are prepared so that no doubt is left for future. Detailed specifications for raw material and finished product should be decided carefully along with the specification of the machines required for their manufacture.

Material Requirement

The list of material required for manufacture is prepared from the drawings. This list is known as "Bill of Material". This bill passes through the storekeeper, who makes the entries of the material available in the store, but in the starting of the project, it directly passes to the purchase organization for the procurement of material.

Operation Planning

The work of planning department is to select the best method of manufacturing, so that the wastage of material, labour, machine and time can be eliminated, to have more production with least fatigue. This work is done in two phases, namely method study and time study.

Method Study

Method study is conducted to eliminate the wastage due to ill-directed and inefficient motions. In this study, work is divided into fundamental elements and then these elements are studied separately and in relation to one another, and then develop a method of least wastage.

Time Study

Exact estimation of time is very essential for correct pricing. Hence time study is required to be performed to find out the correct manufacturing time for the product. Time study is also helpful for production scheduling, machine loading, budgeting and cost control. Time study is performed on average workers and on average machines for the method finalized on the basis of method study.

Machine Loading

Number of machines to be installed in a plant should be decided very carefully, as excess machines will lead to machine idleness, and shortage of machine means difficulty in achieving the target of production. While planning, proper care should be taken to find out the machines time for each operation as correct as possible, so that arrangement for full utilization of machines can be made and machine loading programmer is prepared accordingly.

Sub-contract Consideration

In the past (few decades ago), each and every component of the product was manufactured in the factory. But with the development of technology and specialization, it is difficult to manufacture all the components in the same factory, because specialized machines, plant and skilled workers for each component cannot be afforded by a single concern. The decision about a particular item, whether to purchase or to manufacture, is taken by planning department after making a thorough study of the relative merits and demerits.

Equipment Requirement

Results obtained from the "time and method study" and the "machine loading" helps in calculation the equipment requirement. Specification of equipment should be laid down by considering the drawings. Drawings will help in deciding the necessary requirement of the tools and accessories. After knowing the number of equipments, their accessories and tools required, cost data can be collected to give an idea of capital requirement.

Organization Layout and Staff Requirement

Now with all the available information, layout of organization is decided by considering the nature of work, type of industry, size of industry, etc. Organizational set up should be able to provide the co-ordination among men, material and machine in such a way so as to have the maximum output easily and efficiently under minimum total cost.

Total number of persons required to be employed in the organization and their wages are calculated, which will help in deciding the cost of production.

Material Handling

The material handling problem must be studied before the erection of the factory building and plant layout. Material handling is a prime consideration in designing the new plant building. This problem becomes more important in large scale industries. By proper layout, material handling cost improper handling may cause delays and reduces the efficiency.

Budgeting

Budgeting is a forecasting and preplanning for a particular future period using past experience and market trends. Planning department prepares the budget, i.e. a programme for future operation and expected results about working capital, material, labour, production, etc.

Cost Calculation

Total cost of a product can be calculated by adding the following expenses incurred during a   particular period on a product:

1. Material expenses
2. Labour expenses
3. Factory expenses

4. Administrative expenses
5. Selling expenses
6. Distribution expenses

After calculating the total cost of a product, next step is to decide the profit to be taken on each product, which when added to the total cost gives the selling price of a product. Total cost for a product is fixed, as this is the expenditure actually made on the manufacture of a product, hence only profit is a variable factor which affects the selling price of a product. While deciding the profit fallowing factors should be kept in mind.

1. Whether the business has monopoly or is in competition.
2. Whether to determine on the cost of production or to change what the customers can pay.
3. Whether the substation are available in the market.
4. What is the price of competitive product in the market.

Break-even Point

Break-even point is the level of the production/sales where the industrial enterprise shall earn neither profit nor incur loss. In fact, it will just break even. Break-even level indicates the gestation period and likely moratorium required for repayment of loans.

$$BEP = [F/(S-V)] \times 100$$

Where, F = Fixed cost
S = Sales projected
V = Variable costs

Thus, the break-even point so calculated will indicate at what percentage of sales, the enterprise will break-even.

Critical Report on Feasibility

In the end, a critical report is prepared on the basis of the cost informations available from the above mentioned facts. Generally, rate of return on the invested capital is taken as the criteria for analyzing the feasibility of the project. If the rate of return is too less than some other alternative project may be taken up which may give the highest rates of return on the investment.

CHOOSING THE PROJECT

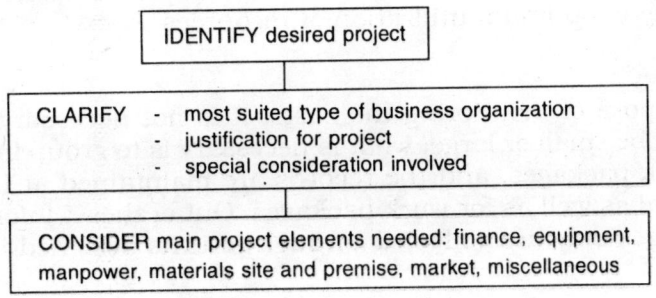

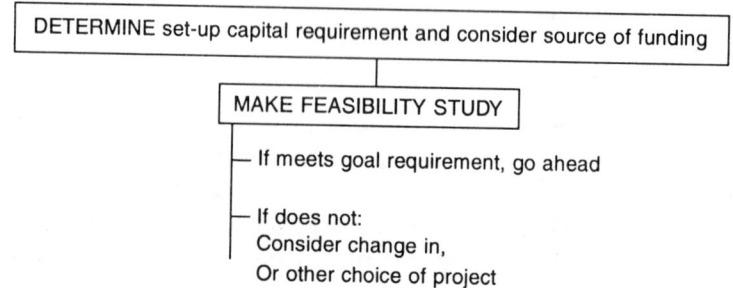

PROJECT IMPLEMENTATION

Next stage in the project cycle is actual implementation of the project for its construction and operation. For proper project implementation, emphasis should be on action as per planning. For this purpose, organization set up and sound project management system should be established so as to manage the projects in a rational and scientific manner, following the latest management principles, tools and techniques. For large international or World Bank aided projects, some times consultants are also appointed.

During the implementation stage of the project, there is need for continuous monitoring to ensure project implementation as per time and cost schedules. For effective monitoring, it is essential to have a good speed and reliability of communication system and establish the dependable information system.

PROJECT MONITORING AND CONTROL

Project monitoring is a system procedure to collect and analyses information related to the implementation of the project. The monitoring provides timely information and feedback to the management regarding vital stage in project implementation. Periodic feedback on the progress of the project helps the management to know the achievement of the project and compare it with the targets in order to take appropriate steps for proper implementation of project. As a corrective step, management can correct the lagging time-schedule, synchronize with other related activities and identify other slippages and take remedial measures.

EFFICIENCY OF THE MONITORING AND CONTROL DEPENDS UPON THE EFFICIENCY OF THE INFORMATION SYSTEM

Monitoring is basically done for parameters, namely project cost originally approved/latest approved estimated cost and project completion/commissioning dates by way of optimum utilization of resources.

Cost Control

For the purpose of monitoring the costs, it is not necessary to consider each activity may be small or large, what is necessary is to group individual activities to form work packages, and the records are maintained at the operating level for individual as well as for work packages. Out of these, information regarding work packages only are collected through returns designed for the monitoring system.

Efficiency of monitoring and control of cost also depends upon the proper reporting format and quality of information supplied. Generally, these formats are the cost status, which enable the monitoring manager to know as to how much work has been done, with what cost, and how much cost should have been incurred for this work as per plan (estimate). The frequency of this report is decided according to the requirement of effectiveness of monitoring. This also enables the management to know shortfalls and surpluses in funds position.

PROJECT EVALUATION

Projects are evaluated and their performance audit is done with idea of gaining experience for subsequent project in their identification, preparation and appraisal. This ex-post evaluation is very useful in providing experience for future work, since during execution process, the attention is more towards the problems being faced at that time.

These evaluation and completion report both re-estimate the economic rate of return on the basis of actual costs and updated information on operating costs and expected benefits. This evaluation system provides very useful information, supplementing and complementing that provided by the project completion reports.

The idea of evaluation is that, past mistakes are not repeated and new approaches, policies, and procedures are adopted to improve the project performance, reduce cost overruns and implementation delays.

Evaluation of the public projects is based on the benefits and costs analysis instead of the rate of return or extent of profit expected to accrue. Public projects are those projects, which are taken up by the government for the benefit of the public, such as public safety, service, health, education, defence, water supply, roads, irrigation, etc. These projects are financed through government exchequer, and are generally of large in magnitude and multiple in purpose. Since there is no financial effectiveness measure available for such projects, their evaluation is difficult. Some of the benefits cannot be converted into money value, and usually they do not pay taxes, therefore the criteria for their economic evaluation is different from the private projects. In such cases, general practice is to identify benefits and costs of the projects, and then consider benefit cost ratio as means of economic effectiveness.

PREPARATION OF PROJECT REPORT

Webster New 20th Century Dictionary defines a project as a scheme, design, a proposal of something intended or devised. In simple words, project report or business plan is a written statement of what an entrepreneur proposes to take up. It is a kind of guide frost or course of action what the entrepreneur hopes to achieve in his business and how is he going to achieve it. In words, project report serves like a kind of big road map to reach the destination determined by the entrepreneur. Thus, a project report can best be defined as a well evolved course of action devised to achieve the specified objective within a specified period of time. So to say, it is an operating document.

Project report is a written statement of what an entrepreneur proposes to take up. It is a kind of guide or course of action.

"It is a well-evolved course of action devised to achieve the specified objective within a specified period of time. It is an operating document".

Significance of Project Report

1. It is like road map.
2. It attracts lenders and investors.

Contents of a Project Report

I. *General Information*

1. Biodata of promoter
2. Industry profile
3. Plant and machinery
4. Product details

II. *Project Description*

1. Site
2. Physical infrastructure
3. Utilities
4. Pollution control
5. Communication system
6. Transport facilities
7. Other common facilities
8. Production process
9. Machinery and equipment
10. Capacity of the plant
11. Technology selected
12. Research and development
13. Raw material
14. Man power
15. Product
16. Market
17. Requirement of working capital
18. Requirement of funds
19. Cost of production
20. Break-even analysis
21. Schedule of implementation.

Project Appraisal

Project appraisal means assessment of a project. It is also a cost and benefit analysis of different aspects of proposed project with an objective to adjudge its viability.

Appraisal of proposed project includes the following:

1. Economic analysis
2. Financial analysis
3. Market analysis
4. Technical feasibility
5. Management competence

Economic analysis: Requirement of raw material, level of capacity, utilization, anticipation sales, anticipated expenses and probable profits.

Financial analysis: Assessment of financial requirement both fixed and working.

a. *Fixed assets*: Tangible and material facilities which purchased once are used again and again, e.g. land, building, plant, machinery.

b. *Working capital*: It means excess of current assessors and current liabilities.

c. *Current assets*: These are those assets which can be converted in cash with a period of one week.

Current liabilities are those obligations which can be payable within a period of one week.

"Working capital is that amount of funds which is needed in day today's business operation."

Working capital works as a lubricant for any enterprise.

Technical feasibility: It is adequacy of the proposed plant and equipment to produce the product within the prescribed norms.

While assessing the technical feasibility of the project: the following inputs corered in the project should be taken into consideration.

1. Availability of the land site
2. Availability of other inputs like water, electricity
3. Availability of servicing facilitator like machine shop electric shop
4. Coping with anti-pollution law
5. Availability of work force-skilled, unskilled
6. Availability of required raw material

COMMON ERRORS IN PROJECT FORMULATION

Project formulation is as not so easy. However, the entrepreneur often makes errors while formulating project reports and business plans. Here, we are highlighting the errors widely noticed in project formulation.

Product Selection

It is noticed that some entrepreneurs commit mistakes by selecting a wrong product for their enterprise. They select the product markets, its future demand, competitive position, lifecycle, availability of required labour, raw material and technology. Hence, when you are selecting a product, take a comprehensive view.

Capacity Utilization Estimates

The entrepreneurs usually make over-optimistic estimates of capacity utilization. Their estimates are based on a completely false premise. The estimates are made in complete disregard of present-enterprise performance, prevailing market conditions, competitive atmosphere, the technical snags, etc. A business plan formulated a such falls prey to financial jugglery. Hence, avoid such temptations while estimating capacity utilization for your enterprise.

Market Study

Product production is ultimately meant for eventual sale. Hence, market study of the product assumes importance. Market study continues to be a grey area. But, there are some entrepreneurs who pass by this component of their business plan completely. Based on their nebulous ideas and scanty and scattered information on demand and supply of their proposed product, they conclude that market is just there waiting to be tapped. This is a wrong attitudinal block. Avoid it.

Technology Selection

The requirement for technology differs from product to product depending upon the nature of products. Swayed by the reported profit margins, the entrepreneurs sometimes plan for a technology not possible to set up within limited financial resources. Thus, in the absence of technology feasibility.

Location Selection

The entrepreneur often makes two types of errors while selecting location for their enterprises. First, they are completely swayed by the government offer of financial incentives and concessions to establish industries in a particular location. This becomes their sole and overriding concern completely disregarding other factors like market proximity, availability of raw materials, manpower and infrastructural facilities. Second, the entrepreneurs select a location for their enterprises merely because it is their home town or they own ancestral land there which is , however, not an appropriate location. Make sure you do not fall prey to such temptations.

Selection of Ownership Form

Many enterprise fail merely because the ownership form of enterprise is not suitable. Hence, select a suitable form of ownership taking a comprehensive view of the factors affecting the selection of a form of ownership.

STEPS IN SETTING UP A SMALL INDUSTRIAL ENTERPRISE

The various steps involved in setting up a business enterprise will be most complex when it relates to an industrial unit. The steps in setting up a small industrial enterprise are as follows.

Deciding to go into Business

This is the most crucial decision a youth has to take, shunning wage-employment and opting for self-employment/entrepreneurship.

Analyzing Strengths/Weaknesses

Having decided to become an entrepreneur, the young person has to analyze his/her strengths/weaknesses. This will enable him/her to know what type and size of business would be most suitable. This will vary from person to person.

Product Selection

The next step is to decide what business to venture into, the product or range of products that shall be taken up for manufacture and in what quantity. The level of activity will help in deciding size of business and form of ownership. One could generate a number of project ideas through environmental scanning, short list a few items, closely examine each one of these and zero on to a final products.

Market Survey

It is easy to manufacture an item but difficult to sell. So it is prudent to survey the market before embarking upon production and satisfy the product chosen is in demand changes in product design required, determining demand-supply gap, extent of competition, your potential share of the market, pricing and distribution policy, etc.

Form of Ownership

A firm can be constituted as proprietorship, limited company, (public or private) co-operative society, etc. This will depend upon the type purpose and size of your business. One may also decide on the form of ownership based on resources on hand or from the point of saving on taxes.

Location

The next step will be to decide on the place where the unit is to be located. Will it be hired or owned? The size of plot and covered and the last one identified. This will be useful in determining the machinery and equipment to be installed.

Machinery and Equipment

Having chosen the technology, the machinery and equipment required for manufacturing the chosen product/s have to be decided, suppliers identified and then costs estimated. One may have to plan well in advance for machinery and equipment especially if it has to be procured from outside the town, state or country that is, have to be imported.

Project Report

The economic viability and technical feasibility of the product selected has to be established through a project report. A project report that may now be prepared will be helpful in formulating the financial, production, marketing and management plans. It will also be useful in obtaining finance, shed, power, registration, raw material quotas, etc.

Finance

Money is no problem for starting scale industry. But an entrepreneur has to take certain steps and follow specific procedures to obtain it. A number of financial agencies will give loans on concessional terms. Under TRYSEM and SEEUY schemes, entrepreneurs are also eligible for subsidies which obviate the need for margin money.

Power Connection

The site chosen should either have adequate power connection or this should be arranged now.

Installation of Machinery

Having arranged finance, work shed, power, etc. the next step is to procure the machinery and begins its installation.

Recruitment of Manpower

Once machines are installed manpower will be required to run them. So the quantum and type (skilled, semi-skilled, unskilled, administrative, etc.) of labour have to be determined, sources of getting desired labour identified and labour/ staff recruited. Possibly, the labour has to be trained either at the entrepreneur's premises or in a training establishment.

34

Need for Literature for Entrepreneurship Development

Kundan Singh, PN Kaul

Farm literature is an important aid to the training of farmers and others connected with rural development. There are three target groups for this literature such as farmers, professionals and industrial entrepreneurs. For farmers and farm women, the subject matter is agricultural production, animal husbandry, home science, and arts and crafts for rural artisans. For professionals, the subjects are veterinary science, recent advances in agricultural and basic science. For industrial entrepreneurs, the subjects are animal nutrition, veterinary pharmacology, veterinary surgery and gynaecology, agricultural engineering, water technology, electronics engineering, and rural engineering. For farmers, the type of literature required is illustrated pamphlets, leaflets and bulletins, experiment can also be done with comics-like literature containing picture stories of important agricultural practices and success stories of farmers. Now the farmers should also be introduced to the scientific method and scientific way of logical thinking. The farmers need less static literature and more dynamic literature like newsletters, newspaper articles, live and recorded telecasts, radio broadcasts, etc. For professionals, more static literature is required; it should be free from references, and the applied aspects should be emphasized. For industrial entrepreneurs, there is a need for more dynamic literature and teleprogrammes of short duration which keeps updating and modernizing itself; it should contain directions for getting additional information; it should contain information on the recent development, innovation and technology of research institutions and universities; it should also contain information about scientific conferences, symposia, etc. and information about institute-industry interface meetings.

Training is an essential ingredient of entrepreneurship development. For training, one of the important visual aids is literature, including the written word in printed either on paper or on electronic media. In rural development, it is important to train farmers and other professionals in various skill-oriented subjects which can lead to an independent way of earning a livelihood for a long time, or for supplementing the family income or for value addition or in any other way contributing to the family economy, keeping in mind the social status of the particular family.

Skills are mostly learnt by practice led by proper guidance. Many skills can be learnt from trainers with the help of suitable literature like manuals, how to-do kits, pamphlets, recorded television programmes, etc. Such literature, being permanent, can be referred to again and again for reference as and when required. Much literature, produced for farmers is made available in a very unsuitable way. The printing is of a very low key. There is a popular notion that farm literature is of little use because most of the farmers are illiterate or semi-literate and thus they cannot understand the printed word. This is not true (Singh, 1981) as most farmers listen to the printed word in groups in which the printed matter is read out to them by a literate person and they understand it to the best of their ability. This was also true in Mahatma Gandhi's time, when the printed word used to spread very fast. At that time, the literacy rate was very low, but now when the literacy rate is much higher, the speed of spread of the printed messages is very high.

TARGET GROUPS

There are basically three groups who may act as the audience for farm literature. One is the farmers including rural farm youth and small farm women. By farmers is meant not only who till the land but also livestock owners, whether they own any land or not, and other rural people whose subsistence is directly or indirectly on agriculture or animal husbandry, like milk vendors, seed dealers, agricultural traders, etc. For farmers, we should have literature on various topics in crop production; e.g. production of major crops of the area such as paddy, wheat, surgarcane, mustard, etc. The literature, should explain all important aspects beginning from preparation of the land and going up to marketing of the product, in a practical manner. The language used should be familiar to the farmer. It is a good idea to first test the material on one or two farmers of the area, and to recast the same wherever necessary. Illustrations should be used freely, because these do not need literacy for understanding, in most cases. The behaviour desired for the changes required, should be emphasized. If available, interviewers of farmers who have adopted the advocated practice, should also be published.

Animal husbandry provides another good subject matter for farmers. The advantages of artificial insemination, prevention and control of important animal diseases like foot and mouth disease, haemorrhagic septicaemia; package of practices for pig rearing, feeding of calves, deworming of domestic animals, backyard poultry farming, hygeinic milk production, balanced feeding of domestic animals, etc. are good subjects for farm literature.

Similarly, home science subjects can also be utilized for writing for farm women. Smokeless chulah, soap making, production of pappads, soap making, candle making, recipes for some delicious foods, etc. can be used for writing. For rural artisans, various arts and like pottery, charpai making, making of toys, tailoring, etc. can be written upon. Basic skills and appreciations like painting can also be taught through literature, and these can be used by farmers in many ways ranging from fabric painting to making of 'rangoli' and designing of houses.

Whereas literature for farmers can directly be used for enhancing farm production or other aspects of agriculture, the literature for professionals can be used indirectly to support the efforts of farmers. These professionals may be professional agricultural graduates, veterinarians, home science graduates, managers of non-governmental agencies working with rural people, etc. Such professionals need literature on recent advances in agriculture science like plant, biotechnology, genetic engineering, production of newer crops, diseases of plants, orchards, packing of flowers, etc.

Veterinarians need literature on recent advances in animal husbandry and veterinary science. The latest trends in veterinary surgery and gynaecology, newer subject like veterinary ethics and animal biotechnology, newer drugs used in veterinary medicine, latest researches in animals feeding, etc. can be written upon.

Professionals engaged in rural development also need information on advances in the basic sciences like biochemistry, biophysics, genetics, bioengineering, electronic, etc. Such professionals are better suited to appreciate such information on the basic sciences.

Another important target group is that of industrial entrepreneurs, i.e. the people who are already producing or plan to produce a product or any equipment relating to rural life and farmers. Such people may be manufacturers of tractors and other agricultural implements, fertilizer factories, water pump manufacturers and repairers, animal feed manufacturers companies manufacturing veterinary medicines and vaccines, manufacturers of veterinary hospital equipment, etc.

The subjects covered for industrial entrepreneurs may be animal nutrition, veterinary pharmacology, veterinary surgery and gynaecology, agricultural engineering, and water technology, electronics engineering, rural engineering, etc. Simple things such as increasing the efficiency of the bullock cart, installation and operation of the biogas plant, etc. are also useful in this category. Under veterinary pharmacology, many new drugs discovered by scientists and found to be useful, have to be popularized for commercial manufacture; even the indigenous drugs tested and found useful, are also included in this category. Tested devices like crystoscope can be included here.

TYPES OF LITERATURE

For farmers, a illustrated pamphlets, leaflets and bulletins are quite useful. In the case of improved techniques, it is a good idea to illustrate the steps one by one, if possible. Each step should be explained to the minutest detail, so that the farmer can be guided properly if he consults the given literature. In the case of new improved equipments, the parts and their working should be explained in detail, accompanied by suitable photographs or line drawings. Pamphlets can be used to present a very small topic, whereas leaflets may give an overall view of what to expect from an organization, or may create awareness about an upcoming event or farmers' fair. For more detailed and thorough treatment of a given topic, bulletins should be preferred. Posters may also be used for passing on information about a forthcoming event of importance to the farmers.

Comics containing illustrations and written material, showing stories or chronological events can also be tried with farmers. These could be used to depict stepwise method demonstrations or success stories of progressive farmers. There is great scope for creativity in such comics.

The time has come when the farmers should be introduced slowly into the world of scientific logic and the method of scientific thinking. Such literature will pave the way for scientific outlook on life and will develop the power of scientific evaluation as opposed to unscientific comments and conclusions. Examples can be taken from the daily life of rural people. Literature may be divided into static and dynamic literature. By static literature, is relatively stable over time and not likely to change much with the passage of time, such as scientific logic, the position of the earth and the stars, etc. By dynamic literature, we mean that literature which is relatively unstable and changes frequently over short time intervals, e.g. agronomic practices for crops, budgeting for domestic purposes, etc. Farmers need more dynamic type of literature like newsletter, newspaper articles, live and recorded telecasts, radio broadcasts and features, etc.

Newsletters inform farmers about various events of their interest, e.g. *Kisan Melas, Kisan Goshthies*, livestock shows, rural markets and fairs, etc. Newsletters may be regular or irregular in periodicity. The news reported should be direct and small sentences should be preferred. Sophisticated language should be avoided. Newspaper articles can carry news as well as opinions of knowledgeable people, forecasts, technological development, problems faced by farmers, etc. Telecasts can cover various events like *Kisan Melas*, rural markets, prize-winning animals, improved methods of farming, etc. Radio broadcasts should obviously be used mostly for those events where the spoken word is of singular importance, e.g. important conversations between scientists and farmers, policy announcements, etc.

For planning how to prepare literature for entrepreneurs, i.e. journal, magazine, manual, newsletter, textbook, farmer's bulletin, pamphlets, etc. five questions who? where? what? why? and when? should be answered first. These components/tools help author/writer in providing guidance for effective literature.

Preparing and finalizing literature for entrepreneurs require with great patience, creativity, care, and efforts. Preparing literature for different type of publication or periodicals, may involve working with several other persons as authors, subject matter specialists, photographers, graphic designers, DTP typesetters and printers/publishers.

While preparing or planning for literature we must keep in mind the following points : Make sure the literature is complete; it should neither be too precise or too lengthy; reorganise the test to make it more effective; ask questions when text is unclear; contents should reach the people or fulfill the objectives; remove errors to reach the facts; improve readability and understandability; check and correct spellings, grammar, punctuations, units of measurement, abbreviations, headings, sub-headings, illustrations, photographs, tables, charts and graphs should match with the text or it may be printed separately as plate.

Literature writing is an important part, however, presentation of literature specially for developmental prgoramme like entrepreneurship of a book are not less important. Even if the text of the of literature is excellent, but if it is not printed with graphics, illustrations, etc., it will not be popular and will not attract the reader. The art work presentation of materials is, therefore, very important. It has several important components, i.e. size of the literature, cover design, illustrations, photographs, selection of type faces and papers, etc.

It is not necessary that all the publications should have illustrations. However, where illustrations are required but are not given, the readers remain unable to explain or make out the sense clear to the readers illustrations are must. These illustrations may be coloured or in black and white. In some literatures, illustrations alone do not serve the purpose, therefore, the text may be combined with illustrations and photographs.

Layout is an essential part of any literature. Unless the layout of the literature is attractive, the presentation of the literature does not appear to be appealing. There are various components of the layout, i.e. selection of type size of the heading, sub-headings, side headings to be used, placement of illustrations/ photographs and space to be left blank. Layout of a publication indicate the setting of page or composition of text and graphics in proper place and focus the attention of the readers. The layout/composition, is the artistic and meaningful positioning of page, balancing of page and a pleasing movement to eye.

Photograph is also an important part of any publication or literature. Sometimes the matter cannot be made clear/without the photograph. Photographs serve both the purposes, i.e. making the sense clear to the reader and making the literature interesting and attractive. The quality of the photograph should be excellent otherwise the very purpose will be defeated. The photographs with poor quality of reproduction are not at all suitable for publication/literatures. Some time the photographs are used as such but at the same time they are used in a cut-out form. Sometimes the photograph is reduced or enalrged keeping in view the printing measure of a publication. Nowadays, digital cameras are used which is compatible with computer and there is no need to develop or print photos. The photo image can directly be taken to the computer for the necessary improvements in any literature. The advance technology with adequate information keeps updating literature which is an important tool to the entrepreneurs.

For professionals like agricultural extension officers, veterinarians, human medical officers, social workers, etc. more static kind of literature is required. That is to say, the applied aspects like what to do, how to do it, and what to avoid, should be emphasized. As far as possible, references to other literature should be avoided, as many of these workers do not have access to libraries nor do they have that much time at their disposal to consult detailed literature. This type of literature should stress on the recommendations, and 'ifs' and 'buts' should be avoided. Only the proven propositions should be highlighted. The advantages of the recommended practices over the existing practices should also be clearly indicated. Illustrations should be used only where necessary to show a new technique or some comparisons.

For industrial entrepreneurs, the need is for information which relates to either updating existing facilities or opening up new facilities. For this purpose, they need project reports, complete with land, buildings, materials, equipment required, as also the manpower and other infrastructure needed and the economic feasibility report, availability of credit facilities, whom to contact for what, etc. The literature needed by them is dynamic; they should know what the latest scientific advances are and should be able to assess for themselves how best they could utilize those advances to their advantage. Nowadays institute industry interface meetings are getting popular; the entrepreneurs should be informed about these so that they can attend these and get face-to-face information from the experts. Similarly, they should also be informed about scientific conferences and meetings, etc. so that they can benefit from attending the same.

Teleprogramme on entrepreneurship development is another important area through which advance information in the shape of live, i.e. visual forms, is found more effective to entrepreneurs and farmers. This is an art which involves consideration on different stages like users (target audience), purpose of the film, duration, data, graphics (maps, diagrams, illustration, supertitle), etc. Data is the back bone or supportive information of a film.

Data including visual/graphics is another important factor for a film. It should be collected and arranged in proper sequence to convey the objective of the film. Visual and commentary should have a smooth flow to convey the meaningful information without any disturbance or jerk. The various shots required for the development programme can be taken in any sequence and re-arranged subsequently. Nowadays television is a powerful medium of mass communication. It plays 3-fold important responsibility in the area of communication/information, entertainment and education. Script writing on different subjects for entrepreneurship development is a complete process of video programming in a suitable form. It can be defined as the previsualised process of the visual and aural elements of a video programme. Selection of shot and visualisation of a scene is a very important step in the writing of script for the teleprogramme. The writer of script for such programmes must have a gamut of imagination and should try to picturise the complete video programme in visual terms by using different visuals and graphics images to make the film/programme more interesting. The total script comprising of video programme is divided into different scenes and shots to create interest and make it more informative. The shots and scenes are composed in such a way that the interest is sustained. Positioning of objects in a video frame in different ways and angles should be marked to achieve a variety of shots like close, short, medium and long shot. Hence, the production part of any teleprogramme is usually done in three stages of script writing, shooting and editing.

The literature for entreprenurship development programmes must have the quality of making other members of a production team understand the requirements of a video programme so that, the best output fulfilling the overall objectives of the film could be made.

We can prepare teleprogrammes on different subject and title. It may be on agriculture, entreprenurship development, animal husbandry, agricultural engineering, water technology, technology integration, documantation and dissemination of technologies, etc. It may be for the use of entrepreneurs, farmers, researchers, field workers, students or for general public. A good script should have complete information supported by visuals, data and graphics. It should be crisp and to the point in simple language which is easily understandable, knowledgeable and should create interest from the beginning to end about the programme. Such film will create awareness amongst the endusers and the film will also helpful to provide them information about the new technique and development in the country.

A script is a mirror to show and reflect the facts to achieve the objective/purpose for which the teleprogramme has been prepared. Script is a guide to a producer for the next step of shooting. But the producer or director may change the sequence of shooting or modify the script or visuals depending on the location and availability of shots at that time of shooting which may vary from the original script. Writing script for a teleprogramme is like preparing a plan of action and is essential for prompt and effective production of a film within the given time frame. Thus the present need of entreprenurs in different area can easily be achieved with the entreprenurship development programmes and these programmes of short duration telefilms considering the aims and objectives can be projected through different mass media channels.

Literature is not a substitute for an expert, but it should be produced as if it were supposed to be so. The ultimate test of literature is how much the knowledge has been translated into practice. At the same time, feedback is also important. Science communicators should know periodically from the readers, as to what improvements are desired in the literature and how it could fulfill its purpose in a better way.

35

Role of Information Technology (IT) in Entrepreneurship Development in Livestock Sector

GS Bisht, YP Singh, Sanjay Kumar

The global challenge the world facing now is staggering 1,300 million people living on less than 50 Rupees per day, 840,000,000 men, women, and children go hungry. The objectives are formidable and conflicting like increasing the productivity, producing an increasing variety of quality, high-value produce to increase their profits and managing natural resources. Increase in agricultural production including the livestock and rural income must derive from intensification, rather than area expansion, knowledge and related information, skills, technologies, and attitudes. For achieving the above said objectives, IT can act as growth engine. In some places, it has provided the opportunity for entrepreneurship development through knowledge centre. It has opened a new vista of knowledge sharing and its utilization. The cooperatives in different parts of the country are using IT as a means of increasing the efficiency and transparency in milk procurement. Gyan Ganga Project is catering the e-governance, health, agriculture and veterinary services to the users. There are evidences that the livestock health advisory services are being provided real-time online through video conferencing and the expert need not have to go to the animal. The owner of an IT Kiosk is not only helping the people but imparting knowledge and information but also generating profit to sustain family and thus giving evidence that the IT can boost the entrepreneurship development.

Today more than 80 low-income developing countries suffer from the chronic food deficits and nearly 800 million people live in hunger. By 2005, the world's population exceeded 8 billion and food requirements in developing countries doubled. Of 1068.6 million population of India, only 28% live in urban areas and rest 72% reside in rural areas. It is estimated that by the year 2050, India will become the largest country in the world with estimated population of 1628 million. This rise in population, especially in the countries that could least afford to support growing number of people, might lead to serious food shortage, social and political unrest. Despite various efforts, India is still looking for reduction of poverty, unemployment and equality of distribution and opportunities. Growing number of people give us increased human hand but might lead to serious problems if adequate and appropriate planning is not done towards engaging the increased manpower properly.

One of the way to link the ever-growing working hand especially in rural areas is to provide them with the opportunity to work. This opportunity can be provided through well thought-out rural development programme where capacity building has to be in the forefront or the concept of entrepreneurship has to be brought into the picture. Rural development is more than ever before linked to entrepreneurship. Institutions and individuals promoting rural development see entrepreneurship as a strategic development intervention that could accelerate the rural development process. Furthermore, institutions and individuals seem to agree on the urgent need to promote rural enterprises: development agencies see rural entrepreneurship as an enormous employment potential; politicians see it as the key strategy to prevent rural unrest; farmers see it as an instrument for improving farm earnings; and women see it as an employment possibility near their homes which provides autonomy, independence and a reduced need for social support. To all these groups, however, entrepreneurship stands as a vehicle to improve the quality of life for individuals, families and communities and to sustain a healthy economy and environment. The entrepreneurial orientation to rural development accepts entrepreneurship as the central force of economic growth and development, without it other factors of development will be wasted or frittered away. What is needed in addition is an environment enabling entrepreneurship in rural areas. The existence of such an environment largely depends on policies promoting rural entrepreneurship. The effectiveness of such policies in turn depends on a conceptual framework about entrepreneurship, i.e. what it is and where it comes from.

There is an ample scope to introduce the entrepreneurship in livestock sector through the information technology. The information technology is a mix of computer and communication technologies and is mainly used for processing, storing and retrieving of information in multimedia format (text, graphics, video and sound). Several success stories are there where the IT has played a crucial role in revolutionizing the development programme.

INFORMATION TECHNOLOGY (IT)

IT has three major components:

1. Computer technologies
2. Communication technologies
3. People

Computer Technology

An advanced electronic technology, which basically helps in processing information or data in an electronic format is called computer technology. The device that carries out the operation is known as 'computer'. This has two major parts—computer hardware and computer software.

1. **Computer hardware:** All mechanical, electrical and electronic physical components of a computer system are known as 'computer hardware'. For example, the monitor, central processing unit and the keyboard.

2. **Computer software:** Computer software is the set of computer programmes, which would carry out particular computer-based applications. Computer

programme is a series of instructions given to a computer to perform a particular task. A fully documented programme, or a set of programmes, designed to perform a particular task is called a 'software package'. Software packages are broadly classified as under:

i. Operating systems: These systems are used to execute the computer application and manage the system.

ii. Application software: These software packages are used to perform a particular application, such as word-processing, database management, information system management, etc. (MS-Office, Oracle, Foxpro, etc.).

iii. Utility softwares: Are used for a specific utility like virus checking, disk management, etc. (e.g. Nash, NC, Red Alert).

iv. Communication software: For online communication like internet and e-mail, a computer needs special software, which is called communication software. By using this software, a user can communicate with another computer user anywhere in the world (e.g. Netscape, Internet Explorer, PC Plus).

Communication Technologies

The technology that helps to communicate data or information (in the multimedia format) in analog as well as digital mode is called 'communication technology'. Communication technology includes telecommunications, satellite technologies, Internet-based technologies and computer networking.

People

The third component of IT is the people—the professionals, who specialise in the field of IT. In fact, the utility of IT will largely depend on the abilities of these professionals. The organisation that create, package and market IT based products and systems must have people who have a high level of technical education and expertise.

TELETEXT, VIDEOTEXT AND TELECONFERENCING

In changing media scenario, we have a wide range of communication technologies for networking purpose that can be effectively used for fast and effective communication. Teletext and videotext are some examples that can provide latest and updated information on various aspects. Teletext is a system that links computer to television through which textual and graphic information can be transmitted on a one-way basis. Videotext links TV set through a telephone line to mainframe computer. It is fully interactive system, by which one can communicate with computer. The developed countries are using teletext and videotext system to provide information at various levels.

Teleconferencing includes video conferencing, audio conferencing and computer conferencing have shown their potential in establishing efficient network among various institutes in India and abroad. To strengthen information and resource sharing mechanism in India, video conferencing network has established connecting 22 institutions including 15 agricultural universities. This multiple site connectivity has helped the participating institutes to have a face-to-face dialogue among renowned scientists, policy makers etc. It is expected that this facility will be used to its full potential by all institutions of this network.

Advantages of IT

Application of IT in various sectors offers many advantages. The important advantages are as under:

1. Save manpower
2. Eliminate human errors
3. Enable faster communication and exchange of ideas
4. Saving time
5. Avoid duplication
6. Quality improvements
7. Total automation
8. Increase productivity
9. Create and expand markets
10. Economic growth

IT APPLICATIONS IN DEVELOPMENT

World over IT is used for a wide variety of applications ranging from simple data processing to complex business and industry information systems, management, e-commerce, instructions and transfer of technology. This can also be utilized efficiently in entrepreneurship development.

Entrepreneurship Development

Defining entrepreneurship is not an easy task. To some, entrepreneurship means primarily innovation, to others it means risk-taking, to others a market stabilising force and to others still it means starting, owning and managing a small business. Accordingly, the entrepreneur is viewed as a person who either creates new combinations of production factors such as new methods of production, new products, new markets, finds new sources of supply and new organizational forms; or as a person who is willing to take risks; or a person who, by exploiting market opportunities, eliminates disequilibrium between aggregate supply and aggregate demand, or as one who owns and operates a business (Tyson, Petrin, Rogers, 1994).

To choose the definition of entrepreneurship most appropriate for the rural area context, it is important to bear in mind the entrepreneurial skills that will be needed to improve the quality of life for individuals, families and communities and to sustain a healthy economy and environment. Taking this into consideration, each of the traditional definitions has its own weakness (Tyson, Petrin, Rogers, 1994). The first definition leaves little room for innovations that are not on the technological or organizational cutting edge, such as, adaptation of older technologies to a developing-country context, or entering into export markets already tapped by other firms. Defining entrepreneurship as risk-taking neglects other major elements, such as a well-developed ability to recognise unexploited market opportunities. Entrepreneurship as a stabilising force limits entrepreneurship to reading markets disequilibria, while entrepreneurship defined as owning and operating a business, denies the possibility of entrepreneurial behaviour by non-owners, employees and managers who have no equity stake in the business. Therefore, the most appropriate definition of entrepreneurship that would fit into the rural development context, argued here, is the broader one, the one which defines entrepreneurship as: *"a force that mobilises other resources to meet unmet market demand"*, *"the ability to create and build something from practically nothing"*, *"the process of creating value by pulling together a unique package of resources to exploit an opportunity"*.

Entrepreneurship so defined, pertains to any new organization of productive factors and not exclusively to innovations that are on the technological or organizational cutting edge. It pertains to entrepreneurial activities both within and outside the organization. Entrepreneurship need not involve anything new from a global or even national perspective, but rather the adoption of new forms of business organizations, new technologies and new enterprises producing goods not previously available at a location (Petrin, 1991). Entrepreneurship is considered to be a prime mover in development and why nations, regions and communities that actively promote entrepreneurship development, demonstrate much higher growth rates and consequently higher levels of development than nations, regions and communities whose institutions, politics and culture hinder entrepreneurship.

Entrepreneurial orientation to rural development, contrary to development based on bringing in human capital and investment from outside, is based on stimulating local entrepreneurial talent and subsequent growth of indigenous companies. This would create jobs and add economic value to a region and community and at the same time keep scarce resources within the community. To accelerate economic development in rural areas, it is necessary to increase the supply of entrepreneurs, thus building up the critical mass of first generation entrepreneurs who will take risks and engage in the uncertainties of a new venture creation, create something from practically nothing and create values by pulling together a unique package of resources to exploit an opportunity. By their example they will stimulate an autonomous entrepreneurial process, as well as a dynamic entrepreneurship, thereby ensuring continuous rural development.

IT and Entrepreneurship Development in Agriculture

Agriculture is considered as the principal engine of growth in many low income developing countries where it accounts for 60–80% of all employment. In India too, agriculture is considered as backbone of Indian economy and 85% population is directly and indirectly associated with this sector. However, efforts for development of agriculture have been made by several institutes and departments by using transfer of technology approach where communication is used as a tool. Extension Directorates of State Agricultural Universities and Government have widely used communication technologies in transfer of technology among farming communities. Technologies like radio, television, print and video have been extensively used, along with interpersonal communication. Farm Forums and Rural Radio Forums are some examples of radio utilization for agriculture and rural development. Many radio stations broadcast programmes exclusively on agriculture. Some slot of time in TV programming is also allotted for agriculture. But with the information explosion, and the availability of various options, this sector is calling for new approach. Diversification of agriculture, promotion of agri-preneurship, precision farming, hi-tech agriculture, post- harvest management, value addition and proper marketing are getting due recognition in agriculture. To fulfill farmers' needs in such areas, a strong communication and information support system is the need of the day. Communication and information technology have great potential in dissemination of information among farming communities. Warna Wired Village project—a collaborative effort of National Informatics Centre, Maharastra Government and Warna Cooperative Society was launched in selected parts of Maharastra to serve the information needs of farmers for cultivation practices, pest and disease control, marketing information, information on processing, etc. through use of ICT. A dedicated website—www.kisan.com of Nagaarjuna fertilizer is using IT for dissemination of information among farmers. Information Village of Pondicherry Project of MS Swaminathan Research Foundation is another effort in that direction which utilized a broad array of modern information and communication technologies for development in general and rural development in particuiar. The agricultural research institutes and universities can also plan to launch the websites where latest information on agriculture and rural technology can be exchanged. Indian Council of Agriculture Research and its institutes, National Institute of Agricultural Extension Management (MANAGE) and State Agricultural Universities (SAUs) through centralized network facilitates the exchange of resources and sharing of knowledge for prompt and effective utilization. Realizing the low coverage of agriculture programmes in mass media, Ministry of Agriculture, Government of India, has decided to start an agriculture channel for farmers and rural people to promote agriculture and rural development.

IT and Entrepreneurship Development in Livestock Sector

Considering the stagnant nature of crop agriculture the livestock sector has emerged as income and employment generating enterprise for many a number of rural households. Livestock is providing secondary source of income to millions of farmers in the rural area. Livestock sector still is not attended well by the input service provider. There is ample scope and opportunity as well as demand for the livestock services in not only in urban areas but also in rural areas of the country. People are willing to pay for the services considering the cash crop like nature of livestock sector. Here lies the opportunity for the person to provide services in the livestock sector with the help of IT. An entrepreneur can establish an internet café/kiosk through which he can provide the information related to the livestock sector. The information is already available with various research organizations in user friendly mode which can be procured and used in the café. Dairy Information System Kiosks software developed by the IIM Ahmedabad which connect to a dairy information portal, it is possible to maintain and access a computerised database that includes all details about the cattle owned, milk production, prices, etc.

The marketing information related to the livestock and livestock products can be posted and retrieved online from various portals. There are many success stories regarding the utility of such portals in providing marketing information not only in crop agriculture but also in livestock sector. Many interested farmers lack information on various aspect of livestock enterprise and an entrepreneur can provide sufficient and authentic information offline from the available sources. The person can act as linkage between the input providers as well as out put purchaser from the far off area also. It can provide genuine product from the input provider and can also get good price for the product thus eliminating the margin of middleman and thus will improve the marketing efficiency of the livestock and livestock product marketing.

Various research institutes are coming out with user friendly expert system related to health and nutrition of the livestock sector. This nutrition expert system can be used for the benefit of the farmers as per their inventory of ingredients which will be cost-effective as well as balanced. The health expert system can act as first aid provider and will be in great demand in the difficult and remote area where even the paravets are not available. These health expert systems work on the basis of symptoms and narrow down to the specific disease and suggest about broad spectrum medicines. The entrepreneur can purchase such system and can provide this service on payment.

The Cyber Cafe/Internet Kiosk as a Business Model

- Average no. of PCs – 1.
- Average charge/hour – Rs 30.
- Average users/day – 30.
- Average time online – 15 mins.
- Potential of Rs 100/day gross.
- **Startup costs:** 15000 Rs/pc, network equipment, UPS/batteries, cabinets– estimated at Rs 50,000.
- **Running costs:** Electricity/rent/cable/dialup/staff/maintenance.

The establishment cost of such cyber cafe/internet kiosk will come around Rs 50000. Only problem with establishment of such venture is facility of electricity in the remote/rural area. In such case, the entrepreneur will have to go for 1KV power generator which will increase the start-up cost. Considering the meagre employment opportunity for the educated youth particularly the rural youth, the establishment of such venture will not only provide the income but also productive employment and will help in reducing the out migration of the rural youth. The financial institution can provide loan and some subsidy component can also be introduced to popularise it.

CONCLUSION

India is still looking for reduction of poverty, unemployment and equality of distribution and opportunities. Growing number of people will no doubt give us increased human hand but might lead to serious food problem and social and political unrest if adequate and appropriate planning is not done towards engaging the increased manpower properly. One of the ways to link the ever-growing working hand especially in rural areas is to provide them with the opportunity to work. This opportunity can be provided through well thought-out rural development program where capacity building has to be in the forefront or the concept of entrepreneurship has to be brought into the picture. The entrepreneurial orientation to rural development accepts entrepreneurship as the central force of economic growth and development. There is ample scope to introduce the entrepreneurship in livestock sector through the information technology. Several success stories are there where the IT has played a crucial role in revolutionizing the development programme. Livestock is providing secondary source of income to millions of farmers in the rural area. Livestock sector still is not attended well by the input service provider. There is ample scope and opportunity, as well as demand for the livestock services in rural areas of the country. The establishment of cyber cafe/internet kiosk providing the information related to livestock sector will provide the entrepreneurship opportunity to the unemployed rural youth at a very low cost.

36

Role of Information Technology (IT) in Entrepreneurship Development in Agriculture

S Islam, HO Agarwal, JP Sharma, Mohd S Farooqui

Agriculture in India has grown from its infancy to a full-fledged science and a complex business as well. It has sailed the nation out of a storm of hunger, malnutrition to a safe shore of food security. Agriculture and allied activities has been the most crucial sector of the Indian economy, making the single largest contribution to the gross domestic product (GDP), accounting for almost 25% of the total. Agriculture provides employment to around 65% of the total work force. To emerge as developed nation by the year 2020, agriculture has to play a vital and significant role. It has to contribute more substantially to the GDP of Indian economy (Table 36.1).

Table 36.1: Growth in food grain production during 1950-51 to 2000-01 (production in million tonnes)

Year	Rice	Wheat	Coarse cereals	Pulses	Total food grains
1950-51	20.58	6.46	15.38	8.41	50.82
1960-61	34.58	11.00	23.74	12.70	82.02
1970-71	42.23	23.83	30.55	11.82	108.42
1980-81	52.63	36.31	29.02	10.63	129.59
1990-91	74.29	55.14	32.70	14.26	176.39
2000-01	84.98	69.68	31.08	11.08	196.81

India has more than 1 billion people with one baby born in every 1.25 sec. We will need the resources to feed 1.3 billion people by the year 2020. The Economic Survey for 1996-97 has revealed that the compound growth rate in food grain production at 1.7% is lower than the annual population growth of 1.9% (Figs 36.1, 36.2).

There has been substantial contribution of agriculture to the GDP during last 25 years and it has reached to Rs 44.39 trillion in 1999-2000 as compared to 4.25 trillion during 1980-81. Although its percentage contribution to total has been decreased from 34.72 to 24.85%. This reveals that other sectors are also contributing significantly to the GDP. This is not a matter of concern, since growth in agricultural GDP has shown a substantial increase (Table 36.2).

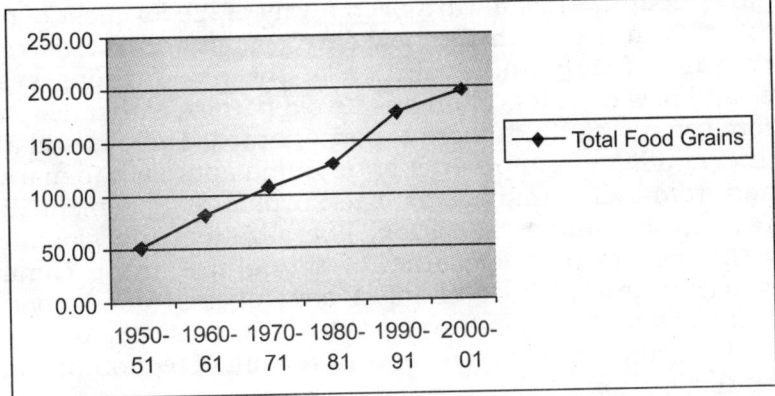

Fig. 36.1: Production growth of food grains

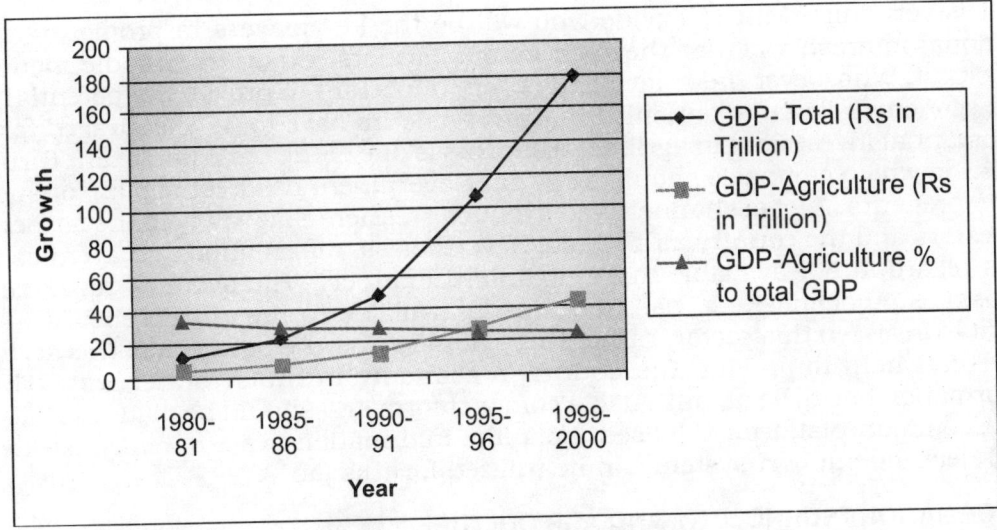

Fig. 36.2: Growth in agricultural GDP

Table 36.2: Share of agriculture and livestock sector in GDP

Year	GDP-Total (Rs in trillion)	GDP-Agriculture (Rs in trillion)	Percentage to total GDP
1980-1981	12.24	4.25	34.72
1985-1986	23.38	7.00	29.94
1990-1991	47.78	13.52	28.3
1995-1996	107.33	27.78	25.88
1999-2000	178.65	44.39	24.85

Traditional agriculture has always been a way of life for most of our farmers, which is losing its impact with the new developments in the current century. With the passage of time and evolution of the new farming systems, new technologies and new tools it is changing its old pattern with a new strategy that makes it more commercialized, more export oriented. There is still a lot of room that shifts the paradigm from production-oriented approach to market-oriented approach and from deficit management to surplus-management. Besides, the economic policies of commercialization, liberalization and globalization have accelerated the pace of transformation of agriculture into a commercial and market-driven enterprise. These changes have opened new opportunities for export and processing of agricultural products and have brought about new challenges in particular that of growing requirement of techno-managerial skills in the agriculture sector.

The agenda for future direction is guided by the implication of these changing scenarios for achieving the goal of sustainable agricultural and rural development leading to rural prosperity in India.

It is very important to decide who will be the key players in promoting the national interest, whether they will be our farmers, exporters, middle men or stockiest. Whosoever they may be, it is very important to project the potential of the economy related to agriculture. Entrepreneurs have to be encouraged for a substantial investment in agribusiness. This is one of the most important thrust areas in which emphasis should be given. Government has a lot of plan for such entrepreneurs. A lot of channels and avenues are there that will help the farmers, investors and the country as a whole. Nevertheless, information and avenues in this regard is not available in an organized manner. The avenues resources, subsidies guidelines, etc. has to be made available to the entrepreneurs who want to invest in this sector, rather they should know the potential of this sector that can help improving the country's economy in much better way. This information has to be organized in a compact form and should be made available at a common platform. IT-based tools like information system, expert system and decision support system can be utilized for this job.

INFORMATION TECHNOLOGY AND AGRICULTURE

Information communication technology is known as the constituent of computers, information processing, computer networks and information transmission on computer networks. A new terminology has emerged with a name agriculture information technology (AIT). This new technology integrates information technology with agriculture. Let us explore the opportunity attached with this technology, its application and its future that gives a new direction to our agriculture and encourages entrepreneurs to invest substantially in this area.

Its potential has been realized by some of the most prominent companies of the country. The most reputed names of business like HLL, Tata, Reliance, Wipro, Infosys, etc. are entering in this field to extract huge benefits. These companies need a significant number of computer professionals who have complete knowledge of agriculture or agriculture professionals that are computer literate also. In most of the cases, these two groups are mutually exclusive. Today's generation is either computer literate or have knowledge of agriculture. It is the need of the hour that our students should take up both of them together so that information technology could be applied in a comprehensive manner in the field of agriculture. These professionals will get a platform and good career opportunities in above-mentioned companies. Considerable opportunities are also emerging in the area of rural development through effective use of information communication technology in agriculture. They are in urgent need of agriculture and allied area graduates who equipped their knowledge and technological skills in order to facilitate the innovation in this field and fill up the demand of market. At present there is much more job opportunities in agriculture information technology and on the other hand there are very few trained professionals to fill the needs. ICAR is generating such type of human resources who are computer and agricultural literate with high level of proficiency as well. The database of the students generated by the ICAR can be passed on to the above-mentioned companies so that they can utilize the services of agri-IT professionals in a fruitful way. This will create a new avenue in the field of agriculture information technology that will bring a significant return to the investors.

Agriculture is a multidisciplinary complex science in which every discipline is studied separately although they are related to each other in one way or the other. Information technology can have its application and significant impact on every discipline. This technology can work directly for the farmers by disseminating the information generated by our National Agricultural Research System.

Our farmers concern is mainly to know the right crop and to get a better yield and after producing it successfully he wants a good return by selling it at right market at right price. Our researchers help them in finding the right variety, suitable method to save the crop from insect/pest/nematodes/weeds, etc. Their concern is also to find the right machinery and save harvest and post harvest losses. All the technologies generated by the researchers should reach the farmers at the right time. Information technology can play a vital role in doing all these jobs, which were earlier done without its application. This will help them in getting better returns and hence open new avenues for the farmers.

Agribusiness

Most of our farmers remain only producers and losers, they never even think of entering into market. There are considerable numbers of organization involved in marketing research. As a result they come with fruitful ideas of market strategy that helps entrepreneurs to involve in expanding their business. A very little encouragement is there for the investors in agriculture. Organizations involved in market research should project agriculture as a big profit-making sector. This generated information should be made available on the web. High quality professional consulting services for agriculture to enhance the understanding of the farmers should be provided for agribusiness and market realities for agricultural products.

Electronic Commerce in Agriculture

Marketing agricultural commodities is one of the most serious problems of Indian farmers. After investing a lot of money, labour and time, farmers hardly get back the return for the best of their efforts. They are being exploited by big investors, middlemen, officials and hoarders. If marketing information systems are developed and made available to the farmers, they will be better informed about the market and can get better return for their products. These marketing information systems on one hand will give the current marketing situations and will predict the market situation in subsequent time. This will help farmers in finding the suitable market for their crop. Farmers can electronically sell out their goods to big investors, industries or directly to the consumers.

For advising the right investment opportunity and avenues, investment analysis should be done by computer-based tools using operation research and statistical tools. These tools can give instant information to the investors to take the right decision in no time.

Sales and Channel Management

Sales and channel can be managed through computers utilizing the available national network. Adequate connectivity of systems across the country with fibre optic cables about 800 thousand kilometer of fibre lines have been already laid out. Every village will be converted to a knowledge centre by 2007 with "National Alliance for Mission 2007". Establishment of information kiosk's and e-chaupal's all over the country is in process. These facilities will establish a better connectivity with farmers, entrepreneurs and consumers.

Production management should also be demand driven based on demand forecast done by IT-based model using statistical forecast techniques and economic analysis. Social and economic profiling at national, state, district and sub district levels using primary and secondary data can be done. Through this analysis farmers should know the demand of an agricultural commodity and can decide what should they produce to meet the demand of the market.

Information service provider in agriculture, food processing, social development and allied sectors will proved to be beneficial that gives a diversified approach from a traditional approach. ICT can provide detailed information about adoption of modern farming system, involving shift in cropping pattern towards crops more in demand like oil seeds, pulses, horticulture, floriculture, medicinal and aromatic plants, etc. ICT can help in synergising through land-based enterprises like livestock and fishery, poultry, etc. It can advise capturing the new market opportunities through enterprises that include post-harvest/value addition.

A computer-based scientific knowledge base can be created that provides information about priorities and target areas giving choice of alternative crops and technology. It should also keep the information about the priority input/credit supply for alternative crops, support given by the government, provides market support and rural uplinking. This knowledge base should contain information about private entrepreneurs and industries, which encourage farmers for contract farming. This guides the farmers to go for a crop asked by the industry. ICT-based entrepreneurship portals should be made available that can suggest area specific crop based on the climate, soil type and market demand.

CONCLUSION

Information communication technology is the technology of the future. If we could integrate it with agriculture it will be proved worthy for the farmers and future of agriculture. It is the need of the hour that we should contribute to agriculture with this powerful technology. It will prove to be central to solve our food problem. It will be a step towards bringing India in the category of developed nations.

37

Role of IT in Micro-entrepreneurship in relation to Livestock Sector

Hemant Yadav

Information technology on date happens to be the most dynamic and robust force in the world of business. As a matter of fact e-commerce is taking on the conventional brick and mortar business in a big way. In India, the rural entrepreneurs are traditionally cash-depleted entities. They do not have enough money to invest for entrepreneurial ventures. In such a scenario, e-commerce and information technology comes as a boon.

Livestock sector has got the potential to rejuvenate the ailing rural economy, as it can provide substantial economic benefits to the micro-entrepreneurs. A variety of livestock products have got the potential to be marketed online. Moreover, the cost of marketing online is lot less than the cost of operating through brick and mortar business model. Whereas, if one decides to have physical premises for its venture it may require several lakhs of rupees; but the virtual premises will only requires few thousands.

The digital revolution across the globe has changed the world of business forever.

DIGITAL ECONOMY

An economy that is based on digital technologies, including digital communication networks, computers, software, and other related information technologies; also called the internet economy, the new economy, or the web.

- The digital revolution accelerates electronic commerce by providing competitive advantage to organizations and enabling innovations.
- Economic, legal, societal, and technological factors have created a highly competitive *business environment* in which customers are becoming more powerful.

Entrepreneurs must not only take traditional actions such as lowering costs and closing unprofitable facilities, but also introduce innovative actions such as customizing, creating new products, or providing superb customer service. That is even more important in the case of agri-based industries. In agricultural-based entrepreneurial ventures such as in the case of livestock, differentiation in the offerings can be created through use of technology and modern processes.

ELECTRONIC COMMERCE (EC)

The process of buying, selling, or exchanging products, services, or information via computer networks is termed as electronic commerce.

Major Business Pressures and the Role of EC

Modern day entrepreneurs face a variety of challenges in the form of environmental factors (Fig. 37.1).

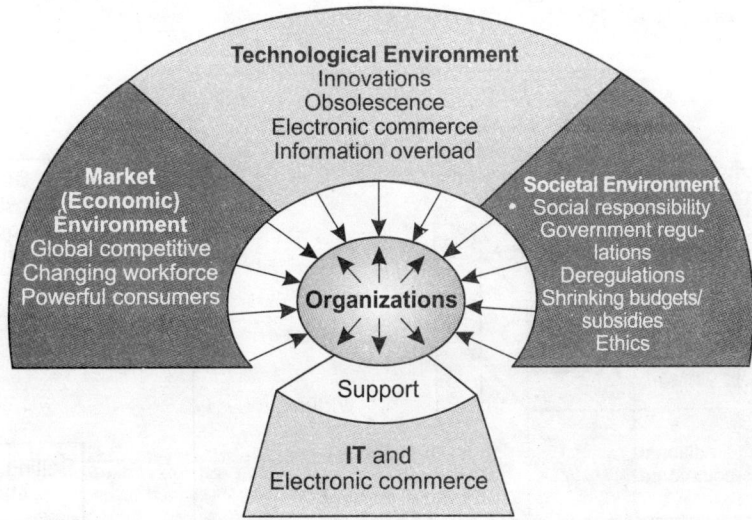

Fig. 37.1: Variety of challenges in the form of environmental factors

The prevailing environmental conditions put every new venture to acid test. The major pressures are economic (market related), societal and technological. The successful entrepreneurs are those who respond well to these pressures. The entrepreneurs can respond by having strategic systems which are agile enough to deal with the prevailing conditions. Information technology and e-commerce is a great help in such cases. Business alliances are a great help irrespective of the type of enterprise. Even issues such as lead time reduction are critical for efficient market response. The role of IT and e-commerce is ubiquitous across all industries and functional areas of business.

E-commerce also allows the decentralization of decision-making and authority via empowerment and distribution systems, but simultaneously supports a centralized control. The supply chain improvement such as reduction in supply chain delays, reduction of inventories and elimination of other inefficiencies can also be achieved through information technology.

IT can also help in creating or capturing knowledge, storing and protecting it and at the same time helps in updating and maintaining the knowledge.

Pure versus Partial EC

Electronic commerce takes several forms depending on the *degree of digitization* (the transformation from physical to digital). It is on the basis of the product sold, the process and the delivery agent or the intermediary. The entrepreneurs can choose the level of digitalization based on the requirements of their project. It is difficult to have pure e-commerce in the case of livestock entrepreneurship, but partial e-commerce is possible in such cases as the process and the agent can be digitalized. A number of brave entrepreneurs are marketing their livestock products ranging from ostrich meat to fur and even the eggshell through internet. In such cases, the process and the agent are digital. It is wonderful for the entrepreneurs as the digital organization can save them a lot of set up cost (Fig. 37.2).

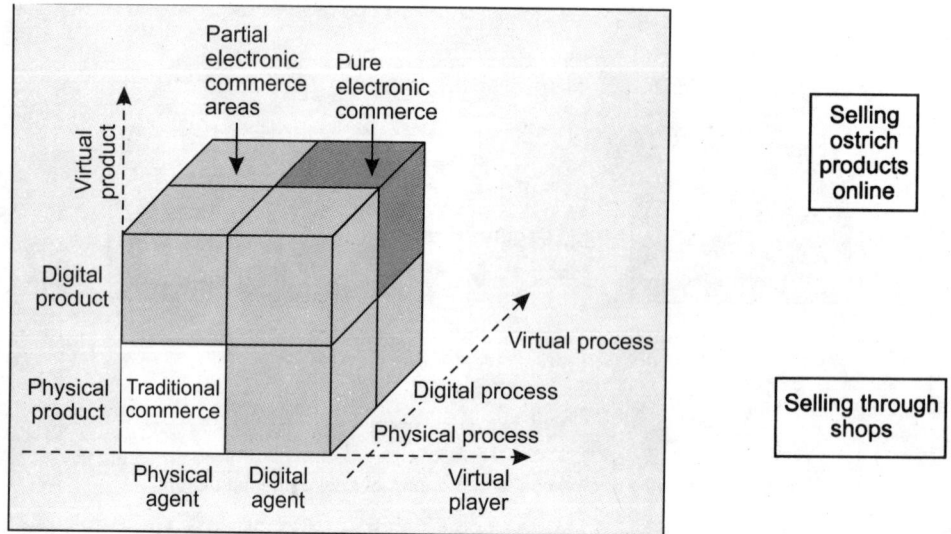

Fig. 37.2: Dimensions of electronic commerce

Electronic Commerce Organization

The entrepreneur should choose the way he/she wants to operate. There can be three different types to choose from initially.

Brick-and-mortar organization: Old-economy organizations (corporations) that perform most of their business offline, selling physical products by means of physical agents. Traditionally, Indian farmers are used to brick-and-mortar form of business organizations.

Virtual (pure-play) organizations: Organizations that conduct their business activities solely online. Virtual organizations are impossible to create with physical products such as meat, milk, etc.

Click-and-mortar (click-and-brick) organizations: Organizations that conduct some e-commerce activities, but do their primary business in the physical world. This form of organizational set-up may be the most preferred one for the budding livestock entrepreneurs in India, as it offers the flexibility and suits the environmental set-up.

INTERNET—BACKBONE OF DIGITAL ORGANIZATIONS

Internet provides the framework on which digital organizations can be erected. The intranet, extranet and internet are the different levels of scope of digitalization (Fig. 37.3).

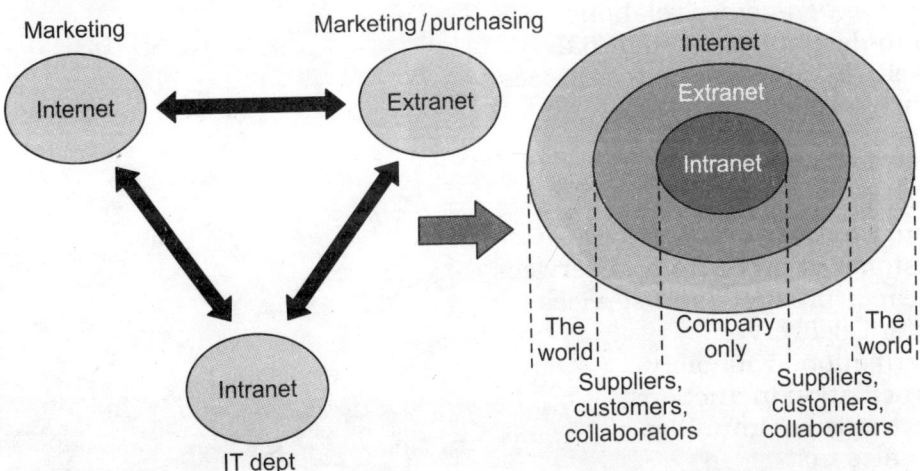

Fig. 37.3: Internet, intranet and extranet provide framework to digitalization

Intranet

An internal corporate or government network that uses internet tools, such as web browsers, and internet protocols.

Extranet

A network that uses the internet to link multiple intranets.

A basic understanding of the digital infrastructure is extremely significant for a new venture. Entrepreneurs can create their own intranets for organization wide connect, but it is insignificant in case of small entrepreneurs. Small entrepreneurs can rather have their website having a brick and click organization to operate efficiently.

THE FUTURE OF EC

- Overall, the growth of the field will continue to be strong into the foreseeable future.
- Despite the failures of individual companies and initiatives, the total volume of EC is growing by 15 to 25% every year.

Benefits of EC to Organizations

- Global reach
- Cost reduction
- Supply chain improvements
- Extended hours
- Customization

- New business models
- Vendors' specialization
- Rapid time-to-market
- Lower communication costs
- Efficient procurement
- Improved customer relations
- Up-to-date company material
- No city business permits and fees
- Other benefits

Benefits to Consumers

- Ubiquity
- More products and services
- Customized products and services
- Cheaper products and services
- Instant delivery
- Information availability
- Participation in auctions
- Electronic communities
- No sales tax

Benefits to Society

- Telecommuting
- Higher standard of living
- Homeland security
- Hope for the poor
- Availability of public services

Some of the limitations of electronic commerce are listed in Table 37.1.

Table 37.1: Limitations of electronic commerce

Technological limitations	Nontechnological limitations
1. Lack of universal standards for quality, security, and reliability.	1. Security and privacy concerns deter customers from buying.
2. The telecommunications bandwidth is insufficient, especially for m-commerce.	2. Many legal and public policy issues, including taxation, have not yet been resolved.
3. Software development tools are still evolving.	3. National and international government regulations sometimes get in the way.
4. It is difficult to integrate internet and EC software with some existing (especially legacy) applications and databases.	4. It is difficult to measure some of the benefits of EC, such as advertising. Mature measurement methodologies are not yet available.
5. Special web servers are needed in addition to the network servers, which add to the cost of EC.	5. Some customers like to feel and touch products. Also, customers are resistant to the change from shopping at a brick and-mortar store to a virtual store.

Table 37.1: Limitations of electronic commerce *(Contd.)*

Technological limitations	Nontechnological limitations
6. Internet accessibility is still expensive and/or inconvenient. 7. Order fulfillment to large-scale B2C requires special automated warehouses.	6. People do not yet sufficiently trust paperless, faceless transactions. 7. In many cases, the number of sellers and buyers that are needed for profitable EC operations is insufficient. 8. Online fraud is increasing. 9. It is difficult to obtain venture capital due to the failure of many dot-coms.

CONCLUSION

Entrepreneurship in India is not a easy job. Because of inadequacy of capital and resources traditionally we could never produce great entrepreneurs in plenty. But, on date the growing digitalization has provided us an opportunity to explore the world. By using IT and working on e-commerce models even the farming community which aspires to have livestock businesses can have global access. Moreover, the cost of having this access is very low. The power of IT is tremendous and it provides us opportunities to create wonderful business models, provided we identify the opportunities intelligently.

38

Interpersonal Skills for Establishing an Enterprise

BP Singh

The capacity of a country for economic growth and development is determined by the three key factors: human resources, physical resources and financial resources. The human resource factor is most strategic and critical in absence of an abundance of natural and physical resources. Machinery and capital may go grossly under-utilized or misused. Human resources need to be trained and build up their personality so that they can achieve beyond their expectations to make the country to bloom in all sphere of social, economical and technological development. Richard Cautillon, a French economist, introduced the term entrepreneur, and since then entrepreneur has been used to describe one who takes the risk of taking a new venture in business or giving the services to the society or introduction of new ideas, products, etc. To establish the enterprise, an entrepreneur has to move through three phases;

i. **Inception phase:** It is related to the perception of an opportunity to establish the enterprise unit,

ii. **Operational phase:** It includes the theory and practice of managerial function required in management of an enterprise,

iii. **Managerial phase:** It includes the profitable application of the mental executive health in taking relevant managerial decisions.

To establish a profitable enterprise unit, an entrepreneur should possess some of the interpersonal skills: human skill, business skill, professional skill, technical skill, legal skill, fund mobilizing skill and innovative skill. Thus, the entrepreneurs are the person of skills, experiences, dexterity, expertise and flair. Interpersonal skills are very critical for successful managing, cooperating, selling, problem-solving and other aspects of one enterprise. Entrepreneurs need to possess the skills to build and encourage productive relationship, even in the most difficult of human relations situations.

Entrepreneur plan the activities for implementation, organize for easy implementation, lead and control the various activities of his enterprise. But they differ in the amount of time devote to each of the activities. These differences depend on the type and size of enterprise for which the entrepreneur works. The entrepreneur of small dairy unit, small livestock service centre, animal health and AI centre, e.g. spend more time quite differently than the manager of large dairy unit, large livestock service centre and large animal health and AI centre. Similarly, the veterinary doctor of a private veterinary clinic spend more time according to his own schedule, by practising medicine and managing the things, than do the veterinary doctors of a large and public veterinary hospital. The type and size of an enterprise require specific skills for manufacturing the specific type of products. Before to conceive the idea to establish the enterprise, one needs to explore the demand and prospects of the product to be made in enterprise, availability of raw material and requirement of manpower. Entrepreneur should have the skills to explore and develop the employee potentials. Further he should have the ability to listen intelligently and carefully to those with whom he work. Listening skill helps the entrepreneur to gain clear understanding of their situation.

Robert L. Katz, a business executive, has identified following basic kinds of skills, viz. technical skills, human skills, conceptual skills and administrative skills which are required for an entrepreneur for successful establishment of the enterprise. These skills are needed to create and maintain a network of contact with people outside one's own chain of command.

TECHNICAL SKILLS

To establish the enterprise, an entrepreneur required to use the procedure, technique and knowledge for manufacturing the specialized products. To establish a milk and milk product processing unit, an entrepreneur has to be upgrade his knowledge regarding the various methods and techniques to prepare various types of milk products at low cost by visualizing the scope in nearby market. Similarly, the specific technical skills are also required to establish a cross-bred farm, wherein he is need to be well equipped regarding the knowledge about scientific management of cross-bred cows so as to minimize the risk of health to which a cross-bred is more susceptible like mastitis, foot and mouth disease and other contagious diseases. The technical skills of an entrepreneur helps in following aspects to establish an enterprise:

1. Skills for searching the idea to establish an enterprise.
2. Skills for processing, selection, assembling the necessary inputs and establishment of enterprise.

Searching the Idea to Establish an Enterprise

An entrepreneur should have the skills to search the innovative idea to establish an enterprise based on the very much demand of certain products in area or in country. The idea should be sound and workable so that it may be exploited. Idea should yield a reasonable return on investment. Huge scope is available to establish a livestock based enterprise, viz. milk product processing unit, meat product processing unit, buffalo-based dairy farm, desi cow-based dairy farm, livestock services and animal health centre, piggeries, goattery, poultry (layers and broilers) enterprise, etc. But, to establish a livestock-based enterprise, the entrepreneur should have the skills to discover the idea from following sources.

Market Observation

Entrepreneur should be skilled in observing the market to reveal the business idea. Since the market survey can reveal the demand and supply position of various livestock-based products. Entrepreneur should be skilled in estimating the future demand of the products and anticipated technological changes. Entrepreneur should determine the trend of demand, composition and the pattern of potential users of the products. Advice of professional experts like dealer of certain products, financing agencies, information from advertising agencies and the personnel from consumer affair ministry/APEDA may also be obtained to supplement the product analysis and market survey. Market survey will give clear picture about the products which are in demand and needs immediate supply. Example: in urban area there is huge demand of milk and milk products, so to increase the milk availability cross-bred cow-based dairy farm/high yielding buffalo-based dairy farm as an enterprise may be established.

Survey of Ultimate Clients/Perspective Consumer

Consumer has variety of needs and taste about the products. Contact with prospective consumer reveals the feature that can be built in a product and services. Keeping in view the consumers demand, a meat product of different flavours by adding green vegetables/spices can be made, a good bulls or AI may be provide for breeding in a specific area.

Study of Project Profile

The entrepreneur should be skilled in studying/reading the various project profile, research journals, magazine in depth to analyze the opportunity of an enterprise. The reports of various government and non-government firms publish the annual report and profiles that describe in detail the technical, financial and market requirement to open an enterprise. A carefully scrutiny of such project profile is very helpful in choosing the line of business to establish an enterprise.

Village Survey

To establish a livestock-based enterprise in rural areas, it is essential to survey the village and accordingly idea should be put into action on the basis of demand of specific services/product. If the farmers are using too much quantity of chemical fertilizers in cultivable land, then opening the vermi-compost unit is the best option as an enterprise in village.

Visit of Trade Fair/Exhibition

Trade fair and exhibition also provide the following opportunities to an entrepreneur, to collect the ideas to establish a potential enterprise:

a. Assessing the market trends in terms of demand potential and type of products, viz. vegetarian/non-vegetarian products, organic/inorganic product.
b. Meeting a large diverse type of customers, viz. agriculture farmer/livestock owners/veterinary doctor/feed dealers/general consumer, etc.
c. Comparing the price and quality of similar products.

d. Establishing the personal contact with different dealers for opening the outlet of the products to be manufactured in enterprise.

Skills for Processing, Selection, Assembling Essentially required Inputs and Establishment of Enterprise

Preliminary Evaluation and Testing of Ideas

After selection of idea to establish an enterprise, its screening and testing is essential. One should consider following points while screening and testing of idea for enterprise.

Technical feasibility: Technical feasibility of an idea is judged in terms of availability of necessary technology, machinery and equipment, labour skills and raw material to manufacture the products for establishing an enterprise. At this stage, one should take into account the necessary technical advise of an expert to judge the technical feasibility of the enterprise to be establish. For example, if the idea is to establish the enterprise on piggery, the availability of feed materials, veterinary facilities in the area and the marketing opportunities should be insure.

Commercial viability: To get the reasonable profit through an enterprise, entrepreneur should analyze the cost-benefit analysis. The demand of the products in market, selling price, cost of production, etc. should be analyzed.

Detailed Analysis

It is the thorough analysis about the enterprise from all angles, by analyzing its strength, weakness, opportunities and threats. Full investigation is carried out in the technical feasibility and economic viability of the proposed enterprise. At this stage, a lot of information is required and due care should be exercised at this stage because the idea is finally accepted or rejected at this stage. Every entrepreneur has to develop a sound system for regular collection, procuring and dissemination of the required information. Such a system is called management information system.

Idea Selection

Following considerations influence the selection of idea for the product to be manufactured for which enterprise is to be establish.

  i. Products whose import are banned or restricted by the govt. For example, the products should contain only permissible quantity of chemicals.
 ii. Product which can be exported easily and profitably (making of less bacterial count in milk products). The products have sufficient shelf life.
iii. Products whose demand exceed their supply, to make the ready availability of the product.
 iv. Products prepared by utilizing the available natural resources.

Requirement of Inputs

After the selection of idea to establish an enterprise, the requirement of inputs/ resources is analyzed. One should collect the information about requirement of finance, land and building, plant, machinery and manpower, etc. for the proposed enterprise. Finance is the life-blood of business and it serves as the lubricant for the wheel of business machinery. Entrepreneur has to take decision about the type, size, location, layout, etc. of the enterprise to be established. For example, to establish a livestock enterprise, one should explore the information about number of animals (cow/buffalo/goat/pig/poultry), type of the breeds (indigenous/improved/cross-bred), place (rural area/breeding farm/research institute) from where animal can be procure, location of dairy unit(urban/rural area), layout about manger, shed, drinking water, disposal of dung, shed for sick animals, calf, milking bar, feed unit, veterinary facilities, availability of fodder, feed. Manpower/personnel are most valuable asset of an enterprise and this asset does not depreciate. An entrepreneur has to make the following decisions concerning the personnel:

i. Number of personnel required for management, technical and other position in the enterprise.
ii. Qualification and experiences required for the employee to perform the jobs effectively.
iii. Sources of recruitment from which the needed staff will be procured.
iv. Procedure and methods of selecting the best candidates.
v. Methods of orientation and training to be employed for the selected personnel.
vi. System and criteria for evaluating the performance of employees.
vii. Policies and procedures for the promotion of staff.
viii. Facilities to be provided for the safety, health and welfare of the staff.
ix. Participation of personnel in the management of enterprise.

HUMAN-RELATION SKILLS

It is required to get the work done by the employees to motivate them by introduction of some human welfare scheme for them. For example, for the enterprise of milk and milk product processing unit, the manpower whoever work in that, needs to be deal with carefully by taking into account their welfare. Human relations skill is required for an entrepreneur so that he can coordinate and integrate all the activities for successful management of his enterprise. Human relation skills consist of the many abilities required to understand other people and to interact effectively with them. For example, interpersonal skills are needed in leading, motivating and communicating (thinking, empathy, speaking, writing, using electronic media, reading and listening) with other person working in enterprise and even outsider. These skills are explained as under.

Leading

Leading involves, directing, influencing and motivating the staff to perform essential tasks. While planning and organizing the activity of enterprise is very concrete. It involves working with people. By establishing the proper atmosphere, entrepreneur helps their employee to do their best. For the best leading the enterprise, an entrepreneur should have various skills, viz. intelligence, charmisa, decisiveness, enthusiasm, bravery, integrity, self-confidence and these should be concern for people and production.

Motivating

Psychologists have described the terms 'motivation' as the immediate influence on the directing, vigour and persistence of action. It is the process of arousing action, sustaining the activity in progress and regulating the pattern of activity. Motivation in general is an important determinant for entrepreneurial growth and development in society. Motivation can be explained, that people who are 'motivated' exerts a greater efforts to perform than those who are ' not-motivated'. Motivations are the factors that cause, channel and sustain an individual behaviour to get the satisfaction. An unsatisfied need creates tension which stimulates, derives within the individual. These derives generate a search behaviour to find a particular goal that, if attained, will satisfied the need and lead to the reduction of tension.

There are two models of motivation which should be known to an entrepreneur to motivate their employees for success management and growth of enterprise.

Traditional Model

The entrepreneur determined the most efficient way to perform repetitive task and then motivated the worker with a system of wage incentive—the more worker produced, the more they earned. The underlying assumption is that entrepreneur understood the work better than the workers, who were essentially lazy and could be motivated only by money. Under the traditional model, worker has been expected to accept managerial authority in return for high wages.

THE HUMAN RELATION MODEL

Elton Mayo and other human related researches found that the boredom and repetitiveness of many tasks actively reduced motivation, while the social contact helped create and sustain motivation. An entrepreneur could motivate employees by acknowledging their social needs and by making them feel and important. This model urged the entrepreneur to give employees some freedom to make job-related decision as well as more information about the goal of an enterprise. A motivated person plays following roles in an enterprise:

1. Motivated person likes to shoulder the responsibility.
2. He likes to take moderate risk.
3. He wants to know the results of his efforts.
4. He wants to persist in the face of adversity.
5. He tends to be innovative.
6. He demonstrates some interpersonal competitiveness.
7. He is oriented towards the future.
8. He shows tolerance to ambiguity.
9. He tends to be mobile.

Communication

Communication skill is required for an entrepreneur so that he can demonstrate himself to his environment. It is use in resolving some of the difficult business situations through role-play. Effective communication is important for entrepreneur for two reasons: first, it is the process by which entrepreneur accomplish the function of planning, organizing, leading, and controlling. Second, communication is an activity to which an entrepreneur devote an overwhelming proportion of their time. Communication has been characterized as the "life-blood" of an enterprise and miscommunication has caused the equivalent of cardiovascular damage to the enterprise. Communication can be defined as the process by which people attempts to share meaning via the transmission of symbolic message.

CONCEPTUAL SKILLS

The entrepreneur should have conceptual skill that will enable them to see what goes on in their work environment and help them to react appropriately. In essence, it is the ability to "see the by picture", to plan ahead rather than to react. Conceptual skills enable the entrepreneur to look for best livestock enterprise. For example, dairying with crossbred cattle and high yielding buffaloes is a remunerative business in rural areas and if it is in urban area, it will be more profitable.

ADMINISTRATIVE SKILLS

It refers to the whole range of skills associated with **planning, organizing, staffing** and **controlling** of the enterprise. These skills include administrator abilities to follow framed policies and procedure, process paperwork in an orderly manner, and manage expenditure within the limit set by a budget. In this sense, administrative skills are an extension of conceptual skills, they implement those decision by using administration skill. **Decision-making and feedback** are the most important part of the administrative skills.

Planning

It implies that entrepreneurs think through their goal and action in advance, that their action are based on plan or logic rather than on hunch. Plan gives the enterprise its objectives and set up the best procedure to achieve them. It can be defined as planning " the choosing course of action and deciding in advance what is to be done, in what sequence, when and how. Good planning attempts to consider the nature of the future environment in which planning, decision and actions are intended to operate, as well as the current period when plans are being made". Planning is done because it confers a number of advantages to the enterprise. To be more specific it:

- helps enterprise to adapt and adjust to changing environment
- assists in reaching agreement on major issues
- enables entrepreneur to see the whole operating picture more clearly
- assists in achieving the coordination among various parts of the enterprise
- tends to make objective more specific and better known
- saves time, effort and money
- helps reduce error in decision-making

Organizing

It is the process of arranging and allocating work, authority and resources in enterprise so that goal can be achieved efficiently.

Staffing

It is the process of analyzing the jobs of an enterprise in terms of manpower needs, recruiting and selecting suitable employee. R. Anderson has defined that "staffing begins with the strategic plan for the organization that defines what different kinds of people will have to do. Staffing is concerned with fitting people to these jobs-matching the skills and abilities of the person with the requirement of the jobs. It is also concerned with training people as job requirement change and managing their careers over their work life." Following steps are required in staffing process:

- Strategic and tactical plans
- Human resource planning
- Job analysis
- Job description
- Recruiting, screening and interviewing
- Selection
- Job orientation
- Career management
- Performance appraisal
- Employment decision and separations

Controlling

The entrepreneur must be sure about the action of the employee to move towards the stated goal of an enterprise. It involves the following main elements:

a. Establishing the standards of performance
b. Measuring current performance
c. Comparing the performance to the established standards
d. If deviations are detected, taking corrected measures.

Decision-making

Decision-making may simply be defined as a rational choice among alternative or as the conscious selection of a course of action from among available alternatives to produce a desired result. An entrepreneur has to make decisions constantly while performing the functions of planning, organizing, staffing, directing and controlling. There are various steps involved in decision-making:

a. Understand and define the problems.
b. Generate potential alternatives.
c. Evaluate alternatives.
d. Make the decision and implement it.
e. Evaluate the decision results.

Understand and Define the Problems

Defining the problems is the critical step. The clear-cut and accurate definition of a problem affects all the step that follow: if a problem is inaccurately defined, every other step in the decision-making process will be based on that incorrect point. An entrepreneur need to focus on the problem, not the symptoms. This is accomplished by asking the right questions. According to Peter Drucker, " the most common source of mistake in management decisions is the emphasis on finding the right answer than the right questions". After identification of proper problem, the entrepreneur needs to develop critical factors of the problems. Critical factors are those factors that rule out certain alternative solutions. One common limitation is, of course, time. If, for instance, a new product has to be on the dealer shelves for one month, any alternative which takes more than one month will be eliminated

Generate Potential Alternatives

At this stage, several alternatives need to be developed for problem-solving, if there is no choice of alternative, then there is no decision to be made.

Evaluate Alternative

At this stage it is important to understand not only the benefits of each alternative and how such benefits may influence the decision objective but also the potential negative side and cost of each alternative. The purpose of this step is to decide the relative merits of each of the alternative. What are the positive and negative sides of each alternative? Do any alternatives conflict with the critical factors that one identified earlier? If so, they must be automatically discarded.

Make the Decision and Implementation

Evaluate the Decision Results

After making and implementing the decision, one must perform the "control" function of management. That is one must evaluate whether the implementation is proceeding smoothly and the decision is attaining the desired results. Final stage in decision-making process is to create a control and evaluation system.

To establish a successful enterprise, Khan (1992) has introduced three tier scheme **to infuse the various skills amongst the entrepreneurs,** required in establishment of an enterprise.

i. **Careful selection of potential entrepreneur:** Careful selection of entrepreneur through an assessment of psychological traits, sociological background, technological knowledge and managerial and business aptitude with the help of intensive screening of personal history.

ii. **Right type of entrepreneurial training:** Development of requisite characteristics through a suitable and structural training programme designed to provide the necessary psychological reinforcement and an awareness of the fundamentals of enterprise management.

iii. **Pre- and post-implementation follow-up support:** Continuous support in the form of counselling, liaison with supporting agencies, provision of finance, conducting surveys to identify opportunities which would assist in choice of product, etc. during the course of establishment of enterprise as well as thereafter.

In any of the area of our country, it is not the interpersonal skill and the spirit of an enterprise that is lacking in the inhabitants. It is the lack of opportunity in keeping with their skills. The entrepreneurs are not able to market their skills. They are not able to reach market themselves because middle men are making the huge profit. An entrepreneur should know how to synchronize their skills with what the market demans. He should have the skills to add values to their products by way of finishing, packaging and advertising.

Katz suggests that all these skills are essential to an entrepreneur in establishing an enterprise. Their relative importance depends mainly on the role an entrepreneur plays in enterprise. Technical skill is the most important to monitor the various activities to be carried out in an enterprise, whereas human skill is important to coordinate the activities and motivate other employees at all levels for smooth functioning of an enterprise.

INTERPERSONAL ROLES OF ENTREPRENEUR

Basically, an entrepreneur requires to play three types of interpersonal roles (figurehead, leader and liaison) for which he has to acquire the interpersonal skills that help to keep an enterprise running smoothly. Three types of interpersonal roles are described below.

Figurehead

As a figurehead, the entrepreneur performs ceremonial duties as a head of enterprise unit, meeting different stakeholders, greeting various visitors, attending customers. More importantly, the entrepreneurs are symbol and personify for both of his enterprise unit and outside observers and for the enterprise success and failure. The manager is himself/herself responsible for any kind of loss in enterprise.

Leaders

Since the entrepreneur works as manager of his enterprise and he works with and through other people, he is responsible and accountable for their employees action as well as for their own. In fact, the employees success or failure is a direct measure of their own success or failure. On the availability of resources, the entrepreneurs are able to accomplish more than their expectations.

Liaison

Like politician, the entrepreneur must learn to work with everyone inside or outside their enterprise unit, who can help them to achieve their enterprise goals. All successful entrepreneur "play politics" in the sense that they develop the network of mutual obligation with the entrepreneur of another enterprise unit.

To sum up, there are various interpersonal skills which one entrepreneur should have like:

1. **Critical cognitive skills:** Understanding behaviour of self and others in social and work relationship, understanding feeling and reaction of others, understanding interpersonal and group dynamics and effective social behviour and behviorual management.

2. **Critical behavioural skills:** It promotes social competence and social skills, those are further responsible for effective relationship management in enterprise such as effective listening, responding and empathy skills.

3. **Team-work and group relationship skills:** These are very important for effective team-building so as to enhance productivity of the enterprise, such as empower others, cooperative group skills, collaborative skills, group presentation skills and relationship skills.

4. **Productive workplace skills:** These are important for effective interpersonal management to increase productivity in the workplace, such as productive team habits, creative contributive, positive impacting.

5. **Effective conflict management skills:** An entrepreneur should have the conflict-resolution skills, problem-solving and negotiation skills, pro-social skills, emotional intelligence and interpersonal stress-management.

6. **Effective leadership skills:** An entrepreneur should have quality of personal leadership, group facilitation skills, influencing motivating skills, visioning skills by offering creative idea, inspiring and motivate the employees.

7. **Effective community skills:** One should have the skills to develop an understanding of diversity/pluralism in the world community and an awareness of civic and social participation and ethical and informed decision-making, such as cultural intelligence, global citizenship awareness, personal ethics and local/global impact, social/cultural/historical knowledge, interpersonal respect and empathy/valuing diversity, civic and social responsibility, social action skills, change catalyst in society, pro-social attitude/behviour and helping/service orientation.

ABILITY AND SKILLS OF ENTREPRENEUR TO RECOGNIZE THE BARRIERS

These ability and skills an entrepreneur should have to identify the basic barriers in smooth running of enterprise. In smooth running of enterprise, the main reasons may be "lack of viable concept" and lack of market knowledge. Sometimes it is hard to attract the people with best information because they have already attractive jobs. A certain number of entrepreneur fail after starting up their own enterprise because they lack general know-how about enterprise. Some of the barrier faces by entrepreneur are given below.

Barriers

i. Lack of viable concept
ii. Lack of market familiarity
iii. Lack of technical skill
iv. Lack of seed capital
v. lack of business know-how
vi. Complacency, non-motivation
vii. Social stigma
viii. Time pressure, distraction
ix. Legal constraints, regulation, red tape
x. Protectionism, monopoly of a particular entrepreneur

Ability of Entrepreneur to Overcome the Barrier

1. Market contact
2. Local incubator companies
3. Technical education and support
4. Suppliers assistance and credit
5. Local venture capitalist
6. Capital local advisor
7. Entrepreneurial education
8. Successful role models

Through interpersonal skills an entrepreneur can improve their skills in building rapport, influencing other and encourage the team work. *Building rapport* is an effective means to get introduced the product in market. *Influencing others* is an important skill and identifies effective behaviours for influencing others. *Teamwork skill* is essential for an entrepreneur that requires to work effectively together with the people and employees of diverse culture to reach a common goal, since they operate in a joint-venture with their counterparts of other enterprise. Entrepreneur should be skilled in identifying the factors that impede or enhance team performance. To give and receive the feedback from employees, or to seek the assistance from other needed agencies (bank, processing unit, marketing network, transport, audit and account) in establishment of an enterprise, an entrepreneur should be skilled in presenting the facts and figure before the required agencies. Entrepreneur should establish goals and objectives and accordingly he should monitor the productivity and make decisions as they operate enterprise in an emerging product making field. Entrepreneur should also be skilled in identifying the strength, weakness, opportunity and threat for the enterprise to be established.

Index